Register Now for ~~Online~~ ~~Access~~ to Your ~~Book!~~

SPRINGER PUBLISHING
C⏻NNECT™

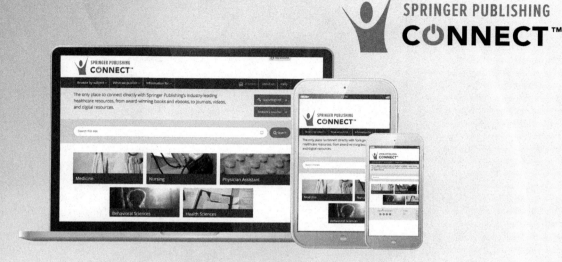

Your print purchase of *Frameworks for advanced nursing practice and research: Philosophies, theories, models, and taxonomies* **includes online access to the contents of your book**—increasing accessibility, portability, and searchability!

Access today at:
http://connect.springerpub.com/content/book/978-0-8261-3323-6
or scan the QR code at the right with your smartphone. Log in or register, then click "Redeem a voucher" and use the code below.

4Y59DHGD

Scan here for quick access.

Having trouble redeeming a voucher code?
Go to https://connect.springerpub.com/redeeming-voucher-code

If you are experiencing problems accessing the digital component of this product, please contact our customer service department at cs@springerpub.com

The online access with your print purchase is available at the publisher's discretion and may be removed at any time without notice.

Publisher's Note: New and used products purchased from third-party sellers are not guaranteed for quality, authenticity, or access to any included digital components.

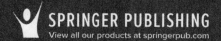

SPRINGER PUBLISHING
View all our products at springerpub.com

MW00838102

Frameworks for Advanced Nursing Practice and Research

Rose Utley, PhD, RN, CNE, is a professor at Missouri State University, where she teaches research, nursing theory, learning theory, and health policy in the master's and doctor of nursing practice (DNP) programs. She is a graduate of the University of Minnesota in Minneapolis, Minnesota (BSN and master's), and Wayne State University in Detroit, Michigan (PhD). She has been a certified nurse educator (CNE) since 2007. Her clinical background is in intensive care, emergency, postanesthesia, and faith community nursing. Her scholarly interests and publications relate to emergency care, geriatrics, nursing education, and nursing theory. She is the author of the book *Theory and Research for Academic Nurse Educators: Application to Practice*, which seeks to connect theoretical knowledge and research with nursing practice.

Kristina Henry, DNP, RN, NE-BC, received her BSN from the University of Central Missouri, Warrensburg, Missouri, and her master of science in nursing (MSN) and doctor of nursing practice (DNP) in organizational leadership from the University of Kansas, Kansas City, Kansas. Dr. Henry has been a board-certified nurse executive since 2009. Her clinical background includes critical care and operating room and mental health nursing. She was the BSN program director and an assistant professor at Missouri State University from 2012 to 2016. Her practice and research focus is leadership, change, and quality improvement.

Lucretia Smith, PhD, RN, CDE, holds a master of science in nursing (MSN) from the University of Missouri, Columbia, and a PhD in family studies from Loma Linda University, Loma Linda, California. She has taught medical–surgical nursing, community nursing, pediatric nursing, and culture-based nursing courses for nearly 20 years. Her clinical experience spans nearly 25 years and includes medical–surgical acute care, pediatric acute care, and pediatric home care. She is a certified diabetic educator (CDE) with current research exploring how family dynamics affect diabetes and the effects of diabetes on the family. Her interest in theory began in her master's program and continues to be the underpinning for both teaching and practice.

Frameworks for Advanced Nursing Practice and Research

Philosophies, Theories, Models, and Taxonomies

Rose Utley, PhD, RN, CNE

Kristina Henry, DNP, RN, NE-BC

Lucretia Smith, PhD, RN, CDE

SPRINGER PUBLISHING COMPANY

Springer Publishing Company, LLC
11 West 42nd Street
New York, NY 10036
www.springerpub.com

Acquisitions Editor: Joseph Morita
Compositor: Newgen KnowledgeWorks

ISBN: 978-0-8261-3322-9
ebook ISBN: 978-0-8261-3323-6
Instructor's Manual ISBN: 978-0-8261-3455-4
Instructor's PowerPoints ISBN: 978-0-8261-3454-7

Instructors Materials: Qualified instructors may request supplements by emailing textbook@springerpub.com

17 18 19 20 / 5 4 3 2 1

The author and the publisher of this Work have made every effort to use sources believed to be reliable to provide information that is accurate and compatible with the standards generally accepted at the time of publication. Because medical science is continually advancing, our knowledge base continues to expand. Therefore, as new information becomes available, changes in procedures become necessary. We recommend that the reader always consult current research and specific institutional policies before performing any clinical procedure. The author and publisher shall not be liable for any special, consequential, or exemplary damages resulting, in whole or in part, from the readers' use of, or reliance on, the information contained in this book. The publisher has no responsibility for the persistence or accuracy of URLs for external or third-party Internet websites referred to in this publication and does not guarantee that any content on such websites is, or will remain, accurate or appropriate.

Library of Congress Cataloging-in-Publication Data
Names: Utley, Rose A., author. | Henry, Kristina, 1971- author. | Smith, Lucretia, 1954- author.
Title: Frameworks for advanced nursing practice and research : philosophies, theories, models, and taxonomies / Rose Utley, Kristina Henry, Lucretia Smith.
Description: New York, NY : Springer Publishing Company, LLC, [2018] | Includes bibliographical references.
Identifiers: LCCN 2017030013 | ISBN 9780826133229 (paperback) | ISBN 9780826133236 (ebook) | ISBN 9780826134554 (instructors manual) | ISBN 9780826134547 (instructors powerpoints)
Subjects: | MESH: Advanced Practice Nursing | Nursing Theory | Nursing Research | Models, Nursing
Classification: LCC RT73 | NLM WY 128 | DDC 610.73072—dc23
LC record available at https://lccn.loc.gov/2017030013

Contact us to receive discount rates on bulk purchases.
We can also customize our books to meet your needs.
For more information please contact: sales@springerpub.com

Printed in the United States of America by Gasch Printing.

This text is dedicated to the scores of nurses pursuing advanced education in nursing or other health care fields who may be unaware of the value and usefulness of theories in their nursing practice. We hope this text provides nurses in all areas of practice, in all types of professional roles, with new insights and understandings about our patients and their families; about the roles and relationships of the nurse, patient, and other care providers; and about the complex environment and circumstances in which we live.

CONTENTS

CONTRIBUTORS

Rhea Faye Felicilda-Reynaldo, EdD, RN
Associate Professor
School of Nursing and Dental Hygiene
University of Hawaii-Manoa
Honolulu, Hawaii

Kristina Henry, DNP, RN, NE-BC
Healthcare Education Consulting
Sole Proprietor
Waynesville, Missouri

Maria Kenneally, DNP, FNP-BC
Family Nurse Practitioner
Premier Medical Group
Gilbert Center for Family Medicine
Gilbert, Arizona

Lucretia Smith, PhD, RN, CDE
Certified Diabetic Educator
Heath Education Consultants of the
   Ozarks
Springfield, Missouri

Rose Utley, PhD, RN, CNE
Professor
Certified Nurse Educator
Missouri State University
Springfield, Missouri

PREFACE

This text provides a review of selected philosophies, models, grand theories, middle range theories, and taxonomies relevant to nursing, collectively referred to as *frameworks*. We use the term frameworks for two reasons: (a) for the economy of expression when referring to multiple types of theoretical structures; and (b) to convey the inherent usefulness of these theoretical structures to nurse educators, clinicians, leaders, and researchers. In the context of this textbook, frameworks imply an underlying structure, connectedness, and organization of knowledge about a topic that is capable of shaping our awareness and guiding our actions.

THE UNIQUE ORGANIZATION OF THIS BOOK

If you are familiar with nursing theory textbooks, especially those that survey theories such as ours, you will notice that we take a different organizational approach from others in several ways. First, the content in most theory textbooks is organized by theoretical level; for example, grouping all grand theories together and all middle range theories together, regardless of subject matter. Our text is not organized by theoretical hierarchy levels but instead organized conceptually by subject matter. Another common organizational strategy is to group the frameworks by origin (i.e., separating nursing theories and "borrowed" theories developed by other disciplines). In our text, both nursing and non-nursing frameworks in a similar conceptual area are grouped together in the same chapter. Grouping chapter content by conceptual category allows the reader to become familiar with frameworks in a concentrated area of study and facilitates easy comparisons of the frameworks, thereby enabling the nurse to determine which ones are most useful for practice or research.

The text includes 24 chapters organized into four parts. Part I: Foundations of Theoretical Knowledge includes three chapters. Chapter 1: Understanding Theoretical Concepts explores such questions as: What are theories? How are they structured? Why are they important? How are they developed, analyzed, evaluated, and tested? Chapter 2: Strategies for Using Frameworks explains the implicit and explicit ways we use theoretical knowledge in our practices. Topics such as theoretical thinking, analogy, and forms of reasoning are covered, and the practical guidance that frameworks provide is explained. Chapter 3: The Relationship Among Theory, Research, and Practice focuses on understanding these interrelationships, how each informs the other, and how each is needed to enhance the development of the nursing profession.

The heart of the text is found in Part II: Frameworks for Individuals and Families and Part III: Frameworks for Communities, Populations, and Organizational Systems. As previously mentioned, each chapter in Parts II and III provides a survey of frameworks grouped by conceptual areas. However, in this text, we added another organizational layer by grouping the conceptual categories according to the focus of practice as either emphasizing individuals and families or communities, populations, and organizational systems. Part II contains chapters related to individuals and families in the following conceptual areas: behavioral change, care and caring, human development, teaching and learning, moral and ethical perspectives, health and illness, interpersonal and family relationships, human needs, physiological needs, psychological needs, and roles. Part III focuses on frameworks relevant to working with communities, populations, and organizational systems, such as economics, community and population health, leadership, evaluation, and sociocultural conceptual areas. This dual level of organization, first by practice area and then by conceptual areas, permits the reader to easily explore and compare frameworks in a given concentration that may be relevant to specific practice and research interests. We recognize that many of the frameworks (especially those originating in nursing) are comprehensive and holistic, which means they fall into more than one conceptual category, or may be relevant to both the care of individuals and populations. In those cases, we have sought to remain true to our conceptual organization and have grouped the framework where it has the strongest emphasis. In several cases, however, we discuss a framework in more than one chapter. For example, Roy's Adaptation Model is covered in Chapter 9: Health and Illness Frameworks; however, the role function mode of her adaptation model is also reviewed in Chapter 14: Role-Related Frameworks. In cases where a framework is discussed in more than one chapter, we provide cross-referencing to facilitate further understanding.

Another way in which our text differs from others is its emphasis on the application of frameworks to the roles of nurse educator, clinician, leader, and researcher. In each chapter in Parts II and III, we integrate explanations of how selected frameworks are used in practice. We also provide synopses of studies that have used some of the frameworks presented. Then in Part IV: Application of Frameworks to Nursing Roles, we provide individual chapters on the application of frameworks to the nursing roles of educator, clinician, leader, and researcher. In these chapters, we emphasize how frameworks are used by the individual nurses in that role, and how the frameworks provide knowledge that underlies nursing's scope of practice, standards, competencies, and best practices, as relevant to each role area.

We recognize that although a nurse may have a professional title that denotes a primary role as an educator, clinician, leader, or researcher, each nurse also relies on theoretical knowledge relevant to other roles. For example, an acute care clinician will find individual and family frameworks presented in Part II useful and relevant in day-to-day practice. However, clinicians also draw on knowledge associated with the other roles when they provide education to patients and families, assume charge nurse responsibilities, mentor new staff, integrate research evidence into practice, and participate in quality improvement research. Thus, nurse clinicians also use knowledge and skills common to nonclinical nursing roles. This integration and overlap of role-related knowledge and skill are not unique to clinicians; they exist at some level for each nursing role. Therefore, we encourage the reader, regardless of his or her primary role in nursing, to explore each chapter in Part IV.

○ INTENDED AUDIENCE

This text is designed for nurses who are pursuing graduate education at the master's or doctoral level in nursing or a related field. The text is useful in any graduate-level nursing science or nursing theory course to gain an overview of both general theoretical knowledge and specific theoretical perspectives. Students engaged in doctoral and master's research will find the text helpful for providing theoretical perspectives and for guiding data collection and analysis. The text may also be useful as an adjunct to graduate-level clinical courses that encourage the application of theory. Finally, the emphasis on the application of frameworks to advanced nursing roles can provide supportive content for courses that explore the advanced nursing roles of nurse educator, clinician, leader, and researcher.

FEATURES THAT FACILITATE LEARNING

The content in each chapter is organized consistently to facilitate student learning. The frameworks covered and terms defined in the text are listed at the start of each chapter, under "Key Terms." Names of the frameworks also appear in the body of the chapter as subheadings. New terms are italicized in the body of the text, when defined. Learning objectives are provided for each chapter and can be used to promote self-review of the content. At the end of each chapter, a bulleted summary is provided, titled "Key Points." The student should find this format helpful in guiding and reinforcing learning and encouraging further exploration.

The instructor may also find the chapter structure helpful. For example, the instructor can use terms defined in each chapter as sources for basic test items. The chapter objectives can be used to form discussion questions or as a basis for short written response assignments. **Each chapter is summarized in PowerPoint slides that can be adapted for use in seated and online classroom settings. An Instructor's Manual provides test items, discussion and self-reflection questions, and Resources for Additional Learning to locate supplemental information, such as websites, articles, and books, for classroom activities. Qualified instructors may request these supplements by emailing textbook@springerpub.com.**

FOR THE INSTRUCTOR

This text can be used in a variety of graduate nursing courses, including those focused on nursing science/nursing theory, master's, doctor of nursing practice (DNP) and PhD research projects, clinical practice, leadership, and nursing roles. The use of the textbook in these areas is described subsequently.

Using This Text in Nursing Science Courses

This text provides a combination of foundational theoretical knowledge and a survey of nursing and non-nursing frameworks. The text covers a wide range of frameworks and concludes with chapters on the application of frameworks to the nurse educator, clinician, leader, and researcher roles. For nursing science courses, which emphasize familiarizing the student with philosophies and theories, following the order in which the content is covered will result in progressive understanding.

Part I provides an excellent overview of basic theoretical knowledge: how it is developed and used, and why it is important in nursing. Chapter 1 introduces and clarifies terminology in discussing concepts such as theoretical perspective, philosophy, theoretical hierarchy, paradigm, worldview, and more. The chapter is structured to answer the questions, What is the role of philosophy? What is theory? How are theories categorized? How are they developed and tested? An overview of the criteria used to analyze and evaluate models and theories is provided to answer the question, What makes a well-constructed model or theory? Chapter 2 emphasizes the implicit and explicit ways frameworks are being used to shape the nurse's perspective. Frameworks can guide assessment and sensitize the nurse to important factors and circumstances that influence nursing practice. Engaging in theoretical thinking through conceptualizing, philosophizing, and using inductive, deductive, and abductive reasoning are also explored. Questions are addressed such as, Why are theories important? What purpose do they serve? And analogies are provided to facilitate this understanding. The chapter concludes with sections that explore the implicit and explicit uses of frameworks in the nurse educator, clinician, leader, and researcher roles. Chapter 3 explores the reciprocal relationships between these three areas and how each area informs the others. Building on concepts of theoretical hierarchy, theory development, and theory testing, the student is guided through these interconnected relationships. To broaden the student's understanding and appreciation of research and its relationship to practice, Boyer's Model of Scholarship is explored. The value of theory, research, and clinical practice is acknowledged in Boyer's five types of scholarship and in the subsequent addition of clinical scholarship and reflective practice scholarship. The emphasis on evidence-based practice provides additional support for the integration of theory, research, and practice.

After exposure to the foundational knowledge in Part I, students can then explore the framework categories in Part II, which focus on concepts relevant to individuals and families. Chapter 4 addresses behavioral change frameworks used to promote change in the individual. Frameworks focused on care and caring are covered in Chapter 5, followed by frameworks focusing on human development (Chapter 6), teaching and learning (Chapter 7), and moral and ethical perspectives (Chapter 8). Understanding of the patient's and family's experiences is enhanced by Chapters 9 through 13, which cover health and illness and interpersonal and family needs-based, physiological, and psychological frameworks, respectively. Clustering the frameworks with each chapter by conceptual categories allows the student to learn about the major perspectives and frameworks in each knowledge area, and compare and contrast frameworks that focus on a single conceptual area.

Part III explores the needs, issues, functions, and structures of communities, populations, and organizations. Individual chapters cover economics (Chapter 15), community and population health (Chapter 16), organizational systems (Chapter 17), leadership (Chapter 18), evaluation (Chapter 19), and sociocultural frameworks (Chapter 20). Clustering of these topics enhances the appreciation of their interconnectedness to the overall health and functioning of communities, populations, and organizations.

Part IV, the last section of the text, enhances the student's awareness of how frameworks are applied at both a micro (daily practice) and a macro (professional practice) perspective. One chapter is devoted to the application of frameworks to each role (i.e., educator, clinician, leader, and researcher). Although recognizing the overlap that exists among these role functions, these chapters focus on the ways the frameworks are used by nurses whose primary role is in education, clinical practice, nursing leadership, or research.

Using This Text in Nursing Research Courses

Being explicit in identifying frameworks used in nursing research is essential for building knowledge. Research can be theory generating, theory testing, or translational in nature. Theory-generating research is typically qualitative and may or may not acknowledge the influence of preexisting perspectives or frameworks. For theory-generating research in which the researcher does not engage in bracketing of preconceived ideas, the chapters in Part II and Part III may help the student identify and clarify the perspectives from which the study is being conducted.

For theory-testing research, the researcher is involved in testing a specific theory to expand its generalizability to different circumstances and settings. Specific frameworks from Parts II and III can be identified and selected for testing. If the researcher has not identified a specific area of interest, then the chapters that are related most closely to the researcher's area of interest can be explored to uncover potential frameworks that could be tested.

For translational or application research, the researcher uses an existing body of evidence and applies it to a real-world setting. Translational research takes the findings from original research, which were obtained under controlled circumstances using controlled samples, and applies them to a natural, uncontrolled clinical setting. As translational research involves implementing and evaluating a systems-level change, several types of frameworks are typically used, including change, organizational, leadership, educational, and quality-improvement frameworks. Additional frameworks related to concepts and variables are identified using the PICO framework (patient/population, intervention/interest area, comparison group, and outcomes). For example, if an intervention or change is being implemented for older adults, a framework related to aging or geriatrics could be used to explain the researcher's perspective and identify potential issues. If the change is implemented in a cultural group such as the homeless, sociocultural, needs-related, and economic frameworks may be relevant.

Using This Text in Clinical, Leadership, and Nursing Roles Courses

In clinical courses, the text can be used to promote the explicit use of frameworks in nursing at a micro level, in day-to-day practice. Reading Chapter 2 provides the student with an understanding of and appreciation for ways in which nurses use frameworks. Reading the chapters in Parts II and III broadens the student's awareness and sensitizes him or her to more nuances in the patient care situation. This broadened awareness enhances the nurse's understanding and may augment the nurse's development of rapport, communication, assessment, intervention, and evaluation skills.

For nursing leadership courses, several chapters in Part III are relevant. The organizational system frameworks in Chapter 17 are used to describe and aid in understanding the organizational processes and structures essential for selecting and applying the most appropriate leadership and management frameworks. Chapter 18 addresses leadership styles and processes, mentoring, and communication within the health care system. Chapter 19 provides frameworks that nursing leaders may use to evaluate individual performance, quality improvement initiatives, and educational programs. In addition, Chapter 23 explores how nurses in formal leadership roles use frameworks in practice. Four formal nursing leadership roles are highlighted, including the nurse executive, academic nurse leader, clinical nurse leader, and policy and advocacy leader. The competencies and expectations for each leadership role and the frameworks that underlie those competencies are acknowledged.

For courses emphasizing nursing roles, the text explores four categories of advanced nursing roles: the educator, clinician, leader, and researcher. Chapter 21 highlights the academic nurse educator and the nurse professional development educator roles and explores the micro- and macro-level application of frameworks in educational practice. The scope of practice standards and competencies for these roles and the underlying frameworks that support and inform them are identified. The role of the clinician and ways in which frameworks are applied on micro and macro levels are also identified. Frameworks underlying the scope and standards of nursing practice and the core competencies of the National Organization of Nurse Practitioner Faculties are also discussed. Chapter 23 focuses on four nursing leadership roles: the nurse executive, academic nurse leader, clinical nurse leader, and policy and advocacy leader. Credentialing, competencies, and how frameworks support the nurse leader's functioning in these roles is also addressed. The final role chapter is focused on the nurse researcher and emphasizes the researcher's responsibilities in adhering to research ethics and ensuring research rigor and competency.

In closing, we have provided a unique organizational structure for this text with an emphasis on conceptual organization of content and application of frameworks in the nursing roles of educator, clinician, leader, and researcher. It is our hope that graduate students and faculty alike find this approach user-friendly, practical, and meaningful for a variety of courses and experiences in their programs.

Rose Utley
Kristina Henry
Lucretia Smith

ACKNOWLEDGMENTS

We would like to recognize the support and contributions of many colleagues and students in the development of this book. Our reviewers include:

- Brian Wagoner, APRN, FNP-BC (Chapter 1)
- Jo Ellen Branstetter-Hall, PhD, RN (Chapter 3)
- Kathy Adams, MSN, RN (Chapters 5 and 6)
- Allison Anbari, PhD, RN (Chapter 7)
- Louise Bigley, PhD(c), RN (Chapter 15)

Their feedback added valuable insights and perspective to our work.

Scattered throughout the final chapters in Part IV are quotations from our students that reflect their understandings and perspectives about the value of theory and research in nursing practice. We thank them for granting permission to add their words to the text. We also thank Monique Fahy, bachelor of secondary education student, for her work in creating PowerPoint presentations from the chapter content.

Foundations of Theoretical Knowledge

Truth can be stated in a thousand different ways, yet each one can be true.
—Swami Vivekananda

In this part, you will become familiar with terminology and key concepts for understanding frameworks used in nursing practice and research. *Framework* is a broad term that encompasses the range of theoretical structures, including philosophies, models, theories, and taxonomies. In Chapter 1, you will find information basic to understanding the types, scope, and purposes of theory, and an overview of criteria for analyzing and evaluating theories and models. The focus of Chapter 2 is on the usefulness of frameworks in nursing practice as educators, clinicians, leaders, and researchers. Frameworks provide guidance, perspective, and structure needed to develop knowledge and facilitate communication and theoretical thinking within the discipline of nursing. In Chapter 3, the emphasis is on understanding and appreciating the interrelationships among theory, research, and practice and the development of nursing knowledge.

Understanding Theoretical Concepts

Rose Utley

If you talk to a man in a language he understands, that goes to his head. If you talk to him in his language, that goes to his heart.
—Nelson Mandela

⬤ KEY TERMS

abductive reasoning	generality	philosophy
aesthetics branch of philosophy	grand theories	practice theory
	hypothesize	pragmatic adequacy
clarity	inductive reasoning	propositional statement
concept	internal consistency	significance
concept analysis	internal validity	simplicity
conceptualize	metaparadigm	social significance
conceptual model	middle range theory	social utility
construct	model	theoretical hierarchy
deductive reasoning	ontology	theoretical substruction
derivable consequences	paradigm	theory
empirical adequacy	parsimony	theory analysis
empirical precision	phenomena	theory evaluation
epistemology	philosophize	worldview
ethics branch of philosophy	philosophizing	

⬤ LEARNING OBJECTIVES

1. Define and differentiate key terms used in theory-based literature.
2. Describe processes used, refining nursing knowledge, including conceptualization; concept analysis; hypothesizing; theory analysis; theory evaluation; theoretical substruction; and inductive, deductive, and abductive reasoning.
3. Compare and contrast theoretical structures in terms of scope and abstractness.
4. Compare approaches to scientific reasoning, concept analysis, theory analysis, and theory evaluation.
5. Explore the purposes, categories, and ways to analyze, evaluate, and test theories.

In this chapter, you are introduced to terminology needed for understanding and using frameworks in nursing education, clinical practice, nursing leadership roles, and research. Frameworks are structures used to describe a perspective, organize thinking, and/or guide actions. In this text, the term *frameworks* includes philosophies, models, theories, or taxonomies that structure and sensitize how we think about and perform in practice.

The terminology used when discussing frameworks can be confusing. However, this problem is unique to neither nursing nor theoretical knowledge. Even common words used in our everyday language can have multiple meanings. Throughout this text, the terms are italicized when first defined.

Some of the questions answered in this chapter include: What is the role of philosophy in nursing? Why is understanding philosophical foundations valuable? What is theory? How are theories classified and organized? What are the criteria for a well-constructed theory? Understanding the answers to these questions will help you appreciate the importance and usefulness of philosophies, models, theories, and taxonomies as frameworks for nursing practice and research. Finally, we explore how theories are developed, analyzed, evaluated, and tested, and why these processes are needed in nursing.

◉ THEORETICAL PERSPECTIVES

A major purpose of frameworks, whether a philosophy, model, theory, or taxonomy is to guide, shape, and delineate a perspective. A *perspective* is how we view people, events, situations, and behaviors. It is influenced by ideas to which we are exposed, life experiences, education, and the unique internal attributes of the person. Each of us operates from a unique perspective that has differences and shares commonalities with other perspectives.

A classic example of differing perspectives is that of the elephant and the blindfolded people. In this example, each person "sees" the same object from a different perspective; however, when asked to describe what they "see," each gives a different rendition based on his or her perspective. One person describes something like a tree trunk; another says it is like a snake; another says it is a fan; and yet another says it is like a wall. All are correct from their perspectives, but the key to seeing the whole elephant is to see it from broad and multiple perspectives. Similarly, our awareness of multiple frameworks helps us appreciate and achieve a broader and more comprehensive perspective. The more aware we are of multiple perspectives, the easier it is to view the patient's situation holistically and comprehensively.

What Is the Role of Philosophy?

Understanding the importance of philosophy has often been obscured by the need to wade through confusing terminology, multiple definitions, and by failing to make the importance and usefulness of philosophy explicit. In its simplest form, *philosophy* is a perspective about something in our world formed from values, beliefs, and experiences. Philosophy can be defined in several ways, including the study of knowledge; a school of thought; and a set of ideas, values, and principles that frame our *worldview* (i.e., our perspective, the way we view the world). Philosophy is broad, abstract, informs our worldview, and influences the types of frameworks we value. Each of us has a worldview that is synonymous with our personal philosophy or the "general conception of the nature of the world in which [we] live and of [our] place in it" (Honderich, 2005, p. 702). Therefore, a nursing philosophy describes the nurse's basic beliefs, concepts, and attitudes about nursing and nursing practice and can illuminate potential biases as described in Box 1.1. A close examination of your nursing philosophy will likely reveal that it describes and explains aspects of the *metaparadigm* (i.e., person or patient, nurse, health, and environment), and either implicitly or explicitly articulates the underlying values and beliefs related to your nursing practice.

BOX 1.1 Research Application of the Post-Positivism Feminist Perspective

Routledge, a cardiovascular nurse, describes the positivism and post-positivism philosophical perspectives and discusses why and how she used post-positivism as a research methodology (Routledge, 2007). She explains feminist philosophies and how empirical feminism provided a foundation for her research into nighttime blood pressure dipping patterns in women and how that related to women's cardiovascular risk. She credits the feminist perspective as increasing her awareness of the gender bias that exists in research and health care.

TABLE 1.1 Branches of Epistemology

Branch	Definition
Empiricism	Knowledge is based on perceptual experiences
Idealism	Reality is mentally constructed, and knowledge is innate
Rationalism	Knowledge is derived from deductive reasoning or evidence
Constructivism	Knowledge is constructed from social experiences and perceptions

As a study of knowledge, philosophy is composed of subbranches including epistemology, ontology, and axiology. *Epistemology* is the study of knowledge or theory. In nursing, epistemology is concerned with understanding and examining how nurses acquire clinical, conceptual, and empirical knowledge. It is the study of the nature, scope, and sources of knowledge. Several branches of epistemology have developed, including (a) *empiricism,* (b) *idealism,* (c) *rationalism,* and (d) *constructivism* (Table 1.1). *Ontology* is the study of being, which focuses on questions about the nature of being, reality, and causation. *Axiology* is the study of value and is subdivided into *aesthetics*—the study of values in the arts and *ethics*—the study of values and moral behavior in humans. The word *ethics* is derived from the Greek word *ethos,* which translates as *custom* or *habit.* As a branch of philosophy, ethics asks questions about how people ought to act and what constitutes right actions. Ethics encompasses the moral ideals that guide behavior and one's philosophy of life. Ethical perspectives are covered in Chapter 8.

Philosophy, though intangible, has value and usefulness to the nursing profession. It has intrinsic and educational worth, as it satisfies our intellectual desire for knowledge and understanding. We approach the world with unconnected beliefs, preferences, and behaviors acquired from experiences and observation. However, there is a natural desire to *philosophize* or systematically organize knowledge and to discover how things are related (Honderich, 2005). Thus, *philosophizing* is a cognitive and self-reflective process in which the individual explores the underpinnings of his or her beliefs, values, and actions. For the profession, philosophizing has direct educational value by illuminating the core values and beliefs of our discipline and clarifying the reasoning processes used in decision making.

Philosophical Perspectives

When examining classical philosophies one can see the gradual overlap in the evolution of the philosophies as influenced by predominant worldviews or *paradigms*. According to Thompson (2012), "Science can never be absolutely 'pure.' It can never claim to be totally free from the influences of thought, language, and culture within which it takes place" (p. 7). Our philosophical perspectives, assumptions, and values influence the types of questions that interest us and influence our choice of ways to explore, study, and validate phenomena. Historically, the terms *analytical* and *continental* have been used to classify philosophical perspectives. These labels have generated much discussion and disagreement in terms of true distinction. Although each classical school of philosophical thought differs in perspective, assumptions, and values, there is overlap, making the true distinctions blurred in some cases (Table 1.2).

Although an in-depth discussion of specific philosophical schools of thought is beyond the scope of this text, an appreciation of the major values, assumptions, reasoning processes, and perspectives of the major schools of thought is helpful in clarifying one's personal philosophy of nursing. *Analytic philosophy* values empirical, observable, and measurable data and is aligned with quantitative research methods. It is based on the assumption that the researcher's role is, and should be, objective and detached from the data collection and analysis process, whereas, *continental philosophy* values the subjective experiences and meanings of experiences and is aligned with qualitative research methods. Phenomena viewed from a continental perspective are not directly measurable, and the meaning of the data must be inferred from what is said or observed. The social and cultural context of the situation is considered relevant as is the role and influence of the observer or researcher. Observation and research conducted from a continental perspective acknowledges the influence of the observer's values, beliefs, and experiences on data collection and analysis.

Understanding philosophy is valuable because it influences scientific thought, the types of questions of interest, the types of data we value and collect, how we conduct research, and our interpretation of findings. For further exploration of philosophy see the works of Cody (2006) and Dahnke and Dreher (2016).

TABLE 1.2 Comparison of Analytic and Continental Philosophy		
Comparative Factors	**Analytic Philosophy**	**Continental Philosophy**
Values	Objectivity	Subjectivity
Perspectives	Empiricism Objectivity	Rationalism Cultural and contextual sensitivity
Reasoning	Deductive	Inductive
Research methodology	Quantitative Empirical analysis	Qualitative Subjective synthesis
Philosophers	G. E. Moore Bertrand Russell	Hegal Heidegger
Philosophies	Positivism Empiricism	Idealism Marxism Hermeneutics Phenomenology

What Is Theory?

The layman's use of the word *theory* commonly refers to something not proven, an idea or statement that explains something, such as, "I have a theory about why Harry is so secretive about his work." However, in professional circles, theory is a description, explanation, or prediction of things or ideas in our world, a statement of the relationship between two or more concepts. Fawcett (2015) defined theory as "concepts and propositions about a phenomenon" (p. 594). *Concepts* are words we use to label or identify people, objects, events, situations, experiences, beliefs, and values.

These concepts or word labels are necessary for communication, developing and sharing information, and describing relationships. An example of a relationship or *propositional statement* is, "increased anxiety is associated with increased pain intensity." We create propositional statements whenever we *hypothesize* or try to explain behavior or experience, or when we attempt to describe or explain a situation or event. Hypothesizing about the relationships among people, events, and circumstances is a pervasive process in daily living and in nursing practice. We are continually generating and testing propositional statements (i.e., theory) in our day-to-day lives and when we provide patient care.

Theories can be depicted by words and graphic representations of concepts and relationships between those concepts. For example, Maslow's Hierarchy of Human Needs Theory is graphically represented as a triangle with the physiological needs at the base followed by safety, love and belonging, with self-actualization at the peak (Maslow, 1943). The relationships between needs are inferred by building one need upon the other until the pinnacle is reached. The size and placement of the levels represent the importance and foundational nature of the physiological needs.

Conceptual models represent relationships between abstract concepts and are more general or broad in scope than grand, middle range, and practice theories. Conceptual models are often criticized for being too broad and abstract to be applied to specific nursing practice situations. Nonetheless, *models* provide useful frameworks examining and observing the phenomena of interest and provide ways to structure and classify our perceptions. Models are also sources for developing theories used in nursing practice. For example, Rogers's Science of Unitary Human Beings is a conceptual model that has been used to formulate Parse's Theory of Humanbecoming, Newman's Health as Expanding Consciousness (see Chapter 9), Watson's Theory of Caring, and Anderson's LIGHT Model (see Chapter 5).

Given that the concepts are the word labels we use to identify things we see, feel, or experience (i.e., *phenomena*), the more clearly a concept or phenomenon is defined, the more clearly and accurately we communicate with others. The process of *concept analysis,* discussed later in this chapter, is helpful in defining the attributes and boundaries of a concept and in differentiating similar concepts such as anxiety and restlessness. Concepts can be concrete objects that are detected or measured with the senses (e.g., temperature, body mass index, blood loss), or abstract. Abstract concepts are nontangible things whose existence is inferred from what is observed (e.g., family, parenting, spirituality, grief, resilience). Both concrete and abstract concepts can be difficult to define. Take the concrete concept of "cup." What comes to mind is probably a mental picture of a drinking cup or coffee cup. However, the mental picture of the concept of cup can differ from person to person, depending on the context in which the term cup is used and the person's past experience with the concept. Even after agreeing that "cup" refers to a container from which you can drink, it can be visualized in a variety of ways (Figure 1.1). This points to the importance of defining concepts and exploring the boundaries of the concept through the process of concept analysis. The term *construct* refers to a combination of two or more concepts to describe a unique, abstract phenomenon. In nursing, there are many constructs such as caregiver burden, cancer survivorship, or nursing theory.

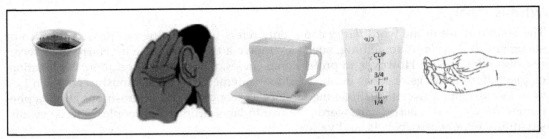

FIGURE 1.1 Examples of the concept of cup.

HOW ARE THEORIES CATEGORIZED?

A common way to visualize categorization of theories is using a *theoretical hierarchy* or continuum with conceptual models as the broadest and most abstract, followed by *grand theories,* middle range theories, and practice theories, which are progressively more narrow in scope and more concrete. In this text, the theoretical hierarchy is conceptualized within the content of the metaparadigm concepts and philosophies (see Figure 1.2). Unfortunately, definitions of these categories vary which has resulted in confusion. However, conceptualizing these theoretical structures as ranging from more abstract to less abstract and from broad in scope to more narrow in scope is helpful.

Theoretical structures range from broad and comprehensive (i.e., *conceptual models*), to narrow in scope (i.e., *middle range and practice theories*). They vary in their level of abstraction ranging from highly abstract concepts that are more difficult to measure, to concepts that are more concrete, and easier to define and measure. Middle range and practice-level theories typically provide more concretely defined concepts compared to conceptual models and grand theories.

In another way, theories are categorized in terms of their origin or source as either "nursing theory" or a "borrowed theory." *Nursing theory* in this text refers to theories developed by nurses for nurses. Florence Nightingale is often cited as the first nursing theorist as she identified common aspects of nursing care such as hygiene, nutrition, light, and air as improving patient outcomes (Nightingale, 1860/1969). Following Nightingale, some nurse theorists developed conceptual models (e.g., King, 1997; Rogers, 1970), others developed grand theories (e.g., Peplau, 1952; Roy, 2009), and still others developed middle range and practice theories (e.g., Kolcaba, 1991; Swanson, 1991). A *grand theory* is broad in scope and is composed of abstract concepts that cannot be directly tested or measured. In contrast, *middle range and practice theories* are related to specific areas of nursing practice or are concerned with certain phenomena in nursing. A testable hypothesis can be derived from the relational statements that form a middle range or practice-level theory.

Borrowed theories were initially developed by non-nurses for use in other disciplines such as education, child development, communication, psychology, and sociology. Nurses commonly use borrowed theories to appreciate and understand the patient's processes and experiences. As nurses use all types of theories, we have deliberately organized the theories in this book by subject matter rather than by type or by level. This intentional organization by subject matter will facilitate the understanding of similarities and differences between frameworks that relate to a common concept.

HOW ARE THEORIES DEVELOPED AND TESTED?

Theories are created or developed by theoretical thinkers and researchers who observe and study certain phenomena, experiences, and events and put their observations into words or diagrams. Volumes have been written about how theories are developed (Fawcett, 2013;

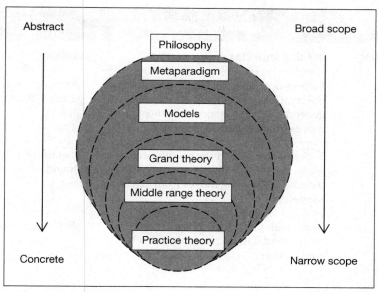

FIGURE 1.2 The continuum of theoretical structures.

Newman, 1975; Reed & Shearer, 2012; Walker & Avant, 2011) and how researchers test theories (Fawcett, 2015; Tappen, 2011). Developing a theory generally begins with observation and uses *inductive reasoning*, wherein specific observations are generalized or applied to broader situations. Inductive reasoning is used to find patterns in what was observed and draw conclusions or generalize about those observations. An example of theory development using inductive reasoning is found in Kübler-Ross's Five Stages of Grief (Kübler-Ross, 1969). She reasoned inductively by clustering similar behaviors, feelings, and perceptions expressed by terminally ill clients. From observation and interviews, she identified five stages of clients' experience in response to learning they have a terminal illness: (a) denial and isolation, (b) anger, (c) bargaining, (d) depression, and (e) acceptance.

It is unknown when the first theory was developed from empirical observation, but once developed, it likely served as a foundation for developing additional theories. Examples of theory development from combining aspects of multiple existing theories are common. For example, the Health Belief Model (HBM; see Chapter 4) was developed by Rosenstock et al. in the 1950s (Rosenstock, 1974). They described a set of factors that influence the person's likeliness to engage in healthy behaviors. These factors include demographic characteristics, four types of perceptions (perceived susceptibility, sensitivity, barriers, and benefits), self-efficacy, and cues to action. Based on the HBM, nurse theorist Lola Pender developed a theory of health promotion (Pender, 1975). She expanded on the HBM by including the concept of activity-related affect, which influences perception, and identified situational and interpersonal influences and competing demands, which can affect the desired outcome. Other theorists have combined concepts and ideas from several theories with their own ideas to create a new theoretical perspective. Newman's Theory of Health as Expanded Consciousness (Newman, 1994) incorporates aspects of Martha Rogers's Science of Unitary Human Beings (see Chapter 9), Prigogine's Theory of Dissipated Structures, and Young's Theory of Human Evolution, to develop a new conceptualization of health and person/environment interaction.

Deductive reasoning, used for testing theories, is based on laws or general principles (Table 1.3). When deductive reasoning is used, a general principle is applied to an example in the real world. This is often referred to as the *top-down* approach because the researcher

TABLE 1.3 Types of Reasoning, Attributes, and Examples		
Type of Reasoning	**Defining Attributes**	**Example**
Inductive	Bottom-up approach. Combines multiple observations, notes the patterns, and generates an explanation (i.e., theory); moves from specific to general.	Qualitative research to generate theory
Deductive	Top-down approach starts with general ideas, then forms and tests hypothesis or theories. Reasoning moves from general to specific.	Scientific method Quantitative research to test theory
Abductive	Starts with incomplete observations or data and determines to most likely explanation.	Medical diagnosis

starts at the top and reasons his or her way down to a deduction or conclusion. The process of theory testing in quantitative research relies on deductive reasoning, in which the researcher starts with broad concepts and determines if and under what circumstances the concepts apply to populations. Deductive reasoning occurs when something that is true of a class of things is applied to all members of that class. For example, based on the generalization or hypothesis, "Conscious patients undergoing an invasive procedure experience anxiety," deductive reasoning would result in the statement, "My patient is conscious and undergoing a needle biopsy, which is an invasive procedure, therefore my patient is experiencing anxiety." For this to be a sound deduction, the original hypothesis or generalization must be true. Therefore, for sound deductive reasoning to occur, it is necessary to accurately identify members of the class, because incorrect categorizations will result in unsound conclusions.

The third type of reasoning, *abductive reasoning* or *abductive inference*, plays a part in logic and belief formation and has received growing attention in the nursing literature (Haig, 2008; Lipscomb, 2012; Råholm, 2010). According to Lipscomb (2012), "Scientific literacy entails awareness of or engagement with the processes of belief formation and belief justification. . . . Abductive inference is a part of reasoning and abduction thus underpins aspects of belief formation/justification and, in consequence, action/behavior" (p. 245). Unlike deductive reasoning in which the premise guarantees a conclusion, *abductive reasoning* uses inference to reach the best possible explanation. The abductive reasoning process is often intuitive, creative, and characterized by incomplete evidence, incomplete explanation, or both. An example is when a patient does not report all relevant symptoms. As a result, the diagnosis or conclusion is based on incomplete evidence. Similarly, when a diagnosis is reached but it does not account for some of the symptoms or empirical findings, the diagnosis or the explanation may not be complete.

Developing Theory Through Research

Qualitative research, which uses inductive reasoning, is often the precursor to developing a theory. Because of the inductive, descriptive focus of qualitative data, virtually any qualitative research method can provide foundational data for theory development. The grounded theory process was developed specifically to generate theory from interview data through coding, categorizing, and clustering of data (see Glaser & Strauss's 1967 seminal work describing the process). Then, categories in other comparison groups are explored, which may support the researcher's grouping or may suggest revisions that will enhance the generalizability of the conceptual categories. Once patterns and themes from qualitative data are identified, the findings can be tested using quantitative instruments developed to determine the limits and boundaries of the phenomena.

Quantitative researchers observe and/or measure concepts (i.e., variables). *Independent variables* are believed to influence or be related to outcomes called *dependent variables*. One of the tasks of a quantitative researcher is to measure the concepts or variables of the study. Making the concepts of a study measurable involves moving from a *conceptual definition* of the concepts to a measurable or *operational definition* of the variable. Making a consistent connection between the conceptual and operational definitions of research variables and carrying this connection to the research questions and data analysis process is referred to as *theoretical substruction* (Dulock & Holzemer, 1991; McQuiston & Campbell, 1997; & Wolfe & Heinzer, 1999). When there is a connection between conceptual and operational definitions, it supports *internal validity* of the study, meaning the study is likely to be measuring what was intended to be measured. However, when there is a disconnect between the conceptual and operational definitions, the variables that were intended to be observed, tested, or measured, as described in the study's theoretical framework, are not actually being observed, something else is. Therefore, the lack of theoretical substruction will result in findings that lack internal validity.

WHAT MAKES A WELL-CONSTRUCTED MODEL OR THEORY?

Determining how well a model or theory is constructed involves a process of analysis, in which the aspects or parts of the model or theory are explored. Direct examination of the primary sources written by the theorist should be conducted. Secondary sources written by someone other than the theorist would not be a reliable nor valid source for analysis.

Analysis of Models and Theories

Model analysis examines three components; (a) the origin, (b) the focus, and (c) the content of the model (Fawcett & DeSanto-Madeya, 2012). Origin of the model considers how the model evolved, what factors, other scholars, philosophies, and worldviews influenced the model. Determining the focus of the model is next. Although the two models may deal with similar populations, problems, or situations, each will look at the phenomena of interest somewhat differently. This is similar to the idea of the differing perspectives of the blind people and the elephant described earlier. Each individual is viewing the same phenomenon but looking at different aspects of it. The final component is an analysis of the content. This can be accomplished by using the *metaparadigm* concepts of person, environment, health, and nursing as an organizational framework. The content related to each metaparadigm concept can then be identified, along with statements that define the concepts and the relational statements that describe relationships between concepts.

Theory analysis involves a structured breakdown of the parts and purposes of a theory and provides an objective framework for studying a theory. Chinn and Kramer (1998) have identified criteria for analyzing theoretical structures, including (a) clarity, (b) simplicity, (c) generality, (d) empirical precision, and (e) derivable consequences. *Clarity* refers to defining the concepts in the theory and may involve diagramming the theory. *Simplicity* is related to clarity but refers to the lack of complexity. If there are numerous interacting factors, the relationships between concepts become unclear. The *generality* of the theory is important for applicability. It is important that the theory not be too limiting. It should be general enough to apply to a broad group of people or situations. A criterion important to researchers is the *empirical precision* of the theory concepts. To be valid, a theory must have research that supports its premises. To be testable, the concepts in a theory must be measurable, and that requires empirical precision. *Derivable consequences* address the importance of the theory and whether the theory should be adopted. Consequences of theories can be explored in terms of client outcomes and social, political, and environmental consequences.

For practitioners, the key attributes of a good theory are obvious relevance to common clinical situations, relative simplicity, and ease of understanding concepts and relationships. This is the point where nurse theorists and clinicians must understand and appreciate the perspective of the other, so that a common understanding is achieved. Clinicians can benefit from looking deeper into the attributes of theories and theorists can develop easily understood and readily used theories by considering the practical application to nursing practice, education, and leadership roles.

Evaluation of Models and Theories

Analysis of a model or theory provides a foundation for evaluation. *Theory evaluation* involves asking and answering a series of questions about the model or theory based on predetermined criteria. The criteria used to evaluate models and theories have been well described in the nursing literature. Fawcett (2013) distinguished between evaluation criteria for models and theories. In this section, key components of the process are highlighted. Moving from broad to specific, the evaluation of models is discussed followed by the evaluation of grand and middle range theories.

Evaluation of Models

Evaluation of nursing models, which are by definition broader in scope and more abstract than theories, is based on examining the content of the model in terms of six criteria. The criteria address the model's origins, comprehensiveness, congruence, credibility, theory-generating ability, and contributions to nursing (Fawcett, 2005, p. 53).

When evaluating the origins of a model, the philosophical foundations, sources of knowledge, and the underlying values and beliefs of the developer are examined. Fawcett (2013) notes that most nursing models have been derived from existing knowledge and include a synthesis of models from other disciplines. The comprehensiveness of content considers both the scope and the depth of content. Models with a comprehensive scope of content address each of the four metaparadigm concepts, provide guidance in diverse health care settings, and will be useful in one or more of the major practice areas (i.e., education, clinical practice, leadership roles, and research). Models with depth include explicit relationships between the metaparadigm concepts and identify multiple sub-concepts and interrelationships. A comprehensive model provides the nurse with guidance on what to observe, types of questions to ask, and actions to take in a given practice area or situation.

The third criterion for evaluating a model is to determine the congruence between the content of the model and the philosophical foundation. As most models reflect a blending of concepts and perspectives from other disciplines, it is important that the merging of ideas is logical and consistent. There is no explicit gauge for determining congruence as it relies on the judgment of the evaluator.

The idea of congruency is foundational to the fourth criteria, which is the ability of the model to generate grand or middle range theories. For a model to generate a theory, consistency between the concepts of the model and the concepts which have been deduced from the model is necessary. Thus, a model is evaluated as high in congruency if it has generated grand and or middle range theories.

The credibility of the nursing model involves determining its social utility, social congruence, and social significance. *Social utility* is determined by asking if the model is appropriate for use in certain settings, situations, and with certain people. It involves reviewing the literature to determine if practice protocols based on the model have been developed or are feasible, or if research protocols have been developed. *Social congruence* relates to meeting societal and cultural expectations. It is concerned with questions about the nature of actions and activities that stem from the model and whether the actions and activities meet the expectations of the community members being served. The value of the nursing model is used to determine if the model meets the criterion of *social significance*. The evaluator reviews the outcomes of published research to determine if research using the model has had a positive impact on society.

The final criterion for evaluation of models is the contribution of the model to nursing. As with previous criteria, this involves a review of the literature. Regardless of the model's focus, the expectation is that it expands our understanding of and our ability to interact with the phenomena of interest. Fawcett (2013) emphasizes that models should not be compared to one another, but evaluated on their unique merits and on the scope and worldview each encompasses.

Evaluation of Theories

As with evaluation of nursing models, evaluation of theories is based on the results of theory analysis and requires judgments to be made about the theory. Six criteria have been identified: (a) significance, (b) internal consistency, (c) parsimony, (d) testability, (e) empirical adequacy, and (f) pragmatic adequacy (Fawcett, 2013). These criteria share some commonalities with the criteria for evaluation of models yet provide more emphasis on aspects that are important for determining usability and application of theory in practice.

The first criterion, *significance,* refers to how explicit the published accounts of the theory are in terms of the philosophical and conceptual origins and use of metaparadigm concepts. Second, *internal consistency* is concerned with congruency between the philosophical and conceptual models on which the theory is based. Common questions include: Are terms clearly defined and semantically consistent? and Do propositional statements reflect structural consistency (i.e., theoretical substruction)?

As an understanding of the theory is required for it to be accepted and used in practice, the criterion of parsimony is important. Evaluating *parsimony* involves determining if the content and structure of the theory are presented in a clear and concise manner. This requires limited use of complex jargon and the use of explicitly defined terms and relationships. Although the theory does not need to be graphically depicted, the evaluator should be able to easily diagram the relationships and underlying structures of a parsimonious theory.

The fourth criterion, *testability,* is regarded as the most essential for determining if a theory is scientifically useful (Fawcett, 2013). This is especially true for interventions delineated in a middle range or practice theory. Because middle range theories are more concrete than grand theories and conceptual models, they should be able to generate operational definitions and relationship statements that can be tested. Therefore, when evaluating testability, the evaluator looks for tools, instruments, or successfully developed and tested research protocols for the theory. In the case of grand theories where it is not possible to provide precise operational definitions that enable variables to be measured, a qualitative approach using induction can be used. Silva and Sorell (1992) discuss a qualitative approach called the *description of personal experiences,* which can be used to collect data that can then be generalized to form the structure of a middle range nursing theory.

Determining *empirical adequacy* necessitates a review of all studies guided by the theory to determine if the findings are congruent with the assertions of the theory. Processes of meta-analysis and meta-synthesis can be used to combine findings from multiple quantitative or qualitative studies and reach conclusions about groups of related studies. The result of determining empirical adequacy is to decide if aspects of the theory need to be changed or modified.

The final step in evaluating a theory is determining *pragmatic adequacy,* which is how useful the theory is for nursing practice. To achieve pragmatic adequacy, the theory needs to be understood by nurses and they need to have the skills to apply the theory. The evaluator can look into published research to find evidence if the theory has been applied in the real world and the studies have produced consistent findings.

◉ CONCLUSION

Frameworks are essential for developing nursing knowledge, communicating that knowledge, and shaping our perspective. They guide our observations, thinking, and actions often on an implicit level. However, they are also used explicitly by educators, clinicians, nurse leaders, and researchers to guide nursing practice. Frameworks shape our worldview and serve as lenses that filter our perceptions and shape our values and beliefs about the world. The implicit uses of frameworks are pervasive in nursing practice and in daily living. However, explicit use is necessary for the growth and development of the discipline of nursing.

The importance of philosophies, models, and theories in developing and communicating nursing knowledge has necessitated organizing and classifying our knowledge into taxonomies. Nursing has also developed criteria for analyzing, evaluating, and testing theories that are useful for enhancing our understanding and determining the strengths and limitations of specific theories.

Models and theories are influenced by the theorist's worldview and philosophy. The theoretical continuum depicts philosophies, the metaparadigm, and models as the most abstract and broad in scope (Figure 1.2). As users of models and theories, we tend to be most comfortable with the theories and models that are congruent with our own worldview and philosophy. Therefore, understanding theory, as described in this chapter, can help nurses to recognize and articulate their philosophy and worldview. Nurses can use the information provided in this chapter to explore the frameworks covered in Parts II and III in more depth.

◉ KEY POINTS

- Frameworks consist of philosophies, models, theories, and taxonomies that structure and guide our observations, thinking, and actions.

- Philosophy is the love of and study of knowledge. It describes the values, ideas, and principles that frame our worldview and perspective.

- Branches of philosophy include epistemology, ontology, and axiology, which are focused on the study of knowledge, being, and value, respectively.

- Analytical school of philosophy is characterized by objectivity, empiricism, and quantitative methodology.

- Continental school of philosophy is characterized by subjective and qualitative methodology.

- Concepts are word labels used to identify people, events, situations, behaviors, experiences, and beliefs or values.

- Concepts and relationships between concepts provide the foundation for developing a theory.

- Theoretical structures exist on a continuum or hierarchy of abstraction and scope.

- The purpose of theory is to describe, explain, and/or make predictions about phenomena.

- Conceptualization involves thinking about and envisioning a phenomenon to better clarify and understand concepts.

- Hypothesizing involves using observation and reasoning to propose relationship statements and generate hypotheses between variables.

- The metaparadigm is a set of overarching concepts of concern to the discipline of nursing (i.e., person, health, environment, and nursing).

- Theories are generally formed through inductive reasoning and tested using deductive reasoning.

- Abductive reasoning is used to arrive at a reasonable conclusion or diagnosis of clinical situations.

- Theoretical substruction refers to the congruence and linkage between concepts being studied, measured, and analyzed. Lack of theoretical substruction affects the internal validity of the study.

- Analysis of a theory or a model involves examining each aspect without judgment, using predetermined criteria. Analysis is the foundation for evaluation.

- Evaluation of a theory or model is judgment based and looks at how well the theory meets predetermined criteria.

REFERENCES

Chinn, P. L., & Kramer, M. K. (1998). *Theory and nursing: A systematic approach.* St. Louis, MO: Mosby.

Cody, W. (2006). *Philosophical and theoretical perspectives for advanced nursing practice.* Sudbury, MA: Jones & Bartlett.

Dahnke, M., & Dreher, M. (2016). *Philosophy of science for nursing practice: Concepts and applications.* New York: Springer Publishing.

Dulock, H., & Holzemer, W. (1991). Substruction: Improving the linkage from theory to method. *Nursing Science Quarterly, 4*(2), 83–87.

Fawcett, J. (2013). *Contemporary nursing knowledge: Analysis and evaluation of nursing models and theories.* Philadelphia, PA: F. A. Davis.

Fawcett, J. (2015). Theory testing and theory evaluation. In J. Butts & K. Rich (Ed.), *Philosophies and theories for advanced nursing practice* (Chapter 24, pp. 593–611). Burlington, MA: Jones & Bartlett.

Fawcett, J., & DeSanto-Madeya, S. (2012). *Contemporary nursing knowledge: Analysis and evaluation of nursing models and theories* (3rd ed.). Philadelphia, PA: F. A. Davis.

Glaser, B. G., & Strauss, A. L. (1967). *The discovery of grounded theory: Strategies for qualitative research.* Chicago, IL: Aldine Publishing.

Haig, B. D. (2008). An abductive perspective on theory construction. *Journal of Theory Construction & Testing, 12*(1), 7–10.

Honderich, T. (2005). *The Oxford companion to philosophy* (2nd ed.). New York, NY: Oxford University Press.

King, I. M. (1997). The King conceptual system and theory of goal attainment. *Nursing Science Quarterly, 10,* 180–185.

Kolcaba, K. (1991). A taxonomic structure for the concept of comfort. *Image: Journal of Nursing Scholarship, 23*(4), 237–240.

Kübler-Ross, E. (1969). *On death and dying.* New York, NY: MacMillan.

Lipscomb, M. (2012). Abductive reasoning and qualitative research. *Nursing Philosophy, 13*(4), 244–256. doi:10.1111/j.1466-769X.2011.00532.x

Maslow, A. H. (1943). A theory of human motivation. *Psychological Review, 50*(4), 370–396.

McQuiston, C., & Campbell, J. (1997). Theoretical substruction: A guide for theory testing research. *Nursing Science Quarterly, 10*(3), 117–123.

Newman, M. (1975). *Theory development in nursing.* Philadelphia, PA: F. A. Davis.

Newman, M. (1994). *Health as expanding consciousness.* New York, NY: National League for Nursing.

Nightingale, F. (1860/1969). *Notes on nursing*. New York, NY: Dover Publications.

Pender, N. J. (1975). A conceptual model for preventive health behavior. *Nursing Outlook, 23*, 385–390.

Peplau, H. E. (1952). *Interpersonal relations in nursing*. New York, NY: G. P. Putnam & Sons.

Råholm, M. (2010). Abductive reasoning and the formation of scientific knowledge within nursing research. *Nursing Philosophy, 11*(4), 260–270. doi:10.1111/j.1466-769X.2010.00457.x

Reed, P., & Shearer, N. (2012). *Perspectives on nursing theory*. Philadelphia, PA: Wolters Kluwer Health/ Lippincott Williams & Wilkins.

Rogers, M. E. (1970). *An introduction to the theoretical basis of nursing*. Philadelphia, PA: F. A. Davis.

Rosenstock, I. (1974). Historical origins of the health belief model. *Health Education Monographs, 2*(4), 328–335.

Routledge, F. (2007). Exploring the use of feminist philosophy within nursing research to enhance postpositivist methodologies in the study of cardiovascular health. *Nursing Philosophy, 8*(4), 278–290.

Roy, C. (2009). *The Roy adaptation model* (3rd ed.). Upper Saddle River, NJ: Prentice Hall.

Silva, M. C., & Sorrell, J. M. (1992). Testing of nursing theory: Critique and philosophical expansion. *Advances in Nursing Science, 12*(4), 12–23.

Swanson, K. M. (1991). Empirical development of a middle-range theory of caring. *Nursing Research, 40*(3), 161–166.

Tappen, R. M. (2011). *Advanced nursing research: From theory to practice*. Sudbury, MA: Jones & Bartlett.

Thompson, M. (2012). *Understand philosophy of science*. London, UK: Hodder.

Viswanathan, B. (n.d.). Lessons from the blind men and the elephant. Retrieved from https:// balajiviswanathan.quora.com/Lessons-from-the-Blind-men-and-the-elephant

Walker, L., & Avant, K. (2011). *Strategies for theory construction in nursing*. Upper Saddle River, NJ: Prentice Hall.

Wolfe, Z., & Heinzer, M. (1999). Substruction: Illustrating the connections from research question to analysis. *Journal of Professional Nursing, 15*(1), 33–37.

Strategies for Using Frameworks

Rose Utley

There is nothing quite so practical as a good theory.
—Kurt Lewin

Everything that happens to us leaves some trace behind; everything contributes imperceptibly to make us what we are.
— Johann Wolfgang von Goethe

KEY TERMS

analogy
conceptual definition
conceptual framework
conceptualization
explicit use

frameworks
implicit use
Magnet® status
operational definition
Synergy Model

theoretical thinking
theoretical definition
theorize

LEARNING OBJECTIVES

1. Appreciate the importance of philosophies, models, theories, and taxonomies in daily living and in nursing practice.

2. Explore the concepts of conceptualization; philosophizing; and inductive, deductive, and abductive reasoning used in theoretical thinking.

3. Identify and differentiate implicit and explicit uses of frameworks in nursing practice.

4. Clarify how theories are used in nursing education, clinical practice, nursing leadership, and research roles.

The title of this chapter may be somewhat misleading because it conveys the idea that using frameworks, such as conceptual models and theories, must be a deliberate event that requires forethought or strategies. Theory does have obvious practical ramifications as alluded to by Kurt Lewin's quote or its use may be less obvious as von Goeth suggested. Although the use of theory can be explicit, it may also be less obvious, less preplanned, referred to as *implicit*. Using theory in the research process, such as with theory-testing research, demands forethought and attention to the theoretical substruction linkages as discussed in Chapter 1. That is *explicit use*. However, in teaching, clinical, or leadership roles, the use of theory is often implicit. The *implicit use* of theory is often unrecognized unless an effort is made to explore our thinking. The aim of this chapter is to bring both types of usages to your awareness.

The premise of this chapter is that we all operate with certain attitudes, values, beliefs, perceptions, and philosophical perspectives. These are formed from our ongoing experiences and education. By exploring and articulating our attitudes, values, beliefs, perceptions, and perspectives, underlying concepts important to nursing practice can be identified and linked, and relational statements can be established. This is theory making in its simplest form, a propositional statement that describes, explains, or predicts the relationship between two or more concepts. Theory is created by developing relationship statements between two or more concepts. Then, these relationship statements can be used to guide our actions and behaviors. In addition to creating a theory, concepts and relationships from existing theories can be used to guide our day-to-day activities, actions, and predispositions in nursing.

The goal of this chapter is to increase awareness of and appreciation for the explicit and implicit ways we develop and use philosophies, models, theories, and taxonomies (collectively referred to as *frameworks*), specifically, to increase the understanding and appreciation of the use of frameworks in the development of knowledge and theoretical thinking in nursing. This chapter also introduces ways in which frameworks are used by nurse educators, clinicians, leaders, and researchers. The application of frameworks to these nursing roles is addressed in greater depth in Part IV.

 ## WHY ARE THEORIES IMPORTANT?

Theories provide description, explanation, and/or prediction about phenomena in our world. To understand why theory is important to the profession of nursing, it is helpful to appreciate the definition of a profession. The key characteristics of professionals include being educated in institutions of higher learning; use of a specialized body of knowledge, expansion of the body of knowledge, and development of standards of practice (Johnson & Webber, 2001). Nursing frameworks, including philosophies, models, theories, and taxonomies, represent our specialized body of nursing knowledge. This knowledge can be expanded through research that tests existing theory or develops a new theory.

A profession's theoretical body of knowledge is a foundation for developing standards of practice and competencies of the profession (see Part IV, for applications of frameworks to the nurse educator, clinician, leader, and researcher roles). By definition, the use of and development of theory and research are necessary for professional status and distinguish professions from nonprofessions. Without theory and research, there can be no organized body of knowledge from which professionals act. The importance of the relationship between theory and research is explored further in Chapter 3.

Theories are also important to nursing because they provide perspectives for viewing and understanding phenomena we encounter in our work. The perspectives we develop as nurses come from our experiences, values, beliefs, and education. When we approach a patient care situation from a distinct, specific, perspective, we use that perspective as a *theoretical framework*. An example of using a theoretical framework is when a hospital, or a specific unit within a hospital, adopts a nursing theory such as Orem's Self-Care Theory or Roy's Adaptation Model to guide patient care and documentation. We can also combine aspects of several theoretical perspectives to form a broad, unique perspective called a *conceptual framework* or conceptual model. Fawcett notes that, "Conceptual models have existed since people began to think about themselves and their surroundings … everything that human beings see, hear, read, and experience is filtered through the cognitive lens of some conceptual frame of reference" (2005, p. 16). Therefore, theories and conceptual frameworks have intrinsic value by virtue of shaping our perceptions and molding our interactions within the world.

USING THEORIES FOR THINKING

Another characteristic of the nursing profession is that we think about, analyze, and evaluate our domain of interest and the body of knowledge that affects our practice. These processes rely on *theoretical thinking*, which includes conceptualizing, philosophizing, hypothesizing, analyzing, evaluating, and using various forms of reasoning. *Conceptualization* is the mental process of development and clarification of concepts. To conceptualize involves forming an idea or picture (concept) of something in your mind; seeing the characteristics, attributes, and/or the context in which the concept exists; and identifying the linkages and relationships of the concept to other concepts. Conceptualization is both a process of thinking about phenomena and the outcome of that thinking, which results in greater understanding of the concept. We develop definitions of concepts from our observations, experiences, and perspectives. For example, knowledge, personal experience, and the context of grief will shape how an individual conceptualizes grief. Grief can be conceptualized within a specific context such as grief related to miscarriage, or grief related to loss of a spouse, or it can be a feeling related to a perceived loss.

Theoretical thinking is an umbrella term that involves abstract thinking and uses conceptualization. It incorporates creative cognitive actions, such as inventing, defining, redefining, judging, and concluding. Additionally, theoretical thinking may involve the application of logic, contemplation of ideas, analysis of phenomena, and metacognitive functions such as reflection. Theoretical thinking is used in formal processes of theory development, theory analysis, and theory evaluation. However, it is not restricted to those processes. Nurses, whether educators, clinicians, leaders, or researchers, all engage in some degree of theoretical thinking. According to Meleis (2011), the nurse uses theoretical thinking when deciding what to assess and when to assess a patient. The clinician "develops hunches, pursues some, accepts others, and refutes others ... develops priorities, modifies them, and reorders them in the process, making some 'automatic' decisions and others that require careful consideration and deliberation" (p. 25). Clinicians use these processes and engage in theoretical thinking though they may not be aware of these underlying processes.

WHAT PURPOSES DO THEORIES SERVE?

One criticism of theories is they are not useful in clinical practice. However, in reality, theory serves many useful purposes. The problem is we have not examined theory and the contributions theories make to our lives. Theories describe, explain, and predict things that happen in our world, and to people in our world. Awareness of a theory expands our perspective and sensitizes us to observe the world differently, and more comprehensively. Theories provide the scaffolding or framework around which we observe, think, and explain things; and they help us understand our patients and the situations that affect them. The more theories to which we have been exposed, the more likely we can make sense of life, see more connections, and interpret events and situations with greater sensitivity.

According to Gopnik and Meltzoff (1997), theories have *structural, functional,* and *dynamic* qualities. Structural and functional qualities are linked to the basic purposes of theory, while the dynamic qualities provide us an understanding of the general nature of theory. Structurally, a theory is an abstract but interrelated set of concepts and relationships between concepts. The concepts of a theory provide a structure or framework around which we can expand and develop knowledge. Functionally, theories describe, explain, or make predictions about phenomena in our world. Thus, they enhance our awareness and understanding of phenomena. Finally, theories are dynamic and change, as do the concepts on which they are based.

Examples of the structural, functional, and dynamic qualities are seen in the *metaparadigm* concepts of person, environment, health, and nursing. The metaparadigm concepts provide a framework for nursing as a discipline. Nursing models and theories emphasize one or more of the metaparadigm concepts and provide a unique perspective related to those concepts. As our profession and our world have changed, so have the structure, function, and the interaction between these concepts. Changes over time give theories a dynamic quality and result in a gradual shift in our theoretical understanding and perspectives. Theories exhibit dynamic qualities by evolving and mirroring changes in our perspectives, concepts of emphasis, and definitions.

One thing nursing generally agrees on is our focus on knowledge and theory, which addresses the metaparadigm concepts of person, environment, health, and nursing. Examination of conceptual models, grand theories, and middle range theories reveal that nursing frameworks are concerned with the metaparadigm concepts but differ in the *conceptual definitions* or meanings of those concepts. For example, Roy's Adaptation Theory acknowledges the client's internal physiological and mental environment and the external stimuli (physical environment and society) as they affect the client's health and adaptation. The nurse is part of the client's external environment and is responsible for the assessment of the client's ability to adapt and modify stimuli to enhance homeostasis (see Roy's Adaptation Theory in Chapter 9). In comparison, King's Theory of Goal Attainment (see Chapter 9) focuses on the client–nurse interaction to determine and achieve health goals. The difference between any two frameworks is a matter of perspective and emphasis. In nursing, the metaparadigm concepts of person, environment, health, and nursing grounds the theories and provides a common structure.

Frameworks provide a body of knowledge used to carry out our key nursing roles in education, clinical practice, leadership, and research. Nurse educators not only teach nursing students about theories for patient care such as Orem's Self-Care Deficit Theory (Chapter 11) and Roy's Adaptation Theory (Chapter 9), but also use learning style theories (see Chapter 7) to develop their teaching approaches and guide their interaction with students. Nurse managers and administrators use leadership theories (see Chapter 18) to guide their actions and decisions. They also use theories about organizational systems and organizational change (see Chapter 17) and economics (see Chapter 15) to develop structural and procedural foundations within the work unit. Researchers conduct studies to generate new theory, test existing theory, and/or determine situations and populations in which a theory best applies (see Chapter 24). In addition, researchers may use theories as a framework for approaching the study of phenomena and may define and observe phenomena from a specific conceptual, theoretical, or philosophical perspective. Quantitative researchers may use theory to develop survey questions or research tools, and qualitative researchers may develop interview questions or conduct data analysis using certain frameworks as a guide.

Although this chapter provides merely an overview of strategies for using frameworks, more depth is provided throughout the text. In Part II of this text, philosophies, models, theories, and taxonomies related to individuals and families are reviewed; and in Part III, frameworks related to communities and organizations are discussed. The application of frameworks to the roles of the nurse educator, clinician, leader, and researcher is explored in Part IV, as well as the importance of frameworks in supporting existing standards, competencies, and expectations related to each role.

Theory as a Map Analogy

An exercise that may help to uncover the uses of theory in practice is to identify analogies between theories and maps (Fontes, 1994). This *analogy process* helps us to identify commonalities between an abstract concept (theory) and a concrete, useful object (a map) and, as a result, the nurse may see more concrete uses of theory.

So how are theories and maps similar? Both theories and maps guide us to a goal or destination. Specifically, practice theories may point out concepts that are important to consider or assess in patients, families, and in the environment. For example, when conducting health promotion activities, awareness of the main concepts in the Health Belief Model (see Chapter 9) can be used to assess the client's readiness to engage in health-promoting behavior. Asking about the client's perceptions can help anticipate perceptual barriers to change. In other words, theories can point out important things to observe as we progress on our journey and can guide us to an outcome or destination, just as a map can.

Both maps and theories have a defined scope. They are focused on specific aspects of our reality, from a particular perspective. For example, a map may be broad in scope such as a world map or narrow in scope such as a city street map. Maps that are broad in scope do not provide enough direct guidance for navigating from city to city but do provide us with awareness of major important concepts. Similarly, conceptual models are broad in scope but do not explain or guide day-to-day nursing practice. Likewise, a map with a narrow scope such as a map of biking trails in a specific city is most helpful if we are navigating that city on a bicycle. Thus, a middle range/practice theory is most helpful when working with specific types of patients or specific health care settings.

Another shared characteristic is that both theories and maps are abstract representations of reality. A map merely depicts places in our reality and shows how these places are related and connected to one another. Likewise, theories depict key concepts in our reality and identify how the concepts are connected and related to one another.

Analogy of Theoretical Structures to a Building

Theoretical structures may be visualized as a continuum comprising philosophies, the metaparadigm, conceptual models, grand theories, middle range/practice theories, and micro-theories (Figure 1.2). Duff (2011) uses the analogy of a building, explaining how the parts of a building relate to one another and how they are similar to theoretical structures within the theoretical continuum. Expanding on Duff's analogy, the philosophical perspective is added to provide the foundation for the building, and the metaparadigm concepts are added to form the four walls of the building.

Like the walls of a building, the metaparadigm concepts provide the structure for building a conceptual model or rooms of the building. There can be several conceptual models within our metaparadigm (building), and each will have a different shape, size, and/or perspective. However, each shares a connection with the metaparadigm concepts, and each is supported by a foundation or philosophical perspective. Each conceptual model may be divided into smaller rooms, which are likened to grand and middle range theories generated from a conceptual model. Each room has a purpose, a unique perspective, and uses one or more aspects of the conceptual model.

The use of the map and building analogies can be a way for students to develop understanding and appreciation of theories and see the connection between specific theoretical components. Analogies in general may facilitate movement from dualistic to conceptual thinking and from concrete to abstract thinking. The process of analogy helps us make connections between existing knowledge and new, abstract information.

USING FRAMEWORKS IN NURSING PRACTICE

Many nursing students as well as nurses in clinical practice have lamented they do not see the value of theory. Theory is abstract, which unfortunately for many nurses translates to "not practical." As many theories are concerned with things we cannot directly see, touch, or measure, and things difficult to empirically define, many nurses feel time is better spent on "practical" information. However, abstract phenomena, such as caring, comfort, therapeutic communication, self-care agency, and emotional support, are common occurrences in patient care settings and need to be understood.

Indeed, theories *are* practical precisely because they describe, explain, or predict abstract phenomena in our world. Frameworks encompassing the spectrum of theoretical structures (i.e., philosophies, models, theories, and taxonomies) expand our worldview and enable us to see things differently and more comprehensively. They provide a framework for our thinking and actions; and they sensitize and broaden our perspective. This broader perspective enables the nurse to understand others better and to interact more compassionately and effectively with others. When we realize that the multiple purposes of frameworks are to guide, describe, explain, and/or predict phenomena in our world, then their value is realized and the illusion of uselessness fades.

In the nursing roles of educator, clinician, leader, and researcher, common ways of using theory can be categorized as explicit (deliberate and formal) and implicit (nonintentional and informal). Part of the reason theory is perceived as abstract, not useful, and impractical may be related to our limited awareness of our implicit uses of the theory. This chapter explores both implicit and explicit uses of theory in teaching, clinical, leadership roles, and research practice and strategies to enhance our appreciation and use of frameworks.

Engaging in Theoretical Thinking

The importance of theory to the foundation of the nursing profession is evident in our research and in our thinking processes. According to Meleis (2011), "Theory is the goal of all scientific work. *Theorizing* is a central process in all scientific endeavors and theoretical thinking is essential to all professional undertakings" (p. 23). *Theoretical thinking* is something that all nurses do, yet may not be aware of. We think about concepts important to nursing and about how those concepts are related, and we wonder about other factors that influence the relationship between concepts. In other words, we *conceptualize* (i.e., form a mental idea) and *theorize* (i.e., generate or use theories) about events and situations in nursing.

As nurses, we engage in theoretical thinking when we use the processes of analysis and deductive, inductive, and abductive reasoning in patient care decision making, and when we use problem solving to diagnose and treat patients. Analysis occurs when we break down a concept, situation, or experience, and examine the components, processes, and relationships involved.

Various forms of reasoning are used in daily living and in nursing practice. A deductive argument claims that if the premises are true, the conclusion must be true, whereas an inductive argument claims that if its premises are true, its conclusion is probably true. When forming hypotheses or explanations about our world, inductive reasoning is typically used. This results in relationship statements that are the foundation for theory construction. When testing a hypothesis or testing theory, we engage in deductive reasoning, in which we take a generalized statement and explore its fit with instances in our world.

Though the term *abductive reasoning* may be less familiar, it also describes a process regularly used in nursing practice. Abductive reasoning involves drawing conclusions from the best available evidence. In other words, the facts are examined and compiled to arrive at the most likely conclusion (see Box 2.1 for an example of abductive reasoning). These processes are essential for decision making and problem solving in all phases of the nursing process for nurse educators, clinicians, leaders, and researchers. Engaging in theoretical thinking is common, pervasive, and typically an implicit way frameworks are used in nursing. The following sections explore more specific ways in which frameworks are used in the role of educator, clinician, leader, and researcher.

Using Frameworks in the Nurse Educator Role

Nurse educators face the tasks of helping students learn and apply theory to patient care situations, use theory to guide their teaching approaches, and use theory to structure the nursing program's philosophy and curriculum. Frameworks may be used in a formal manner,

---

BOX 2.1 Research Application of Abductive Reasoning

In the article titled, *Launching the Tidal Model: Evaluating the Evidence,* Gordon, Morton, and Brooks (2005) describe the process used to evaluate the effectiveness of the Tidal Model for achieving positive outcomes in mental health settings. They discuss a criticism that the research did not provide conclusive evidence that the implementation of the model was directly responsible for reported improvements in violence, harassment, and other adversarial behaviors. Gordon et al. point out that although a theory can be disproved through one well-designed study, no amount of research is able to provide conclusive evidence to prove a theory. Therefore, the use of abductive reasoning is the most viable alternative. In abductive reasoning, conclusions are drawn based on reasoning that the conclusion provides the best possible explanation for the findings.

---

such as having students complete a theory-based learning style assessment tool and then use the information to guide teaching approaches. Or nurse educators may use frameworks in an informal manner when they apply adult learning theory by emphasizing the usefulness of new information for the adult learner (see Chapter 7).

At the program level, nurse educators use theory to articulate the philosophy of the nursing program by identifying and defining concepts important to the program and explain the interrelationships between concepts. Many nursing programs use a specific nursing model or theory as a basis for the program's philosophy and curriculum. Others draw from multiple theories to create a unique conceptual framework for their program.

On an individual level, nurse educators may be asked to articulate their philosophy of nursing or their philosophy of teaching as part of the tenure or promotion review process. This articulation process involves identifying attitudes, values, beliefs, and perspectives regarding nursing and teaching. It involves identifying concepts and describing relationships between those concepts. Many nurse educators have not mentally nor verbally articulated their philosophy of nursing or philosophy of teaching. However, they still have one, and it just needs to be brought to a conscious level of awareness. Each educational theory or philosophy that is learned and incorporated into the nurse's cognitive structure has the potential to influence attitudes, values, beliefs, and perspectives, and eventually the educator's teaching role.

Using Frameworks in the Clinician Role

A good example of the formal use of theory in clinical practice is when an entire health care facility or nursing unit adopts a framework to guide patient care and documentation. An initiative by the American Nurses Credentialing Center (ANCC) established a program for acknowledging health care facilities for excellence, referred to as *Magnet status* (ANCC, 2016). Standard 12 for achieving Magnet status calls for the use of a quality program and evidence-based practices. To meet this standard, many organizations have integrated the use of a theory or conceptual framework to guide patient care. One example of a facility's integration of theory is the use of Henderson's Definition of Nursing Theory to provide childbirth education (Box 2.2).

The *Synergy Model* is another example of the formal use of theory in clinical practice. In 1994, the American Association of Critical-Care Nurses Certification Corporation developed the Synergy Model to link the certified critical-care nurse's practice to patient outcomes (Hardin & Kaplow, 2005). The model was founded on the idea that when synergy exists between the nurse's competencies and the patient's needs, health outcomes are improved. The nurse's clinical competency and the patient's characteristics are represented on a

---

BOX 2.2 Research Application of Virginia Henderson's Theory

Virginia Henderson's theory was used to develop the educational content for a child-birth curriculum (Waller-Wise, 2013). Using each of Henderson's 14 human needs, content relevant to childbirth was identified. For example, for the first need, to breathe normally, the author identified breathing patterns recommended for various stages of labor. For the second need—eat and drink adequately—the most recent research on the effect of certain foods and fluids on the delivery process and the fetus was identified. Content for the third need—eliminating body wastes—emphasized how the elimination of stool and urine affects the labor process, signals progression of labor, and improves comfort levels. The use of Henderson's theory provided a framework for developing a theory-based curriculum and supported the hospital's quest for Magnet status, which requires the use of evidence-based practices to guide patient care.

---

continuum, making the model adaptable to a wide range of acute care settings. Since 1999, the Synergy Model has been integrated into the Critical-Care Nurse Certification Exam. It also has been used by hospitals as the theoretical framework to guide patient care and to support the designation as a Magnet hospital.

Another example of the formal use of theory in clinical practice is the use of the nursing process. The nursing process is a common framework for providing nursing care and decision making in all areas of nursing practice. Developed by Orlando as the Deliberative Nursing Process, steps for patient care are identified, including observing the patient's behavior, the nurse's reaction, and the nurse's action (Orlando, 1961). Later, the term *diagnosis* was added as the second step in the process, and a taxonomy of nursing diagnoses was developed by the North American Nursing Diagnosis Association. When using the nursing process, assessment cues are clustered and a hypothesis is generated to formulate a diagnosis and plan interventions. Nurses then implement selected interventions and evaluate the effectiveness of interventions using the nursing interventions classification and the nursing outcomes classification systems. Thus, when using the nursing process, we form relationship statements and implement and evaluate the effectiveness of interventions. We essentially create theoretical statements and test them whenever we employ the nursing process. In the early stages of one's nursing career, the use of the nursing process is an example of the explicit, formal use of theory. Later, after the nursing process becomes internalized, it is used implicitly with less conscious deliberation.

When we implement an intervention, make suggestions for new interventions, or try certain approaches to deal with patients, we are using theory. When a postoperative patient experiences pain, we might try a medication regimen. Or if we notice that the patient's position is not optimal, we could assist him or her in changing positioning for greater comfort. When the rationale for these interventions are analyzed, we can see they are based on beliefs about the concepts and the relationships between certain concepts, which is the definition of theory.

Just as using the nursing process in clinical practice can be an informal and internalized process, using other theories may also become internalized. This process is explained by the premise of this text: that our attitudes, values, beliefs, and perspectives are influenced by our knowledge and experiences. In other words, the things we learn sensitize us and shape our attitudes, values, beliefs, and perspectives, which shape our actions or nursing care. For example, nurses familiar with the Kübler-Ross's Fives Stages of Grief are more attuned to patient behaviors that indicate shock, disbelief, anger, bargaining, and acceptance. They are more likely to understand and realize that the patient's response is part of the normal experience of loss and grief. In this example, awareness of and belief in a theory filter the nurse's interpretation of the patient's behavior and influence the nurse's response. This implicit, internalized use of theory operates automatically as part of our cognitive processes. Any theory in which we find value adds to our understanding of the world. Theory sensitizes us, guides our thinking, contributes to our perspective, and shapes our understanding of others and our interactions with others. The implicit use of theory plays a significant role in our nursing practice as clinicians, educators, leaders, and researchers.

Using Frameworks in Nursing Leadership Roles

Advances in health care technology, medical therapeutics, and emphasis on cost containment, safety, and quality of care require innovative and evidence-based practices. The use of sound clinical, administrative, and managerial theories and care delivery models enable the nurse leader to achieve desired outcomes for patients, staff, and the health care system. The scope of an administrative role in nursing practice necessitates familiarity with diverse theories in education, nursing care, organizational systems, leadership, communication, and change.

The Magnet Recognition Program®, discussed earlier, has resulted in increased motivation with health care facilities to integrate theory into the daily operations of the organization. One example of such application is the use of the Synergy Model to guide nurse/patient care assignments. Nurse administrators, managers, and charge nurses may use the Synergy Model to structure patient care assignments to align the strengths and temperament of each nurse with the needs and temperament of the patient. The nurse administrator may also help the staff apply nursing care theories to improve patient care situations or apply educational learning theories to staff developmental programs implemented within the unit.

Nurse administrators also apply leadership theories and leadership styles to the management of the unit, and they may subscribe to specific organizational, communication, and change theories when navigating changes in policies or procedures. The use of frameworks from a variety of disciplines is essential for effective administrative nursing practice. Additional uses of frameworks for nurse leader role are discussed in Chapter 23.

Using Frameworks in the Researcher Role

Research is a process used to study and generate knowledge about our world. Research is used to test existing theories or develop new theories. Nursing research is focused specifically on studying the concepts of concern to the discipline (nursing, person, environment, and health). Interestingly, the purpose of nursing research is the same as the purpose of theory: to describe, explore, explain, and/or predict things. There is a cyclical relationship between theory-generating and theory-testing research. Research generates theory and the theory provides the focus of further research. Theory-testing research examines a theory's applicability to people in certain health situations, or those who live in specific environments. Research and theory are intertwined and interdependent as discussed further in Chapter 3.

Similar to the use of frameworks by educators, clinicians, and leaders, the use of frameworks by researchers may be explicit or implicit. Explicit uses of theory occur when the researcher is testing a theory or using a framework to guide a study. In well-designed theory-testing research, the variables (concepts) are clearly defined. The *theoretical* or *conceptual definition* provides an abstract description or meaning of the variable being studied and the *operational definition* provides a definition of how the variable will be measured in the study. The congruence between the operational and theoretical/conceptual definitions is referred to as *theoretical substruction* (Dulock & Holzemer, 1991; McQuiston & Campbell, 1997; Trego, 2009). An example of inaccurate substruction would be a study of anxiety in nursing students, where anxiety was viewed as a subjective mental state of uneasiness (theoretical definition) but where anxiety was measured by increased pulse rate or inability to concentrate (operational definition). To demonstrate strong theoretical substruction, it would be necessary to change the operational definition of anxiety to a subjective mental state such as the self-reported rating of uneasiness.

Concept Analysis

Concept analysis is a foundational theory development strategy, which results in the clarification of a concept and its definition. Several processes for conducting a concept analysis have been published and used in the nursing literature. Wilson originally popularized the concept analysis process in 1963. Later, Walker and Avant (1988) presented a modified concept analysis process. More recently, Rodgers (1989, 2000) developed an evolutionary approach to concept analysis. Each of these methods is reviewed in the following.

Wilson's concept analysis method begins with asking questions about the concept (Wilson, 1963). These can be questions of fact that would be answered with empirical knowledge, or questions of values that would be answered with the use of moral principles, or questions of the meaning of the concept within the cultural context. The next step involves finding right answers by determining elements that are essential or not essential to the core of a concept. Wilson notes that questions concerning the core of a concept may not have a single right answer. The articulation of examples of the concept then follows. A model case is an example of the concept and contains all elements essential to the concept. Contrary cases are the opposite, an example of a concept that does not share any of the essential attributes. Related cases describe a similar concept that shares attributes but does not share all essential attributes. Borderline cases are missing an attribute of the concept. When concepts are rare or are very unfamiliar, an invented case is created to demonstrate the essential attributes. Wilson's method emphasizes the language used to describe the concept, the meanings derived, and the social–cultural context of the concept.

Walker and Avant (1988) built on Wilson's concept analysis approach giving more attention and details to the processes used. The first step is the selection of a concept to analyze, which should reflect the topic or area of greatest interest. Next, the aims or purpose of the analysis are determined. Concept analysis is performed to (a) clarify the meaning of the concept, (b) develop an operational definition, (c) distinguish between the ordinary and scientific usage of the concept, or (d) satisfy a personal interest in the concept. The third step is to identify all uses and definitions of the concept both in and outside of nursing. The fourth step is to determine the defining attributes of the concept by noting the repeating characteristics of the concept. The next steps are similar to Wilson's method and involve constructing a model, contrary, borderline, related, and invented case. The model case is formed from a real-life example of the concept that includes all the critical attributes of the concept. Walker and Avant added the construction of an illegitimate case, which is an example of improper use of the concept and the identification of antecedents and consequences of the concept. Antecedents are events that must occur before the occurrence of the concept. Consequences are the events that occur as a result of the occurrence of the concept. The process ends with identifying empirical referents of the concept that can be used to identify instances of the concept or provide a means to measure or collect data about the occurrence of the concept.

Rodgers's (1989) evolutionary method of concept analysis builds on previous frameworks but views concepts as dynamic and being influenced by the context of their use. Therefore, the process of analysis is more focused on the uses of the term within the discipline and on the articulation of a real-life model case. The unique aspects that Rodgers adds to concept analysis are the importance of the selection of the sample literature and the development of cases. Both the scope of the disciplines, domains reviewed, and the historical time frame of the concept are considered in the review of literature. Because of the evolving nature of

TABLE 2.1 Comparison of Concept Analysis Methods		
Steps of Rodgers's Evolutionary Method	**Steps of Walker and Avant's Method**	**Steps of Wilson's Method**
Select a concept based on significance	Select a concept	Ask a question
Identify surrogate terms and uses of the term	Determine purpose of analysis	Find the answer
Collect sample for analysis	Identify uses and definitions	Describe a model case
Identify attributes	Identify defining attributes	Describe a contrary case
Identify references, antecedents, and consequences	Develop cases similar to Wilson's method	Describe a related case
Identify related concepts		Describe an invented case
Develop a model case based on experience		

concepts, the need to identify borderline, invented, contrary, and illegitimate cases is not viewed as necessary because those types of cases describe the concept as fixed. Table 2.1 provides a comparison of the phases or steps of these concept analysis methods.

For researchers, concept analysis provides the basis for conceptual definitions of quantitative research variables and clarifies the conceptualization of concepts. Clarifying the conceptual meaning of terms helps discover the limits of our understanding and produces criteria for identifying the concept in research and nursing practice.

CONCLUSION

All nurse educators, clinicians, leaders, and researchers utilize theory in an implicit manner that may be below our conscious awareness. Many also engage in the explicit use of specific frameworks relevant to their role. Nurses may use the analogies of maps and buildings to understand the usefulness of theory and theoretical structures. A major way we use theories is when we engage in reasoning, analyzing, problem solving, hypothesizing, and decision making. These actions require the nurse to engage in theoretical thinking, which requires the use of theoretical knowledge.

KEY POINTS

- Frameworks and specific theories are used in all nursing roles and settings.
- Use of frameworks can be explicit such as using a theory to guide a research study or using a theory to guide nursing care with a health care setting.
- Implicit uses of frameworks (i.e., below conscious awareness) is common.
- The use of analogies between maps and theories and between buildings and theoretical structures can enhance understanding of the uses, purposes of theories, and the relationships between theoretical structures.

- Theoretical thinking is a common activity in nursing that involves analysis, reasoning processes, problem solving, and decision making.

- Nurse educators use frameworks to guide teaching practices, assess students, develop nursing curriculum, develop a philosophy of nursing for the nursing program, as well as develop a personal philosophy of teaching.

- Clinicians use frameworks to guide patient assessment, intervention, and documentation to enhance understanding of, and sensitivity to, the patient's needs and perspectives.

- The nursing process, nursing diagnosis systems, nursing intervention classification, and nursing outcome classification provide the process and frameworks nurses can use to develop and test relationship statements in clinical practice.

- Nurse leaders use frameworks related to organizational systems, leadership, change, management, and communication to navigate change within the nursing unit.

- Researchers design and conduct studies to test or modify existing theories and develop new theories.

- The processes a nurse researcher may use involve establishing theoretical substruction within a study and exploring the meaning of concepts through concept analysis.

- Purposes of concept analysis are to clarify the meaning, develop an operational definition, and/or differentiate uses of a concept.

REFERENCES

American Nurses Credentialing Center. (2016). Practice standards. Retrieved from http://www.nurse credentialing.org/Pathway/AboutPathway/PathwayPracticeStandards

Duff, E. (2011). Relating the nursing paradigm to practice: A teaching strategy. *International Journal of Nursing Education Scholarship, 8*(1), Art. 11. doi:10.2202/1548-923X.2076

Dulock, H. L., & Holzemer, W. L. (1991). Substruction: Improving the linkage from theory to method. *Nursing Science Quarterly, 4*(2), 83–87.

Fawcett, J. (2005). *Contemporary nursing knowledge: Analysis and evaluation of nursing models and theories.* Philadelphia, PA: F. A. Davis.

Fontes, H. C. (1994). Maps: Understanding theory through the use of analogy. *Nurse Educator, 19*(1), 5–32.

Gopnik, A., & Meltzoff, A. (1997). *Words, thoughts, and theories.* Cambridge: Massachusetts Institute of Technology Press.

Gordon, W., Morton, T., & Brooks, G. (2005). Launching the tidal model: Evaluating the evidence. *Journal of Psychiatric and Mental Health Nursing, 12*, 703–712.

Hardin, S., & Kaplow, R. (2005). *Synergy for clinical excellence: The AACN synergy model for patient care.* Sudbury, MA: Jones & Bartlett.

Johnson, B. M., & Webber, P. B. (2001). *An introduction to theory and reasoning in nursing.* Philadelphia, PA: Lippincott Williams and Wilkins.

McQuiston, C. M., & Campbell, J. C. (1997). Theoretical substruction: A guide for theory testing research. *Nursing Science Quarterly, 10*(3), 117–123.

Meleis, A. (2011). *Theoretical nursing: Development and progress.* Philadelphia, PA: Wolters Kluwer/ Lippincott Williams & Wilkins.

Orlando, I. J. (1961). *The dynamic nurse-patient relationship, function, process, and principles.* New York, NY: G. P. Putnam.

Rodgers, B. L. (1989). Concepts, analysis and the development of nursing knowledge: The evolutionary cycle. *Journal of Advanced Nursing, 14*, 330–335.

Rodgers, B. L. (2000). Concept analysis: An evolutionary view. In B. L. Rodgers & K. A. Knafl (Eds.), *Concept development in nursing: Foundations, techniques, and applications* (2nd ed., pp. 77–102). Philadelphia, PA: W. B. Saunders.

Trego, L. L. (2009). Theoretical substruction: Establishing links between theory and measurement of military women's attitudes towards menstrual suppression during military operations. *Journal of Advanced Nursing, 65*(7), 1548–1559. doi:10.1111/j.1365-2648.2009.05010.x

Walker, L. O., & Avant, K. C. (1988). *Strategies for theory construction in nursing* (2nd ed.). Norwalk, CT: Appleton & Lange.

Waller-Wise, R. (2013). Utilizing Henderson's nursing theory in childbirth education. *International Journal of Childbirth Education, 28*(2), 30–34.

Wilson, J. (1963). *Thinking with concepts.* Cambridge, MA: Cambridge University Press.

The Relationship Among Theory, Research, and Practice

Lucretia Smith

The time will come when diligent research over long periods will bring to light things which now lie hidden.
—Seneca, philosopher

The art and science of asking questions is the source of all knowledge.
—Thomas Berger, novelist

KEY TERMS

borrowed theories
Bourdieu's Theory of
  Practice
Boyer's Model of
  Scholarship
nursing theories

scholarship
scholarship of application
scholarship of clinical
  practice
scholarship of discovery
scholarship of engagement

scholarship of integration
scholarship of reflective
  practice
scholarship of teaching
theory-based practice
Transformation Theory

LEARNING OBJECTIVES

1. Define terms related to advanced nursing practice and nursing scholarship.
2. Compare and differentiate the types of scholarships.
3. Describe the interrelationship among research, theory, and nursing practice.
4. Identify the ways frameworks can be used in advanced nursing practice roles to expand nursing knowledge and improve health care outcomes.

Scholarship is defined as knowledge gained from study and research in a field (*American Heritage Dictionary*, 2016). As will become apparent in the following discussion, all nurses engage in scholarship in some way, depending on educational level and practice setting. The interrelationship among theory, research, and practice provides the mechanisms for demonstrating scholarship and building the nursing profession. Unfortunately, scholarship is often viewed as an "ivory tower" activity reserved for nurses prepared at the doctoral level. However, Boyer (1990, 1996) proposed a model that has broadened our understanding of scholarship and the definitions of what constitutes scholarship. His model of scholarship acknowledges and values the interrelationships among theory, research, and practice, which are relevant to scholarship in nursing practice.

Boyer's Model of Scholarship

Boyer (1990, 1996) identified five separate but related types of scholarship easily applicable to the nursing profession: (a) the *scholarship of discovery* or generation of new knowledge (e.g., research and quality improvement projects), (b) the *scholarship of integration* or activities that make knowledge meaningful within and across disciplines (e.g., presentations and publications), (c) the *scholarship of teaching*, which conveys meaningful knowledge to learners, (d) the *scholarship of application*, which evaluates new knowledge against practice experience and connects theory to practice in a tangible way, and (e) the *scholarship of engagement*, which channels the resources of academic disciplines toward solving society's greatest and most difficult problems (Hulsay, Nagelsmith, & Sharts-Hopko, 2015).

Boyer's typology of scholarship has been expanded by others to include two additional and complementary types of scholarship that promote clinical practice changes. Dreher (1999) described *clinical scholarship* as intellectual work that includes systematic inquiry and scrutiny of practice. Freshwater, Horton-Deutsch, Sherwood, and Taylor (2005) described *reflective practice scholarship* as thinking about professional work in conceptual and theoretical ways. These seven types of scholarship provide a solid foundation for the implementation of research and engaging in translational sciences. Additionally, they provide unlimited opportunities for nurses practicing in diverse roles and settings to contribute to nursing knowledge.

 ## THEORY, RESEARCH, AND PRACTICE

It is easy to think about nursing theory, research, and practice as separate, unrelated concepts. Nurses often believe that theory and research are not routinely used in daily practice, when in fact, both are intimately tied to nursing practice regardless of educational level or practice setting. In fact, Sellman (2010) asserted that nursing theory is pervasive in practice and that "the theory-practice division is largely imaginary because nurses cannot practice without a theory base, regardless of how well it is understood" (p. 85). Support for Sellman's assertion is provided by use of the term *theory* to mean the rationale for nursing interventions and as a term referring to the literature that supports specific nursing interventions or skills.

The interrelationship among theory, research, and practice has never been clearer than it is today. The current focus on evidence-based practice and the Centers for Medicare & Medicaid Services (CMS) value-based purchasing system to improve health care (CMS, 2015) necessitates the use of research to generate knowledge and use it in practice.

Evolution of the Nurse's Knowledge and Understanding

Nursing students in pre-licensure programs learn to provide direct nursing care to patients using concepts and evidence generated by theory. However, they are largely unaware of the different types of nursing scholarship, different levels of nursing theory, and the interrelationships among theory, research, and practice. Nursing students are essentially operating from the "ground level." They are focused on the task at hand and are often unable to appreciate broader perspectives.

In contrast, nurses in graduate nursing programs are learning to use *ground level* practice as a springboard for identifying problems relevant to nursing. Through advanced education and practice, they learn to engage in one or more of the seven types of scholarship described earlier. The nurse is able to select appropriate frameworks from nursing or another discipline to inform and guide his or her practice and research. In graduate studies, additional skills in appraising the strength of evidence and applying the evidence to decision making at the individual, community, and organizational systems level are acquired (American Association of Colleges of Nursing [AACN], 2006; Butts, Rich, & Fawcett, 2012; Karnick, 2014). The graduate student in nursing becomes increasingly aware that the interrelationships among theory, research, and practice are vital to the generation of knowledge and that these inter-relationships provide mechanisms for evaluating evidence, refining theory, and enhancing practice. Furthermore, these processes of knowledge generation and testing ensure that nursing is meeting professional expectations and is fulfilling its unique contract with society. Thus, the interrelationships among theory, research, and practice establish nursing as a scholarly discipline with an important and unique knowledge base.

Using the Theoretical Hierarchy to Understand

The levels of nursing theory provide a good way to understand the linkage among theory, research, and practice. Theory is defined as a set of cohesive, interrelated concepts that describe, explain, or predict nursing care; guide nursing practice; and provide a foundation for clinical decision making (Petiprin, 2016). Grand theories are complex and comprise abstract concepts that describe the key concepts and principles of the discipline (e.g., what nursing is and is not). Middle range theories are more precise and describe, explain, or predict a situation or phenomenon using a limited number of variables. Practice theories, also called *situation-specific* theories, are prescriptive for one practice situation, identify specific goals, and describe how the goals will be met (Butts & Rich, 2015).

The different levels of nursing frameworks provide many opportunities to select one that fits the study's purpose and aims at, guides the inquiry, or leads to greater understanding of the research or clinical question. Nursing researchers use frameworks developed by nurses specifically for nursing (i.e., *nursing theories*) or may use frameworks developed by other disciplines (i.e., *borrowed theories*). Whether originating in nursing or another discipline, these frameworks are useful for understanding factors related to nursing's metaparadigm concepts of person, health, environment, and nursing. For example, frameworks relevant to understanding the individual that have been addressed in this text include human development (Chapter 6), human needs (Chapter 11), and psychological frameworks (Chapter 13). Frameworks for understanding health include health promotion (Chapter 4), health and illness frameworks (Chapter 9), and physiological frameworks (Chapter 12). Knowledge of the environment is heightened by frameworks covered in Chapters 15, 16, 17, and 20. Understanding of nursing is facilitated by frameworks covered in Chapters 5, 14, and 18.

The Hospital Supply Room Analogy

Understanding the interrelationships among theory, research, and practice can also be enhanced by an analogy to a familiar concept, a hospital supply area. At the broadest level, the hospital supply room represents conceptual models and grand theories from nursing or another discipline. Within the supply room are the tools (i.e., middle range and practice-level theories, and theoretical concepts or variables) needed by the clinician to provide patient care and explore or answer research or clinical questions. Tools that are well matched to the task (i.e., the research question or nursing care) are selected, and the nurse evaluates how useful each is in completing the task. The nurse also evaluates how well the tools worked or if different tools (i.e., a different theory or theoretical concepts or variables) would be more useful. The nurse who is familiar with the tools in the supply room can easily identify appropriate tools to complete the nursing tasks. However, when the tools in the unit's supply room are not regularly evaluated for efficiency and fit to the task, they may become outdated or unusable and may lead to poor task performance. This analogy provides a view of the interrelationship among theory, research, and practice at a broad level. Once a broad view is understood, the specific relationships between theory and research and theory and practice can often become much clearer.

Theory Development

The usefulness of a framework lies in its ability to add to existing knowledge about the question or problem under study. For example, theory-testing research can identify new concepts or relationships between concepts that advance the theory and make it more meaningful to practice. Sometimes, an entirely new theory can emerge that provides a completely new perspective on the question or problem. Theory development is largely accomplished using qualitative inductive methods and tested using quantitative deductive methods.

Qualitative research, such as that of Alligood and Fawcett (2004), can clarify the definitions and relationships of a theory. They conducted a rational hermeneutic interpretive study of Martha Rogers's use of the terms *pattern* and *patterning*. The process involved five steps: (a) identifying written passages, (b) discussing the interpretation, (c) identifying new insights based on current understanding, (d) discussing insights and conceptual changes in the meaning over time, and (e) discussing Rogers's rationale for those conceptual changes. As a result of the research, they were able to clarify the definitions and distinguish pattern, the noun, from patterning, the verb.

In qualitative research, theory may also guide how phenomena should be studied. In other cases, qualitative research is conducted to generate new theory. In grounded theory, for example, the researcher *grounds* the theory directly in the data without letting previous thinking about the phenomena influence the interpretation of the data. It is the job of future qualitative and quantitative researchers to test and refine theory (Connelly, 2014; Green, 2014).

When research is conducted without a theoretical framework, findings do not advance, and existing knowledge and theory development will stall or come to a complete stop (Connelly, 2014). According to Connelly, although a theory or conceptual framework provides a useful lens through which to study a nursing problem, not all studies or projects require one. Connelly suggested that a study or project should not include a theoretical framework simply to have one. Instead, a theory or conceptual framework must clearly direct the design of the study to maximize the understanding of the problem or question under study. A single theory is seldom adequate to describe nursing practice or thoroughly inform and guide a research study or project. More often, multiple theories, matched to the nursing problem or question, are used as a conceptual framework for a study or project. See Box 3.1 for a review of the use of the Quality Health Outcomes Model as a framework for research.

Relationship Between Theory and Practice

Theory-based practice refers to practice in which theory provides the basis for prediction and prevention (Dale, 1994). The hallmark of the relationship between theory and research is the reflection and critical thinking that results in a clinical question and guides selection of a

---

BOX 3.1 Example of Theory Used in Research

Radwin and Fawcett (2002) described the application of the Quality Health Outcomes Model (QHOM) to past and present research by Fawcett. The QHOM proposes that interventions interact with client characteristics and health care system characteristics to produce outcomes. Use of the QHOM allowed Fawcett to view seemingly disparate studies as a coherent program of research and provided a framework for guiding future research. Aligning with an explicit conceptual model provided a meaningful frame of reference for interpreting previous research and uncovered possibilities for future research.

theory or conceptual framework to drive the study and guide project design decisions. Well-constructed, reliable, and valid theory provides concepts and principles that are capable of directly guiding practice.

The primary consideration in theory selection is the usefulness of the theory for making predictions that guide nursing practice for specific populations, settings, and roles. Studies to test and revise a theory should be conducted before it is used in a new setting or with a new population. Therefore, borrowed theories, as well as nursing theories, should be carefully considered and tested before application to specific nursing contexts. Careful consideration and testing of a theory before clinical application provide support and evidence for nursing actions.

Theory as a Guide to Practice

All levels of nursing theory guide practice in some fashion. However, middle range and practice theories provide the best guide for direct clinical practice. One example is explained by a nurse who used Barrett's theoretical concept of "voluntary mutual patterning." The nurse described it this way:

> As [the client] was speaking, I saw nursing theory unfolding before my eyes. The client's actions were evidence to support Barrett's proposition that "power is knowing-participation in change!" I believe that my responsibility as a nurse is to witness and reflect the positive changes that patients make as they claim their power as human beings. (Reyes, 2013, p. 62)

Another example of using theory to guide practice is demonstrated by the use of the theory-based sharing the patient's illness representations to increase trust (SPIRIT) intervention to facilitate end-of-life decision making (Box 3.2). The SPIRIT intervention was developed based on sound theoretical underpinnings and pilot tested on diverse patient populations.

Practice as a Guide to Theory

Just as theory guides practice, practice often guides theory. For example, nurses are sensitive to the need to support families with young children. There has been a significant impetus at the international level to establish partnerships between professionals and families. Hopwood, Fowler, Lee, Rossiter, and Bigsby (2013) organized a study of this partnership phenomenon using the Family Partnership Model. They found that aspects of advanced nursing practice, such as time, tasks, and facility expectations, often interfered with establishing

---

BOX 3.2 Example of Theory Used in Practice

Authors Song and Ward (2015) explained the theoretical underpinnings of an advanced care planning intervention, called SPIRIT, which stands for "sharing the patient's illness representations to increase trust." The SPIRIT intervention was designed to prepare the patient and his or her surrogate decision maker for end-of-life decision making. SPIRIT developed from the synthesis of an intervention checklist developed by Conn (2012) and an intervention taxonomy called intervention taxonomy, developed by Schulz, Czaja, McKay, Ory, and Belle (2010). The guiding theory of the SPIRIT intervention proposes that individuals have representations of their illness or health problems. Understanding these representations is critical because they affect whether or not an individual will accept or reject information and whether or not new knowledge will be translated into changes in behavior.

nurse–family partnerships and the ability to set meaningful family goals. The resulting theory referred to as *practice architectures* was proposed. Refinement of the theory/framework was conducted to make it usable by advanced practice nurses involved in creating partnerships with families.

Another example of practice guiding theory is the development of a trauma care model that included long-term nursing interventions. The model developed by Richmond and Aitken (2011) depicts a continuum of trauma care, ranging from predefinitive, definitive, and postdischarge phases and their impact on long-term health outcomes.

> All elements of the injury continuum from pre-injury risk through to long-term outcomes of trauma care take place within and are directly affected, both positively and negatively, by all aspects of the socio-economic-cultural environment. The "pre-injury" person and family factors come with the person to all phases of care and these factors directly affect the interventions, structure and intermediate outcomes of care. (p. 2746)

The model that includes all phases of care from emergency through long-term rehabilitation continues to be tested (Richmond & Aitken, 2011).

Relationship Between Research and Practice

The case has been made that theory is both a guide for practice and a result of practice, with research being the link between theory and practice. However, some nursing leaders are attempting to use evidence without a supporting theory or framework (McCrae, 2012). Therefore, it would be appropriate to note the present state of relationships among research, evidence-based practice, and nursing practice. There is discussion that, even if research evidence could be separated from theory, nurses still do not readily base their daily tasks on the researched evidence. In 1998, Rolfe argued there was a significant gap between research and practice. Then Matthew-Maich, Ploeg, Jack, and Dobbins (2009) noted the inconsistent use of research and argued that using research in practice involved not only changing the practices of nurses but changing their beliefs and attitudes.

Interestingly, Matthew-Maich et al. (2010) proposed the *Transformation Theory* as an explanatory theory to account for nurses' failure to engage in research utilization practice. The theory identifies strategies such as critical reflection and critical discourse as helpful in exploring and transforming nurses' attitudes, beliefs, and behaviors so that research may be understood, validated, and used more consciously to guide actions.

Severinsson (2012) reviewed articles on the link between practice and theory. The growing interest in evidence-based practice (EBP) has done much to increase the funding and production of research aimed at guiding nursing practice. Severinsson argued that bringing research to bear on the day-to-day practice of nurses will result in better patient care, increasingly regulated nursing practice, and more cost-effective care. In addition, Severinsson recognized the importance of using research to discover the gaps and the reasons for the gaps between the research evidence and its implementation in practice. Last, but not least, Severinsson noted the importance of theory to guide implementation, develop collaboration between research and practice, and develop relationships between people involved in research and practice.

◉ INTEGRATING THEORY, RESEARCH, AND PRACTICE

In a perfect world, a practicing nurse would have time to notice trends in patient responses to illness and care. These trends would trigger research studies, which when based on replicated findings, would refine the theory. Evidence would accumulate and be translated into practice. Then nursing practice would use the theory, evaluate the effectiveness of the theory in improving patient outcomes, and revise the theory if indicated. In the real world, completion of these complex cycles takes time and expertise, often more than an individual nurse, or even group of nurses is likely to possess. This creates significant barriers to the integration of theory, research, and practice. However, when those barriers are overcome, multiple benefits in the form of development of professional knowledge (i.e., theory), utilization of EBP, and improved patient outcomes can be realized.

As previously mentioned, the complexity and time consumption required may be the most problematic aspects of integrating theory, research, and practice (Bjørk et al., 2013). This process includes three steps in which time and education are essential. First, a thorough understanding of the theory is required, followed by a comprehensive review of the research that supports the theory. Then a clear statement of guidelines for introducing the relationships and definitions into practice needs to be developed (Fawcett, 2009). Despite the barriers, several nursing scholars have developed theories that describe the process and guide nurses in integrating theory and research into nursing practice (Rhynas, 2005; Wilson, 2014). See Box 3.3 for a study by Rhynas, which used Bourdieu's Theory of Practice.

This reciprocal relationship between theory and practice occurs not only at the level of ideas but at the level of people and personal interaction in which collaboration between practitioners and theorists is essential (Chan, Chan, & Liu, 2012; Hatlevik, 2012). The advantage of having multiple nurses involved in the collaboration process is that it often engenders ownership by nurses. Nurses who own the integration of theory, research, and practice are more likely than spectators to build a professional nursing skill set versus a technical nursing skill set.

Another closely related benefit is the ability of multiple nurses in multiple roles to communicate clearly with one another and develop respect for each individual's contribution to the process. Parlour and McCormack (2012) offer the Practice Development Framework to guide nurses in their methods of practice and evaluation. Based on critical realism and emancipatory practice theories, the framework focuses on the influence and outcomes of practice, not only on the client but on nursing's need to implement change. Use of the framework begins with Enlightenment, a stage that contains an in-depth assessment of the macro and micro contexts of the nurses' practice and client environments. In the second stage, Empowerment, themes are developed from the assessment and actions implemented around the need for change. The last stage, Emancipation, contains the evaluation of the changes and relates

---

BOX 3.3 Example of Integrating Theory, Research, and Practice

Rhynas (2005) used Bourdieu's Theory of Practice as a research framework to explore how nurses conceptualize illness and the clients for whom they care. Bourdieu's theory values reflexivity and uses the concepts of field, capital, and habitus to explain the individual's interactions within the social world. The field is the frame of analysis and includes structures, institutions, authorities, and activities. Capital represents the power of a person and can be economic, cultural, or symbolic. Habitus encompasses the history, tradition, customs, and principles that people do not make explicit. According to Rhynas, Bourdieu's framework

could allow nurse researchers to explore the interactions of nurses with the structures, agents, and symbols of illness within the field of care. This work could enhance understanding of how nurses view and react to patients in their care, and promote the development of practice innovations and policy change. (p. 179)

Use of this theory can facilitate knowledge of how nurses view and react to patients in their care, and could guide the development of interventions and policy change.

them specifically to improved practice outcomes. Across all stages is the expectation that evidence will be obtained, applied, and disseminated. The framework contains grids and other tools to aid multiple researchers and practitioners in the development of cohesive and effective nursing.

⬤ CONCLUSION

Theory, research, and practice constitute three inseparable components in the life of a professional nurse and the nursing profession. Using research in day-to-day nursing practice will enhance patient care and nursing practice, and can help to provide safe and cost-effective care. The survival of nursing as a profession depends on nurses' ability to understand and apply theory and the evidence that supports it, and on the efforts of nurse researchers to build and maintain nursing theory and knowledge. The interaction of nursing research and practice is at the forefront of this scholarship. It is the privilege and responsibility of those involved in advanced nursing practice to participate in, and advocate for this scholarship.

⬤ KEY POINTS

- Nursing theory is not static but under continual revision.
- All nurses engage in some form of scholarship.
- Boyer's Model of Scholarship, which incorporates aspects of theory, research, and practice, defines five types of scholarship: (a) discovery, (b) application, (c) integration, (d) teaching, and (e) engagement.
- Dreher described clinical scholarship as involving systematic inquiry and scrutiny of practice.
- Freshwater et al. described "reflective practice scholarship" as conceptual and theoretical thinking about one's professional work.
- Both research and practice act to create and revise theory.
- Theory acts as a guide to both practice and research.
- Integrating theory, research, and practice defines and distinguishes nursing as a profession.
- The process of integrating theory, research, and practice requires understanding the theory, a comprehensive review of the research that supports the theory, and the development of guidelines and definitions to be used in practice.
- Barriers to integrating theory, research, and practice include time, expertise, and complexity of the process.
- Benefits of integrating theory, research, and practice include the development of professional knowledge (i.e., theory), utilization of EBP, and improved patient outcomes.
- The integration and advocacy of nursing scholarship is the privilege and responsibility of nursing in advanced nursing practice roles.

REFERENCES

Alligood, M. R., & Fawcett, J. (2004, January). An interpretive study of Martha Rogers' conception of pattern. *Visions: The Journal of Rogerian Nursing Science, 12*(1), 8–13.
American Association of Colleges of Nursing. (2004). AACN position statement on the practice doctorate in nursing. Retrieved from http://www.aacnnursing.org/DNP/Position-Statement

American Association of Colleges of Nursing. (2006). *AACN position statement on nursing research*. Washington, DC: Author.

American Heritage. (2016). Scholarship. *The American Heritage dictionary of the English language*. Boston, MA: Houghton Mifflin Harcourt.

American Nurses Association. (n.d.). What is nursing? Retrieved from http://nursingworld.org/EspeciallyForYou/What-is-Nursing.

Bjørk, I. T., Lomborg, K., Nielsen, C. M., Brynildsen, G., Frederiksen, A. S., Larsen, K.,...Steinholt, B. (2013). From theoretical model to practical use: An example of knowledge translation. *Journal of Advanced Nursing, 69*(10), 2336–2347. doi:10.1111/jan.12091

Boyer, E. L. (1996). Clinical practice as scholarship. *Holistic Nursing Practice, 10*(3), 1–6.

Boyer, E. L., & Carnegie Foundation for the Advancement of Teaching. (1990). *Scholarship reconsidered: Priorities of the professoriate*. San Francisco, CA: Jossey-Bass.

Butts, J. B., & Rich, K. L. (2015). *Philosophies and theories for advanced nursing practice*. Burlington, MA: Jones & Bartlett.

Butts, J. B., Rich, K. L., & Fawcett, J. (2012). The future of nursing: How important is discipline-specific knowledge? A conversation with Jacqueline Fawcett. *Nursing Science Quarterly, 25*(2), 151–154. doi:10.1177/0894318412437955

Centers for Medicare & Medicaid Services. (2015). Home health value-based purchasing model. Retrieved from https://innovation.cms.gov/initiatives/home-health-value-based-purchasing-model

Chan, E.A., Chan, K., & Liu, Y.W. (2012). A triadic interplay between academics, practitioners, and students in the nursing theory and practice dialectic. *Journal of Advanced Nursing, 68*(5),1038–1049. doi:10.1111/j.1365-2648.2011.05808.x

Conn, V. S. (2012). Unpacking the black box: Countering the problem of inadequate intervention descriptions in research reports. *Western Journal of Nursing Research, 34*(4), 427–433. doi:10.1177/0193945911434627

Connelly, L. M. (2014). Use of theoretical frameworks in nursing research. *MEDSURG Nursing, 23*(3), 187–188.

Dale, L. E. (1994). The theory-theory gap: The challenge for nurse teachers. *Journal of Advanced Nursing, 20*, 521–524.

Dreher, M. C., & Sigma Theta Tau International Clinical Scholarship Task Force. (1999). *Clinical scholarship resource paper*. Indianapolis, IN: Sigma Theta Tau. Retrieved from https://www.nursingsociety.org/docs/default-source/position-papers/clinical_scholarship_paper.pdf?sfvrsn=4

Fawcett, J. (2009). Using the Roy adaptation model to guide research and/or practice: Construction of conceptual-theoretical-empirical systems of knowledge. *Aquichan, 9*(3), 297–306.

Freshwater, D., Horton-Deutsch, S., Sherwood, G., & Taylor, B. (2005). *The scholarship of reflective practice*. Indianapolis IN: Sigma Theta Tau International. Retrieved from http://www.nursingsociety.org/aboutus/PositionPapers/Documents/resource_reflective.pdf

Green, H. (2014). Use of theoretical and conceptual frameworks in qualitative research. *Nurse Researcher, 21*(6), 34–38. doi:10.7748/nr.21.6.34.e1252

Hatlevik, I. R. (2012). The theory-practice relationship: Reflective skills and theoretical knowledge as key factors in bridging the gap between theory and practice in initial nursing education. *Journal of Advanced Nursing, 68*(4), 868–877. doi:10.1111/j.1365-2648.2011.05789.x

Hopwood, N., Fowler, C., Lee, A., Rossiter, C., & Bigsby, M. (2013). Understanding partnership practice in child and family nursing through the concept of practice architectures. *Nursing Inquiry, 20*(3), 199–210. doi:10.1111/nin.12019

Hulsay, T., Nagelsmith, L., & Sharts-Hopko, N. (2015). STTI scholarship defined. Retrieved from http://www.nursingsociety.org/docs/default-source/position-papers/resource_scholarship_definition.pdf

Hutchinson, M., East, L., Stasa, H., & Jackson, D. (2014). Deriving consensus on the characteristics of advanced practice nursing. *Nursing Research, 63*(2), 116–128. doi:10.1097/NNR.0000000000000021

Karnick, P. (2014). A case for nursing theory in practice. *Nursing Science Quarterly, 27*(2), 117. doi:10.1177/0894318414522711

Matthew-Maich, N., Ploeg, J., Jack, S., & Dobbins, M. (2010). Transformative learning and research utilization in nursing practice: A missing link? *Worldviews on Evidence-Based Nursing, 7*(1), 25–35. doi:10.1111/j.1741-6787.2009.00172.x

McCrae, N. (2012). Whither nursing models? The value of nursing theory in the context of evidence-based practice and multidisciplinary health care. *Journal of Advanced Nursing, 68*(1), 222–229. doi:10.1111/j.1365-2648.2011.05821.x

Parlour, R., & McCormack, B. (2012). Blending critical realist and emancipatory practice development methodologies: Making critical realism work in nursing research. *Nursing Inquiry, 19*(4), 308–321. doi:10.1111/j.1440-1800.2011.00577.x

Petiprin, A. (2016). Nursing theory definition. Retrieved from http://www.nursing-theory.org/articles/nursing-theory-definition.php

Radwin, L., & Fawcett, J. (2002). A conceptual model-based programme of nursing research: Retrospective and prospective applications. *Journal of Advanced Nursing, 40*(3), 355–360. doi:10.1046/j.1365-2648.2002.02377.x

Reyes, D. (2013). A composite case study of a woman with human immunodeficiency virus: Integration of nursing research and theory with practice. *International Journal of Nursing Knowledge, 24*(1), 59–62. doi:10.1111/j.2047-3095.2012.01232.x

Rhynas, S. (2005). Bourdieu's theory of practice and its potential in nursing research. *Journal of Advanced Nursing, 50*(2), 179–186. doi:10.1111/j.1365-2648.2005.03377.x

Richmond, T. S., & Aitken, L. M. (2011). A model to advance nursing science in trauma practice and injury outcomes research. *Journal of Advanced Nursing, 67*(12), 2741–2753. doi:10.1111/j.1365-2648.2011.05749.x

Rolfe, G. (1998). The theory-practice gap in nursing: From research based practice to practitioner based research. *Journal of Advanced Nursing, 28*(3), 672–679.

Schulz, R., Czaja, S. J., McKay, J. R., Ory, M. G., & Belle, S. H. (2010). Intervention taxonomy (ITAX): Describing essential features of interventions. *American Journal of Health Behaviors, 34*(6), 811–821. doi:10.5993/AJHB.34.6.15

Sellman, D. (2010). Mind the gap: Philosophy, theory, and practice. *Nursing Philosophy, 11*(2), 85–87. doi:10.1111/j.1466-769X.2010.00438.x

Severinsson, E. (2012). Nursing research in theory and practice: Is implementation the missing link? *Journal of Nursing Management, 20*(2), 141–143. doi:10.1111/j.1365-2834.2012.01387.x

Song, M., & Ward, S. (2015). Making visible a theory-guided advance care planning intervention. *Journal of Nursing Scholarship, 47*(5), 389–396. doi:10.1111/jnu.12156

Wilson, A. (2014). Being a practitioner: An application of Heidegger's phenomenology. *Nurse Researcher, 21*(6), 28–33. doi:10.7748/nr.21.6.28.e1251

Frameworks for Individuals and Families

All that is valuable in human society depends upon the opportunity for development accorded to the individual.
—Albert Einstein, scientist

Call it a clan, call it a network, call it a tribe, call it a family: Whatever you call it, whoever you are, you need one.
—Jane Howard, novelist

The next 11 chapters cover frameworks relevant to individuals and families. Each chapter represents a conceptual cluster of frameworks related to a specific concept pertinent to the individual and/or family. Topics include behavioral change, care and caring, human development, teaching and learning, moral–ethical perspectives, health and illness, interpersonal and family relationships, human needs, psychological frameworks, physiological frameworks, and roles. This clustering allows the nurse to gain an overview of selected frameworks within each conceptual area, compare and contrast these frameworks, and engage in an additional study of the frameworks most relevant to his or her clinical practice or research areas of interest.

Frameworks for Individuals and Families

Frameworks for Behavioral Change

Kristina Henry

If you're in a bad situation, don't worry it'll change. If you're in a good situation,
don't worry it'll change.
—John A. Simone, Sr.

Bandura's Self-Efficacy
    Theory
behavioral change
    frameworks
change
change theories
Common Sense Model of
    Self-Regulation

Health Action Process
    Approach
Health Belief Model
Health Promotion Model
Integrated Behavioral
    Model
Lewin's Change Theory
Lippitt's Theory of Change

self-efficacy
Theory of Planned
    Behavior
Theory of Reasoned Action
Transtheoretical Model of
    Behavioral Change

LEARNING OBJECTIVES

1. Define and explain the process of change.
2. Explore the key elements of theories and models related to individual and personal change, including purpose, application, and evaluation.
3. Describe theories and models as applied to individual and personal change processes.
4. Analyze the application of theories and models used to guide individual and personal change processes.
5. Analyze recent, as well as potential, evidence-based practice of theories and models as applied to individual and personal change.

For many people, change elicits a negative connotation. Others may be excited and invigorated by the notion of change. However, everyone can agree that change is challenging and complicated. The concept of *change* is rooted in the idea of modifying or altering something that exists. Regardless of the positive or negative nature of change, it is by definition a transformation or a difference in what has been considered the norm. Frameworks have been developed and tested to explain, facilitate, and guide this process. This chapter focuses on personal change processes and the roles and responsibilities of the patient and nurse in those processes.

A primary role of the nurse is to facilitate behavioral change to achieve positive health outcomes. To do this, the nurse partners with the patient while collaborating with the health care team to maximize health outcomes. The nurse cannot expect to improve patient outcomes without empowering the patient to change negative behaviors. The caring and compassionate attributes of nurses combined with the ability to navigate a complex health care environment produces nurses who are expert in facilitating change. *Change theories* and models are tools designed to guide the patient, the nurse, and the health care team as they lead and manage this process. Choosing a framework should be based on its applicability to the particular patient situation.

Change frameworks focused on individual behavioral change are based on psychological concepts such as behavior and cognition. As patient teaching frequently involves patient change, learning theories are frequently used in conjunction with change theories (see Chapter 7). The change frameworks related to organizational and system change are addressed in Chapters 17 and 18. However, many change frameworks can be applied at both the individual and organizational systems level as they are easily adaptable or generalizable depending on the topic, project, or population.

 ## BEHAVIORAL CHANGE FRAMEWORKS

Educating and advocating for patients is a primary responsibility of nurses. The approach to patient care is not a "one size fits all" approach. The patient's needs and desires guide this process; therefore, the plan of care must be patient specific. For this reason, it is crucial for nurses to understand and use behavioral change frameworks as guides to develop patient-specific care and optimize patient outcomes.

Behavioral change frameworks represent a general concept used to describe a set of theories and models that explain why people change their behavior and explore the motivation or stimulus behind the change initiative. Many theories and models come under the umbrella term of *behavioral frameworks*. In this chapter, classic behavioral change frameworks are reviewed, including the Health Belief Model (HBM), Lewin's Change Theory, Lippitt's Theory of Change, the Theory of Reasoned Action (TRA), and the Theory of Planned Behavior (TPB). Other more recent frameworks, such as the Integrated Behavioral Model (IBM), Bandura's Self-Efficacy Theory, the Transtheoretical Model of Behavioral Change, Pender's Health Promotion Model (HPM), the Common Sense Model (CSM) of Self-Regulation, and the Health Action Process Approach (HAPA), are also covered. See Table 4.1 for a comparison of behavioral change frameworks in terms of grounding influences, key concepts, and unique attributes.

The Health Belief Model

The HBM was developed in the 1950s by a group of social psychologists to explain the lack of participation in health-related programs offered by the U.S. Public Health Department (Rosenstock, 1974). The HBM is still widely used and has provided a foundation for the development of many other models and theories (Skinner, Tiro, & Champion, 2015).

The model provides a way to discover what motivates people to take specific actions regarding their health. Six beliefs are offered to explain a person's motivation to engage in healthy behaviors. These are four perceptual barriers to motivation to change and two factors related to taking action. Motivation is influenced by the individual's perception of (a) susceptibility to the disease, (b) severity of the consequences, (c) benefits of taking action, and (d) barriers such as costs–benefits. The final two concepts relate to the individual taking action. The individual needs to have cues to action, meaning he or she should know and be

TABLE 4.1 Comparison of Behavioral Change Frameworks

Theory (Theorist)	Grounding Influence	Key Concepts	Unique Attributes and Utilization
Self-Efficacy (Bandura)	Behavioral Change Theory	Perception of ability to change is based on experience, modeling, social persuasion, and physiological factors	Empowering the individual to undergo the self-change process
Theory of Reasoned Action (TRA) (Fishbein & Ajzen)	Behavioral Change Theory	Personal beliefs, societal influences, and consequences of behavior are considered before purposeful behavior or decisions	Used to predict behaviors and decisions
Theory of Planned Behavior (Ajzen)	Behavioral Change Theory, TRA	Addresses the individual's perceived level of control	Used to predict behaviors and decisions
Transtheoretical Model of Behavioral Change (Prochaska, DiClemente & Norcross)	Behavioral Change Theory: Self-Efficacy	Based on six stages: precontemplation, contemplation, preparation, action, maintenance, and termination	Applicable to long-term change processes Acknowledges relapse and reentry into the change process
Health Action Process Approach (Schwarzer)	Behavioral Change Theory: Self-Efficacy	Based on a two-phase process: goal setting (motivation) and goal pursuit (volition)	Explains and predicts change from unhealthy to healthy practices
Change Theory (Lewin)	Social Psychology	Based on three stages of change: Unfreezing, Moving, and Refreezing	Basic change concepts are generalized to any change process
Theory of Change (Lippitt, Watson, & Westley)	Lewin's Change Theory	Based on seven stages: diagnosis, willingness to change, evaluate change agent, plan change, define change agent role, change progress, and terminate change agent	Emphasizes the role of external change agent to facilitate the change process

reminded to take action, and the individual needs *self-efficacy* or the ability to perform the needed actions. Motivating factors can include either positive benefits or avoidance of negative consequences. Each influences a person's perception of a threat and the likelihood that he or she will adopt a new health behavior (see Table 4.2, which highlights concepts within the HBM).

Research, patient care, and most clinical nursing roles can benefit by considering each of the HBM beliefs in the context of their patients. Attention to these beliefs when screening the

TABLE 4.2 Health Belief Model Concepts

Perceptions	Modifying Factors	Likelihood of Action
Perceived susceptibility	Demographic variables	Perceived benefits of action minus perceived barriers to action
Perceived severity	Psycho-social variables	Perceived threat (a result of susceptibility, severity, variables, and cues to action)
	Structural variables	
	Cues to action	

Sources: Bensley and Brookins-Fisher (2009); Skinner, Tiro, and Champion (2015).

products and services offered to patients will benefit both the patient and the nursing profession. In light of the multifaceted nature of these beliefs and the dynamic context in which individuals live and work, research should continue to explore the patient's health behavior, to discover ways to facilitate behavioral change.

Lewin's Change Theory

In 1951, psychologist Kurt Lewin developed what would become a well-known theory of change. According to Lewin's Change Theory, the process of change occurs in three dynamic stages: unfreezing, moving, and refreezing (Figure 4.1). The unfreezing stage involves the preparation for change, including problem analysis and stakeholder identification. The moving stage consists of acceptance of the need for change and implementation of the change process. Patient empowerment and participation are essential for successful implementation. The refreezing stage is the final integration of the modification into practice, in which the change becomes the cultural norm. These stages are fluid and dynamic, as opposed to distinct categories with specific completion markers.

Lewin (1951) explained the presence of driving and resistant forces in the change process. Driving forces are change agents that empower and motivate others to engage in the process of modification. Resistant forces are those that oppose modification and instead strive to abolish the change movement. For change to successfully occur, the driving forces must lead and control the resistant forces.

Lewin's Change Theory is generalizable and lends itself to potential application in individual, family, community, organizational, and system change projects. Many modern change theories have roots in Lewin's Change Theory. For example, Everett Rogers (1995) expanded on Lewin's Change Theory and developed the Diffusion of Innovation Theory for greater applicability to organizations and systems (see the discussion in Chapter 18).

Lippitt's Theory of Change

Lippitt's Theory of Change is based on seven stages and emphasizes the use of an external change agent (Lippitt, Watson, & Westley, 1958). Like many other theories of change, it is based on the original premise of Lewin's Change Theory. However, the focus is on the change agent and not the process of change. Lippitt et al. emphasized that the success of a specific change becomes greater the more widespread the modification. For instance, if an individual can apply the change in more than one aspect of his or her life, the greater the chance of maintenance.

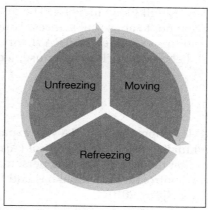

FIGURE 4.1 Lewin's Change Theory.

The first stage is to diagnose the problem and communicate to all members of the team, as well as to begin plan development. The second stage is centered on assessing motivation, establishing willingness or resistance to change, and assessing available resources. It is also a prime time to brainstorm about solutions or possible barriers. The third stage is designed to evaluate the abilities of the external change agent, including knowledge, skills, and expertise. The change agent must be vested in the change and have a genuine desire to succeed in the process. The fourth stage is to design the plan for change, including specific details and timeframes for each goal. This stage also involves organizing and assigning the duties and responsibilities of the team members. During the fifth stage, the change agent's role is outlined and defined. The sixth stage emphasizes team communication regarding a team member's progress in carrying out responsibilities. The final stage involves finalizing the change by establishing guidelines and rules and terminating the relationship with the change agent.

Lippitt's Theory of Change can be used for behavioral change of the individual, as well as for organizational change processes. In the case of behavioral change of the individual, the role of the external change agent is often the nurse caring for the patient. However, for organizational or system change, hiring an external change agent may be beneficial if the change is highly complex, requires specific knowledge or skills, or if the change is controversial and needs an external agent for validity and objectivity.

Theory of Reasoned Action

Based on behavioral psychology, the TRA provides an approach to the study of human decision making. Originally developed in 1967 by Fishbein and Azjen, the TRA seeks to explain and predict the relationship between attitudes and behaviors, specifically the link between personal attitudes and intentions that lead to specific behaviors and actions (Fishbein & Ajzen, 2010). According to the TRA, individuals make decisions or complete actions with the expectation of a specific outcome. This expected outcome is a result of societal norms and personal attitudes (Fishbein & Ajzen, 2010; Maden, Ellen, & Ajzen, 1992).

The TRA is dependent on a person's positive or negative perception of a particular behavior combined with the societal perceptions of the behavior. Based on personal beliefs and societal perceptions and influences, the person considers the consequences before initiating the behavior. An individual's effort is directly correlated with the individual's level of intention, thus the likelihood of success. For instance, when the individual's effort and motivation level are high, his or her intention is high. High motivation and intention result in an increased probability of achievement. More specifically, if an individual's workplace mandates random drug screens as a requirement for employment, the intention of the individual to not abuse substances will likely increase. The intention to remain employed raises the individual's motivation not to abuse substances. Thus, the individual is likely to avoid abusing substances. As in this example, the TRA theory has historically been used to study and predict high-risk behaviors such as drug use, teenage sexual behavior, and college hazing.

Theory of Planned Behavior

Through further research and development, the TRA was expanded to the TPB to address an additional factor: the individual's perception of control (Ajzen, 1991; Madden, Ellen, & Ajzen, 1992). The TPB explains that the factors affecting personal behavior are in direct relation to the amount of perceived control an individual has and his or her desire or intent to perform the behavior (Fishbein & Ajzen, 2010).

Similar to the TRA, the TPB can be applied to predict behavior and decisions based on the primary concept of intention. *Intention* is described as the conscious willingness toward the behavior or action and comprises the individual's attitude, subjective norm, and the perception of control. The TPB is based on the assumption that intention is the foremost predictor of behavior. However, specific attitudes will predict behaviors, as well as the person's beliefs, cultural expectations, and perception of ability to carry out the behavior. If a person is raised to believe that a behavior is good or just, that becomes the person's subjective norm, and it will positively influence the behavioral outcome. Conversely, if the person believes he or she is unable to accomplish the behavior, the negative perception becomes the person's subjective norm and will likely lead to a negative outcome.

The TPB has been applied in education to develop, implement, and evaluate patient educational strategies and concerns. In health care, the TPB can be helpful for predicting patient decision making and behaviors, based on an assessment of the patient's attitudes, beliefs, cultural expectations, and perceived control. Assessing for these factors allows the provider to identify patient-specific content to address and communication strategies to achieve positive behavioral changes. See Box 4.1 for a synopsis of a study that used the TPB.

The IBM

The IBM is a synthesis of the TRA and the TPB (Fisher, Kohut, Salisbury, & Salvadori, 2013). These frameworks are based on the idea that behaving in healthful ways is not only dependent on the individual's health beliefs but on the beliefs of people important to them. These models have been used to predict the likelihood that persons will engage in specific health-related behaviors (Montaño & Kasprzyk, 2008).

Further research on the models revealed the need for integration of additional components from other theories as well. Thus, the IBM emerged. Aspects of the TRA and TPB were combined, which enabled the prediction of health-related behaviors (Montaño & Kasprzyk,

---

BOX 4.1 Research Application of the Theory of Planned Behavior

Parker, Manstead, Stradling, Reason, and Baxter (1992) studied drivers' intentions to commit driving violations based on the Theory of Planned Behavior. Drivers were surveyed regarding the major concepts of the theory, including attitudes, subjective norms, perceived control, and intentions toward specific driving violations. The results of the study supported the use of the Theory of Planned Behavior to predict driving and drinking, excessive speed, tailgating, and passing in risky circumstances.

> ## BOX 4.2 Use of the Theory of Reasoned Action and the Theory of Planned Behavior
>
> Fisher et al. (2013) integrated the Theory of Reasoned Action (TRA) and the Theory of Planned Behavior (TPB) in a single study on the acceptance of the vaccine against human papillomavirus. Students at a Canadian university were asked questions related to the TPB. Specifically, they were asked what their attitude was toward the vaccine, and if they had social support for receiving the vaccine. Their responses were compared to their intent to be vaccinated, which reflected concepts relevant to the TRA. The results indicated that the TPB questions were significant predictors of the intent to be vaccinated ($R^2 = 0.53$ men and 0.44 women). Based on these findings the Integrated Behavioral Model was proposed.

2008). The study that led to the development of the IBM is described in Box 4.2. The integrated model uses the central idea of motivation/intention from the TRA and TPB models, along with the constructs of behavioral control, environmental constraints, and habit. The theory differentiates between behavioral control and self-efficacy. According to Ajzen (2002), "perceived behavioral control is the overarching, superordinate construct that is comprised of two lower-level components: self-efficacy and controllability" (p. 680). Self-efficacy is the perceived ease or difficulty of carrying out an action, while controllability is the person's perception of control and is largely influenced by external factors.

The most important use of the IBM is to find specific ways to intervene in behavioral change by recognizing the interplay between three sets of concepts. These sets of concepts include (a) the patient's experiential and instrumental attitudes, (b) injunctive and descriptive norms or perceived norms, and (c) perceived control and self-efficacy (Montaño & Kasprzyk, 2008). Assessment of the patient's experiential (affective, emotional) and instrumental (cognitive) attitudes includes determining his or her feelings about behaviors and beliefs about behaviors. Asking about the person's expectations (i.e., injunctive norms) and behaviors (i.e., descriptive norms) is used to determine the patient's perceived norms. The third set of concepts is concerned with perceived control and perceived self-efficacy. Perceived control is the person's self-awareness of control over behavioral performance, whereas self-efficacy is the person's belief in his or her effectiveness and skill in performing certain behaviors. When combined, these three sets of concepts influence the intention or decision to perform the behavior and ultimately impact the behavioral outcome.

Bandura's Self-Efficacy Theory

Self-efficacy is defined as the perception of the individual related to his or her personal abilities. The concept of self-efficacy holds a great impact on the person's ability to successfully engage in positive behavioral changes. Although self-efficacy theories such as Bandura's are not typically classified as a behavioral change theory, they are included in this chapter due to their influence on the person's ability to make positive changes. When determining a person's self-efficacy, it is helpful to look at the person's response when presented with a challenging event or task. Does the individual view the situation as something to withstand or something to accomplish? The person's past experiences and prior successes or failures play a role, as do the characteristics and attributes of the individual. Multiple external factors such as the availability of support systems, resources, or communities also impact the person's self-efficacy and ultimate success (Luszczynska & Schwarzer, 2005).

In Bandura's Self-Efficacy Theory, he identified four components influencing self-efficacy: experience, modeling, social persuasion, and physiological factors (Bandura,

1977). Experience is related to prior success or failure. Success in the past results in higher self-efficacy. Failure in the past results in lower self-efficacy. Modeling is the effect of another person's success or failure on the individual. If an individual observes someone succeeding or failing, it is likely to impact the individual's success. Social persuasion is the direct encouragement or discouragement of others. The individual who is encouraged to succeed will have higher self-efficacy than the individual who is discouraged and as a result may be more likely to succeed. Physiological factors are the final component influencing self-efficacy. These include the person's perceptions of physical signs and symptoms. A person with low self-efficacy may interpret the physical signs and symptoms of stress or anxiety as the inability to perform the task, whereas a person with high self-efficacy may simply view the signs and symptoms as a natural response to the situation.

Self-efficacy also affects goal-setting behaviors. A patient with low self-efficacy may avoid setting goals or completing tasks to escape the risk of failure. People with low self-efficacy may feel discouraged, resulting in unreliable or unpredictable behaviors and goal setting. However, those with high self-efficacy may be overconfident in their ability to reach a goal. As a result, these individuals may set lofty goals and struggle to attain them. However, they also tend to be highly motivated and persistent in their attempts to reach personal goals. In the face of failure, those with high self-efficacy are more likely to blame external factors and not take personal responsibility for their inability to achieve success.

Before assisting the patient in setting goals, it is imperative to assess the patient's self-perception of the ability to succeed and accomplish goals. A thorough analysis of the patient's self-efficacy will reveal the person's level of motivation and commitment. The General Self-Efficacy Scale is useful for nurses preparing patient-specific plans of care that require behavioral change. The scale uses a 10-question format with a Likert scale response system. The questions are related to individual perceptions of abilities related to problem solving, goal attainment, resourcefulness, effort, confidence, and coping with the unexpected. The authors recommend that the questions be adapted to include items specifically related to seat belt use, smoking cessation, weight loss, or other topics of change (Schwarzer & Jerusalem, 1995).

Transtheoretical Model of Behavioral Change

The Transtheoretical Model of Behavioral Change is based on patient self-efficacy and empowerment (Prochaska, DiClemente, & Norcross, 1992). This is a flexible model focused on implementing long-term behavioral change. It is frequently used in establishing a contract between the patient and the health care provider with mutually agreed-upon interventions and goals. Through this partnership, the nurse is able to identify the patient's readiness to change and select supportive interventions to match the patient's readiness to change. Accordingly, the nurse–patient partnership is an essential component for successful patient outcomes. The model focuses on change through patient education and advocacy, with the patient ultimately in control of managing the change process.

There are six stages described in the Transtheoretical Model of Behavioral Change: precontemplation, contemplation, preparation, action, maintenance, and termination (Prochaska, Redding, & Evers, 2008). In the precontemplation stage, the patient is not ready to take action or is not aware that a problem exists. Although the individual is unaware of the need for change, others are aware of the need. Regardless of how vocal others are about the need for change, the individual denies the issue and refuses to acknowledge the concern. This stage will continue until the individual experiences a personally persuasive reason to change. Well-meaning advice or coercion is not effective; the experience must be timely, relevant, and powerful to compel the individual to seek change.

The next three stages are action oriented. The contemplation stage is the process of getting ready, mentally and/or physically. Initiation of the contemplative stage may be motivated by a health scare or an intimate conversation between the individual and his or her family members. The patient is starting to recognize a problem or issue and is beginning to consider the consequences of continued behavior. After analyzing all data and consequences, the individual moves forward to the preparation stage. In the preparation stage, the patient sets a goal, is ready to change, and is ready to take action, including minor behavioral changes. Once the preparation stage had been accomplished, the individual enters the action stage. The action stage involves major modifications, including supplementing negative behaviors with beneficial ones and using coping techniques. Next, the maintenance stage consists of continual and consistent changes while working to sustain effective behaviors and prevent relapse. Long-term revisions to behavior mark this stage. Termination is the final stage. During this stage, the individual has no desire to return to previous negative behavior. The changes are integrated into everyday life and have become intrinsic to the individual (Prochaska et al., 1992).

This model is easily applied to smoking cessation or changing other negative habits. For instance, an employee who smokes and is not ready to quit or sees no health risk may be in the precontemplation stage. However, exposure to a new workplace smoking cessation program or to family members who have voiced concern about smoking may motivate his or her movement to the contemplation stage. In the contemplation stage, the individual may recognize symptoms such as shortness of breath with minimal exertion and may become concerned about the risks associated with continued smoking. This spurs the individual to begin thinking about changing unhealthy behaviors. In the preparation stage, the individual may take action in the form of seeing a health care provider to discuss options and resources for smoking cessation or may decrease the number of cigarettes smoked per day. However, in the action stage, the individual takes action to quit smoking, perhaps by attending a smoking cessation class or using nicotine replacement therapies. The maintenance stage is characterized by being free from smoking and having continued success in smoking cessation, day by day. During the termination stage, the individual gradually ceases to rely on medications or other interventions to sustain the new behavior. As with any significant change in habit, relapse may occur. In the case of relapse, the person reverts to contemplation or possibly the action stage to begin the change process again.

The HPM

In 1975, nurse theorist Nola J. Pender defined the goal of nursing as optimal health. Building on this definition and the influence of multiple frameworks, the HPM was developed and published in 1982. Influenced by Bandura's Social Learning Theory (Chapter 7) and the TRA, Pender's model acknowledges multiple dimensions of the person interacting with the multiple dimensions of the environment. An updated version of the model was published in 1996 to provide greater explanatory power and provide a foundation for health-promotion interventions (Pender, 1996). Unlike the HBM discussed earlier, Pender's model accounts for positive factors that impact health as well as negative barriers and beliefs. According to Pender (2011), "emphasis is placed on strengths, resiliencies, resources, potentials, and capabilities rather than on existing pathology" (part 1, para. 5).

The HPM contains three categories; each includes relevant components or factors that influence or explain the individual's health behaviors. The first category is individual characteristics and experiences. This category includes prior behavior, personal factors, habit, self-efficacy, benefits, barriers, and emotions (Pender, Murdaugh, & Parsons, 2006). The second category, behavior-specific cognitions and affect, contains behavior-specific variables with motivational significance such as perceived barriers and interpersonal influences. The third category, behavioral outcomes, contains a commitment to a plan of action and competing demands. The model holds that the outcome of health promotion in nursing is health-promoting behavior (Pender et al., 2006).

Pender has specific definitions for the concept of person, environment, health, and nursing. The concept of person in Pender's model is the unique individual. The concept of the environment includes the physical, interpersonal, and economic circumstances surrounding the person. The concept of health is defined by the individual and is that person's positive, high-level state. The nursing role in health promotion is to raise the individual's consciousness about health-promoting behaviors. Empowering action, controlling the environment, and decreasing barriers are important health-promoting behaviors (Pender et al., 2006).

Pender's HPM is essential to the science of nursing. The diverse roles within nursing enhance the ability of the patient to find ways to manage barriers and increase health-promoting behaviors. Based on the assessment of all three categories of the model—(a) individual characteristics and experiences, (b) behavior-specific cognitions and affect, and (c) behavioral outcomes—specific interventions can be identified. This is a useful model for providers in the current health care environment who have control over resource distribution to encourage health promotion.

CSM of Self-Regulation

The CSM in its current form was published in 2003 (Sonney & Insel, 2016). The CSM was developed from Dollard and Miller's Model of Fear-Driven Action and Leventhal's Parallel Processing Model. These models are based on the observation that although fear can change behavior, the duration of the behavior is directly correlated with having an action plan in place.

The CSM consists of four concepts and specific relational statements (Leventhal, Brissette, & Leventhal, 2003). The first concept, health threat, is a detrimental change related to an individual's perceived health. The second concept is illness representation, which is divided into five domains: identity, cause, consequences, controllability, and timeline (Hale, Treharne, & Kitas, 2007). Identity refers to the descriptive name applied to the condition or the symptoms being experienced. The remaining domains are focused on the person's beliefs about the cause of the condition, consequences or impact of the condition, whether the condition can be cured, and the expected duration of the condition. Subsequent research has added the concept of *illness coherence*, defined as the person's belief that the illness "makes sense" (Moss-Morris et al., 2002). Together these domains define the individual's representation of the illness.

The illness representation component of the model has been used by researchers to develop and test cognitive-based therapies for patients with diverse conditions such as lupus (Goodman, Morrissey, Graham, & Bossingham, 2005), myocardial infarction (Petrie, Cameron, Ellis, Buick, & Weinman, 2002), and rheumatoid arthritis (Evers, Kraaimaat, van Riel, & de Jong, 2005). Hale et al. (2007) note that,

> The core of the CSM is that people with an illness use common sense in constructing their representations based on their knowledge and experiences. People actively test out these common-sense hypotheses by their use of emotion and problem-focused coping efforts. (p. 905)

The third concept in the CSM is self-regulation, which involves carrying out a plan to either complete a specific action or to take no action. The last concept is appraisal, which occurs when the person evaluates his or her plan and as a result accepts or rejects the illness representation. Subsequent threats, representations, and plans will refine the person's illness representations and the actions that flow from them (Sonney & Insel, 2016).

The Common Sense Model can be applied to clinical practice to guide goal development, understand the patient's illness representations, and identify interventions congruent with those illness representations. Use of the model may enable the clinician to predict certain outcomes that are amenable to intervention.

Health Action Process Approach

The HAPA is a model based on behavioral change theories, including the concept of self-efficacy. Developed by psychologist Ralf Schwarzer, it is used as a tool to explain and predict changes in individual health practices such as changing from an unhealthy practice to a healthy one (Schwarzer, 2008).

HAPA is based on five principles that describe the health action process. First is motivation and volition, which reflects the mind-set of individuals who are moving from thinking about taking action and taking action. The second principle involves a two-phase sequential process of goal setting (motivation) and goal pursuit (volition). The first phase, goal setting, examines motivation including self-efficacy perceptions and expectation analysis to predict success. The second phase, goal pursuit, examines the individual's intent for action. In this phase, it is determined whether the individual is actively pursuing the goal or planning to act at a later time. If the individual is not active yet, what are the barriers? The lack of action may be attributed to a deficit in skills or lack of necessary resources. The third principle is concerned with "post-intentional planning," which applies to individuals who are intending to change but lack knowledge or skills needed to take action. Post-intentional planning mediates between the intention and action to provide strategies for implementing change. Two types of planning or mental stimulation are described in the fourth principle. Action planning pertains to the logistics of carrying out the intended action, the who, what, when, where, and how. "Coping planning" involves anticipating barriers and designing alternative actions to take when those barriers arise. The final principle is concerned with phase-specific self-efficacy, which recognizes that self-efficacy is needed in all phases of the change process but differs depending on the phase and the primary focus. Phase-specific self-efficacy has been categorized as "preactional" (i.e., before taking action), coping-, and recovery-related self-efficacy.

This model is designed to address barriers before they impact the change process; therefore, action planning and coping planning are essential components. Both action plans and action control are strongly influenced by perceived self-efficacy and perceived situational barriers and support. Throughout the process and with each new challenge, variations in self-efficacy barriers and support are analyzed (Schwarzer, 2008). HAPA proposes that intention to change fosters planning, which helps the individual address anticipated barriers, cope with others, and produce positive health outcomes.

◎ CONCLUSION

Nurses have many change theories and models at their disposal to assist in planning patient-specific care (Table 4.1). Many of the frameworks have built on one another, yet each brings a new emphasis, or perspective, and understanding of the complexity of behavioral change. Regardless of which framework is used to guide assessment, planning, and intervention, it is crucial to understand the underlying concepts of human behavior, such as motivation, self-efficacy, coping, and support, which are needed for successful maintenance of behavioral changes.

● KEY POINTS

- Change is a complex transformative process.

- A nurse's role is to collaborate with the patient and health care team to develop a patient-specific change plan. Frameworks are used as guides for this process.

- It is crucial for nurses to understand and apply behavioral change theories when planning and implementing patient care plans.

- The HBM stems from psychology. It is based on six beliefs about disease that will motivate action: perceived susceptibility, severity, benefits, barriers, cues to action, and self-efficacy.

- Kurt Lewin developed a general theory of change involving movement through three stages: unfreezing, moving, and refreezing. It may be applied to individuals, communities, or organizations.

- Lippitt's Theory of Change focuses on the role of the change agent. It can be utilized for personal change, as well as organizational change.

- The purpose of the TRA is to explain and predict the relationship between attitudes and behaviors, specifically the link between personal attitudes and intentions.

- The TPB is used to predict behavior and decisions based on the primary concept of intention.

- The IBM is a synthesis of ideas from the TRA and the TPB, along with the constructs of behavioral control, environmental constraints, and habit. The theory differentiates between behavioral control and self-efficacy.

- Self-efficacy predicts the likelihood of success or failure at individual behavioral change. Self-efficacy should be assessed before planning or implementing change.

- Bandura's Self-Efficacy Theory includes components influencing self-efficacy such as experience, modeling, social persuasion, and physiological factors.

- The Transtheoretical Model of Behavioral Change is a flexible model based on patient self-efficacy and empowerment for long-term behavioral change. Each stage is correlated with stage-specific interventions.

- Pender's HPM is organized around (a) individual characteristics and experiences; (b) behavior-specific cognitions and affect; and (c) behavioral outcomes, specific interventions can be identified.

- Major concepts in the CSM of Self-Regulation include health threat, illness representation, beliefs, and consequences or impact of the condition.

- The HAPA is a model based on self-efficacy, and is used to explain and predict changes in individual health practices such as a shift from unhealthy to healthy behaviors.

REFERENCES

Ajzen, I. (1991). The theory of planned behavior. *Organizational Behavior and Human Decision Processes, 50*(2), 179–211.

Ajzen, I. (2002). Perceived behavioral control, self-efficacy, locus of control, and the theory of planned behavior. *Journal of Applied Psychology, 32*(4), 665–683. doi:10.1111/j.1559-1816.2002.tb00236.x

Bandura, A. (1977). *Social learning theory*. Alexandria, VA: Prentice Hall.

Bensley, R., & Brookins-Fisher, J. (2009). *Community health education methods: A practical guide* (3rd ed., pp. 7–8). Sudbury, MA: Jones & Bartlett.

Evers, A. W. M., Kraaimaat, F. W., van Riel, P. L. C. M., & de Jong, A. J. L. (2005). Tailored cognitive-behavioral therapy in early rheumatoid arthritis for patients at risk: A randomized controlled trial. *Pain, 100,* 141–153.

Fishbein, M., & Ajzen, I. (2010). *Predicting and changing behavior: The reasoned action approach.* New York, NY: Psychology Press.

Fisher, W. A., Kohut, T., Salisbury, C. M., & Salvadori, M. I. (2013). Understanding human papilloma-virus vaccination intentions: Comparative utility of the Theory of Reasoned Action and the Theory of Planned Behavior in vaccine target age women and men. *Journal of Sexual Medicine, 10*(10), 2455–2464. doi:10.1111/jsm.12211

Goodman, D., Morrissey, S., Graham, D., & Bossingham, D. (2005). The application of cognitive-behaviour therapy in altering illness representations of systemic lupus erythematosus. *Behavioral Change, 22,* 156–171.

Hale, E. D., Treharne, G. J., & Kitas, G. D. (2007). The common-sense model of self-regulation of health and illness: How can we use it to understand and respond to our patients' needs? *Rheumatology, 46*(6), 904–906. doi:10.1093/rheumatology/kem060

Leventhal, H., Brissette, I., & Leventhal, E. A. (2003). The common-sense model of self-regulation of health and illness. In L. D. Cameron & H. Leventhal (Eds.), *The self-regulation of health and illness behaviour* (pp. 42–65). London, UK: Routledge.

Lewin, K. (1951). *Field theory in social science: Selected theoretical papers.* New York, NY: Harper & Row.

Lippitt, R., Watson, J., & Westley, B. (1958). *The dynamics of planned change.* New York, NY: Harcourt, Brace & World.

Luszczynska, A., & Schwarzer, R. (2005). Social cognitive theory. In M. Conner & P. Norman (Eds.), *Predicting health behavior* (pp. 127–169). Buckingham, UK: Open University Press.

Madden, T. J., Ellen, P. S., & Ajzen, I. (1992). A comparison of the theory of planned behavior and the theory of reasoned action. *Personality and Social Psychology Bulletin, 18,* 3–9.

Montaño, D. E., & Kasprzyk, D. (2008). Theory of reasoned action, theory of planned behavior, and the integrated behavioral model. In K. Glanz, B. K. Rimer, & K. Viswanath (Eds.), *Health behavior and health education: Theory, research, and practice* (pp. 67–96). San Francisco, CA: Jossey-Bass.

Moss-Morris, R., Weinman, J., Petrie, K. J., Horne, R., Cameron, L. D., & Buick, D. (2002). The revised illness perception questionnaire (IPQ-R). *Psychology and Health, 17*(1), 1–16.

Parker, D., Manstead, A. S. R., Stradling, S. G., Reason, J. T., & Baxter, J. S. (1992). Intention to commit driving violations: An application of the theory of planned behavior. *Journal of Applied Psychology, 77*(1), 94–101.

Pender, N. J. (1975). A conceptual model for preventive health behavior. *Nursing Outlook, 23*(6), 385–390.

Pender, N. J. (1996). *Health promotion in nursing practice.* Stamford, CT: Appleton & Lange.

Pender, N. J. (2011). *Health promotion manual. University of Michigan.* Retrieved from https://deepblue.lib.umich.edu/bitstream/handle/2027.42/85350/HEALTH_PROMOTION_MANUAL_Rev_5-2011.pdf

Pender, N. J., Murdaugh, C. L., & Parsons, M. A. (2006). *Health promotion in nursing practice.* Upper Saddle River, NJ: Prentice Hall.

Petrie, K. J., Cameron, L. D., Ellis, C. J., Buick, D., & Weinman, J. (2002). Changing illness perceptions after myocardial infarction: An early intervention randomized controlled trial. *Psychosomatic Medicine, 64,* 580–586.

Prochaska, J., Di Clemente, C., & Norcross, J. (1992). In search of how people change: Applications to addictive behavior. *American Psychologist, 47,* 1102–1114.

Prochaska, J., Redding, C., & Evers, K. (2008). The transtheoretical model and stages of change. In K. Glanz, B. Rimer, & K. Viswanath (Eds.), *Health behavior and health education* (pp. 97–121). San Francisco, CA: Jossey-Bass.

Rogers, E. (1995). *Diffusion of innovations.* New York, NY: The Free Press.

Rosenstock, I. (1974). Historical origins of the health belief model. *Health Education Monographs, 2*(4), 328–335.

Schwarzer, R. (2008). Modeling health behavior change: How to predict and modify the adoption and maintenance of health behaviors. *Applied Psychology: An International Review, 57*(1), 1–29.

Schwarzer, R., & Jerusalem, M. (1995). Generalized self-efficacy scale. In J. Weinman, S. Wright, & M. Johnston (Eds.), *Measures in health psychology: A user's portfolio. Causal and control beliefs* (pp. 35–37). Windsor, UK: NFE-Nelson.

Skinner, C., Tiro, J., & Champion, V. L. (2015). The health belief model. In K. Glanz, B. K., Rimer, & K. Viswanath (Eds.), *Health behavior and health education: Theory, research, and practice* (pp. 75–94). San Francisco, CA: Jossey-Bass.

Sonney, J. T., & Insel, K. C. (2016). Toward parent-child shared regulation. *Nursing Science Quarterly, 29*(2), 154–159. doi:10.1177/0894318416630091

Care and Caring Frameworks

Rose Utley

People will forget what you said, they will forget what you did, but they will never forget how you made them feel!
—Maya Angelou

⊙ KEY TERMS

Andersen's LIGHT Model
carative factors
Duffy's Quality-Caring
   Model
Hall's Core, Care, and
   Cure Theory
Kolcaba's Theory
   of Comfort

Leininger's Cultural
   Care Diversity and
   Universality Theory
Locsin's Technological
   Competency as Caring
prescriptive theory
Ray's Theory of
   Bureaucratic Caring

Smith's Caregiving
   Effectiveness Model
Swanson's Theory of Caring
   in Nursing
Watson's Carative Factors
Wiedenbach's
   Prescriptive Theory

⊙ LEARNING OBJECTIVES

1. Describe the focus, key concepts, and unique attributes of frameworks that emphasize care and caring.

2. Compare frameworks about care and caring in terms of grounding influences, key concepts, and unique attributes.

3. Identify ways in which frameworks on care and caring are used in education, clinical practice, leadership, and research.

The proliferation of nursing models and theories related to care and caring support the importance of these concepts to the discipline of nursing. Many researchers, educators, clinicians, and theorists have expressed growing interest in understanding care and caring. In this chapter, a variety of frameworks relevant to care and caring are explored. Some are descriptive in nature, some explanatory, and others prescriptive and designed to guide nursing interventions. Each offers a differing perspective and emphasis but combined they provide a basis for understanding the art and science of caring.

⦿ CARE AND CARING PERSPECTIVES

The concepts of care and caring are central to nursing practice. Yet, before the 1980s they received little emphasis (Reich, 1995). Reich attributes the growing interest in care and caring as being sparked by Carol Gilligan's classic study of ethical decision making in women. Gilligan found that decision making by women was guided by the value placed on relationships and caring (see Chapter 8).

Although care and caring concepts are not new to nursing, it was not until the 1990s that concentrated exploration of these concepts in nursing became evident. Since then, theoretical and research articles on care and caring have proliferated. Nurses have conducted concept analysis on care (Dalpezzo, 2009; Ranheim, Kärner, & Berterö, 2012), comfort (Kolcaba & Kolcaba, 1991), and reviews of research on care to delineate caring attributes and processes (Potter & Fogel, 2013). Along with this proliferation of literature, numerous frameworks related to care and caring have been developed. In the following section, we explore some of the diverse perspectives of care and caring within nursing.

Leininger's Cultural Care Diversity and Universality Theory

In 1954, while studying the role of the clinical specialist in pediatric mental health, Madeleine Leininger, a nurse and anthropologist, developed the Cultural Care Diversity and Universality Theory (Leininger, 1988). Leininger was interested in differentiating nursing knowledge and practice from medicine and came to realize that "care is the essence of nursing and the central, dominant, and unifying feature of nursing" (Leininger, 1988, p. 152). She noticed that children with differing cultural backgrounds had different expectations and responses to nurses. Leininger's Cultural Care Diversity and Universality Theory views culture and care as interconnected concepts, with *transcultural nursing* defined as care delivered in a culturally sensitive and respectful manner.

Culture was defined by Leininger (1995) as "learned, shared, and transmitted...values, beliefs, norms, and lifeways of a particular group that guides...thinking, decisions, and actions in patterned ways" (p. 60). Under this definition, culture is broadened, and caring behaviors are perceived and manifested. Cultural and social beliefs, values, and practices influence the person's worldview and the perception of care and caring behaviors. Therefore, culture and care are intertwined, and influence care expressions, patterns, and practices used to achieve health and wellness.

To ensure that care provided is culturally congruent with a patient's beliefs and values, Leininger (2002) described three modalities to deliver nursing care: culture care presentation or maintenance; culture care accommodation or negotiation; and culture care repatterning or restructuring. In culture care maintenance, the nurse's role is to assist and support patients to maintain health and wellness, recover from illness, and deal with disabilities or death using their care values, lifeways, and practices. In culture care accommodation or negotiation, nurses enable and support patients in health promotion, health restoration, and dealing with disabilities or death. Nurses accommodate care practices that may differ from their own.

Leininger's concept of culture care repatterning/restructuring is defined as culturally respectful nursing actions that help the patient exchange current unhealthy practices and lifeways for healthier options. By providing nursing care using these culturally sensitive modalities, nurses demonstrate care and caring behaviors and become partners with their patients to achieve the desired health outcomes (Leininger, 2002).

Leininger's Cultural Care Diversity and Universality Theory spurred a growing interest in caring among health care professions. Cultural competence training has been implemented in many nursing programs as well as in public and private health care systems to facilitate caring within the patient's cultural context (Malat, 2013).

Hall's Core, Care, and Cure Theory

Hall first presented her Core, Care, and Cure Theory in the 1960s while at the Loeb Center for Nursing and Rehabilitation at the Montefiore Hospital in Bronx, New York City. Her theory was designed specifically as the framework for nursing care delivery at that institution. She used three interlocking circles to represent the concepts of core, care, and cure, and to provide a visual depicting the nurse's responsibilities to the patient (Hall, 1969).

Hall (1959) identified care as an exclusive role of nurses. When providing care and comfort to patients, she viewed nurses as providing care similar to the nurturing role of a mother. However, she noted that the nurturing role of the nurse was backed by knowledge and practice of the natural and biological sciences, enabling nurses to demonstrate care in a professional manner.

According to Hall, the goal of care is to make patients comfortable and support them in performing activities of daily living. The care concept within the theory includes direct nursing care responsibilities such as hygiene, grooming, and assistance with toileting. By assisting patients with their activities of daily living, nurses have opportunities to introduce health and wellness education during casual conversations with patients.

In the cure aspect, Hall's theory focuses on assisting patients and family members as they deal with the disease process. Nurses, along with other members of the health care team, share responsibilities in the cure aspect. The goal of the cure aspect is to help patients and families adhere to the treatments prescribed. Nursing responsibilities include collaborating with different departments within the health care facility to ensure patients receive the tests and treatments needed and reinforcing education regarding the disease process and treatment procedures (e.g., medications or preoperative preparations).

The nurse's knowledge of human and social sciences is applied when the core aspect is used in patient care (Hall, 1959). The "core" concept focuses on the nurse's development of an interpersonal relationship to help patients express their feelings regarding their disease and the treatment received. When a helping interpersonal relationship is developed, the nurse uses therapeutic communication skills (also known as *therapeutic use of self*) to explore patients' thoughts and feelings about their change in health status. Through this process, the nurse can bring awareness to the emotions and the messages patients send to others. Awareness may bring motivation to take action to promote self-healing. The desired outcome of this sense of self-awareness is the ability of the patient to engage in self-healing actions, which, in turn, motivates the nurse to fully utilize Hall's Core, Care, and Cure Theory.

Wiedenbach's Prescriptive Theory

Ernestine Wiedenbach is credited as the first nurse scholar to present her ideas of nursing as a "theory." Wiedenbach's Prescriptive Theory proposes that nursing care is similar to how a mother cares for her child. In her 1963 article "Helping Art of Nursing," she notes that any caring person can provide nursing care; however, the wisdom of professional nursing is based on one's meaningful experiences of caring.

Wiedenbach (1969) defined *prescriptive theory* as a theory in which the desired outcome is conceptualized, and actions (also known as *prescriptions*) are planned and delivered to achieve the desired outcome. The prescriptive theory comprises three major concepts: central purpose, prescription, and realities. Central purpose refers to the nurse's personal philosophy of caring, which depends on his or her outlook on humanity and the world, and the values held about providing patient care. Therefore, the central purpose of nursing becomes the standard to which care is compared. Prescription is developed once the nurse has a clear picture of his or her personal philosophy of nursing. Prescriptions can be likened to nursing care plans, where actions that fulfill the desired outcome and achieve the central purpose are determined. Once the prescription is set, the nurse is ready to implement actions that are either involuntary or voluntary. Involuntary actions are unintended or unplanned responses to a patient's needs. Voluntary actions are well thought out to provide an intended response to a patient's call for help. The concept of voluntary actions is further categorized into three types. First is voluntary actions that are mutually agreed to, understood, and used by the nurse and patient to plan the care. Then the nurse validates the patient's understanding and physical and psychological readiness to receive the care. The second type of voluntary action is recipient-directed action. This occurs when the recipient directs the nurse to perform the care according to the recipient's preferences. Third is practitioner-directed actions, where the nurse completes the action for the patient.

Wiedenbach's concept of realities includes the factors that could affect how actions are carried out and how the nurse fulfills desired outcomes. She identified five types of realities the nurse should know. The first two include the people involved: the agent or the person who will perform the care, and the recipient of care. The remaining three realities are: the goal or desired outcome, the means or actual actions used to deliver care, and the framework for providing care, which incorporates humanistic, professional, organizational, and systems variables.

In 1977, Wiedenbach explained how her theory works with the nursing process. She described nursing practice as a three-step process that involves identifying the patient's need for help, then administering the help needed, and validating/evaluating that the action was helpful. The nurse uses sensory perception of the environment and observation of the patient to identify the need for help. The nurse then interprets the sensory data and makes an assumption about how the patient feels. These perceptions and assumptions are intuitive and lead the nurse to demonstrate care using involuntary, unplanned actions.

When demonstrating intuition, the nurse engages in realization, insight, and planning based on assessment and decision processes. First, the nurse validates assumptions about the patient's behavior or environment with the patient. Next, the nurse assesses the patient for additional factors that could cause the change, referred to as the *insight step*. Then the nurse and patient plan subsequent care based on additional assessment. In this last step, referred to as *decision*, the nurse takes responsibility to act on the mutually agreed-on plan (Wiedenbach, 1977).

Wiedenbach planned for the prescriptive theory to become a structure for clinical practice and a framework for teaching nursing students on how to care for patients. Because of its similarities, her prescriptive theory can be compared to the nursing process, which uses assessment, planning, implementation, and evaluation for the delivery of nursing care.

Andersen's LIGHT Model

Andersen's LIGHT Model is an intervention model, a set of nursing attitudes and actions that can guide nurses' caring interactions with the patient. LIGHT is an acronym used to identify personalized care that nurses provide for the patient and the actions nurses can assist and encourage patients to perform. The model focuses on enhancing the patient's well-being by supporting patient empowerment. Derived from a synthesis of Martha Rogers's Science of Unitary Human Beings and Aristotle's Theory of Ethics, the LIGHT Model was designed as a prescriptive model to promote well-being.

Using the acronym "LIGHT," personalized care provided by the nurse involves Loving the patient unconditionally, having an Intention to help, Giving care gently, Helping the patient improve well-being, and Teaching the process to the patient. *Loving unconditionally* is defined as the "valuing of another without any expectation of any return"....and bypassing "artificial hierarchies and rigidities" (Andersen & Smereck, 1989, p. 122). Intention to help should not be assumed to be the focus of nursing care. The nurse's attitudes and actions must communicate the intention. Giving care gently involves not only providing soft, tangible, physical touch but providing gentle, intangible touch through an attitude of kindness and the quality of nurse–patient energy exchange. The nurse's gentle care focuses on improving the well-being of the whole person. The "H" of the LIGHT model stands for Helping patients improve their well-being through assessment and planned action. This involves helping the patient receive care by establishing goals that the patient values. The final component involves "Teaching," which should occur after the patient has experienced an improvement in well-being. It begins with exploring why the patient feels better and identifies processes or actions he or she can use to continue to improve well-being.

The LIGHT acronym also identifies five personalized actions for the patient to demonstrate. The first action is for the patients to Love themselves, then Identify a focal concern, and third, to set a Goal. The "H" stands for "Have confidence," and the "T" stands for "Take action to meet the goal." Self-love is believing in one's worth and is facilitated when the nurse assesses and acknowledges the patient's talents and strengths and recognizes something the patient does well. Identifying a focal concern is related to Martha Rogers's principle of resonance, which looks for rhythmic patterns in the interaction between the human and environmental energy fields. Focal concerns are evidence of an unsatisfactory sense of well-being and manifest as patterns of human–environment interaction. The nurse assists patients to identify focal concerns or worries through reflection, questioning, and self-observation. Giving one's self a goal and having confidence are related to Rogers's principle of helicy. With helicy, human–environment interaction or change manifests as diverse and nonrepeating patterns and rhythms. The nurse's role is to assist the patient to develop goals that address the focal concerns, identify new actions to deal with the increasing diversity and complexity of the human–environment patterns, and offer support and encouragement to enhance self-confidence. Taking action (or deliberative inaction) is the final process. It involves exploring the ramifications of action or inaction, so that the best choice for well-being is made.

As an intervention model, LIGHT has been studied in patients dealing with drug abuse and HIV/AIDS (Andersen, 1986; Andersen, Smereck, & Branstein, 1993; Hockman, Andersen, & Smereck, 2000). Andersen developed a nursing practice and research corporation (Personalized Nursing Corporation), in which staff and patients were trained to use the LIGHT model to guide nurse–patient interactions. The model was effective in improving well-being, decreasing substance use, and improving coping with HIV (Hockman et al., 2000).

Watson's Carative Factors

Nurse theorist and educator Jean Watson (1996) proposed that nurses assist patients to achieve holistic harmony (mind–body–spirit connection). The nurse's role is to help patients achieve holistic harmony through human-to-human caring processes and caring transactions or nurse–patient encounters. This harmony helps patients to achieve knowledge, respect, and care for one's self, which results in self-healing. The caring that happens between a nurse and patient is referred to as the *transpersonal caring relationship* (Watson, 1996).

According to Watson (1996), nurses' caring actions are based on carative factors or clinical caring processes. *Carative factors* are the main characteristics of a caring relationship and are based on the nurses' commitment to facilitate healing in their patients. Clinical caritas are guidelines for nurses on applying the carative factors in their caring relationships. Watson (1996, 2001) identified 10 clinical carative processes as the core of the nursing profession. These are:

- Forming a humanistic-altruistic system of values
- Enabling and sustaining faith–hope
- Being sensitive to self and others
- Creating and maintaining an authentic helping and trusting relationship

- Promoting and accepting the expression of feelings and emotions
- Engaging in creative, individualized, problem-solving processes
- Promoting teaching and learning processes
- Promoting holistic connection, comfort, and dignity by manipulating the environment
- Assisting patients to meet their basic human needs
- Being open-minded to alternative ways of caring

These carative factors can be used by nurses to develop a transpersonal caring relationship with their patients. Scholars of caring science have developed assessments and scales that empirically measure these carative factors and processes. One example is the 70-item Caring Nurse–Patient Interactions Scale (CNPI-70), which was developed to collect data on nurse attitudes and behaviors using the 10 carative factors (Cossette, Cara, Ricard, & Pepin, 2005).

Multiple health care systems have adopted Watson's philosophy as a framework for nursing care delivery (Clegg, 2012; Nurse.com, 2010; Rosenberg, 2006). In nursing education, care is often identified as a central concept in a nursing program's philosophy statement. Watson's theory and the 10 carative processes have been implemented as frameworks for many nursing education programs.

Swanson's Theory of Caring in Nursing

Kristen Swanson's interest in the human experience during miscarriage coupled with the encouragement of her dissertation chair, Dr. Jean Watson, led to the development of Swanson's Theory of Caring in Nursing (Swanson, 1991, 2015). Swanson focuses on describing and explaining the processes of caring in the nursing profession (Swanson, 1999). Caring is viewed as relating to a person in a supportive way. The caregiver has a commitment and responsibility to the recipient of care (Swanson, 1991). Swanson proposed that good nursing care happens when nurses address not only the biopsychosocial needs of the patient but also their spiritual well-being (Swanson, 1993).

Concepts central to Swanson's theory are the five basic processes of caring: (a) maintaining belief, (b) knowing, (c) being with, (d) doing for, and (e) enabling. These concepts are often interconnected and usually not completed in isolation. A caregiver may find that one action relates to multiple processes of caring. Maintaining belief is concerned with believing that the patient can surpass difficult life events or transitions and look forward to a meaningful future. Knowing relates to understanding what another person is going through and what particular life events mean. In the process of knowing the person, the nurse asks questions, avoids coming to conclusions without confirmation, and observes the person for cues. The concept of "being with" means the care provider is available and emotionally present to support the person receiving care. "Doing for" is assuming the responsibility for performing activities that the patient would normally do if able. In the process of "doing for," the nurse anticipates the patient's needs, provides comfort, and skillfully and competently performs needed nursing care. Finally, the concept of "enabling" involves aiding the patient during stressful life events or transitions by providing information, being supportive, validating and accepting feelings, providing options, and giving feedback (Swanson, 1991).

Because Swanson's theory depicts a low level of abstraction, it provides an easy-to-use framework for practice. It readily applies to diverse populations across different health care settings. Swanson developed empirical indicators to measure the five concepts central to caring in nursing, which is helpful for researchers (Swanson, 1999). Because of the focus on caring processes, Swanson's Theory of Caring has been adapted and integrated into many health care systems. In 2012, the Virginia Mason Medical Center incorporated Swanson's Theory of Caring into its existing management system, resulting in improvements in staff and patient care outcomes ("New Nursing Model Enhances Care," 2013).

> **BOX 5.1 Swanson's Theory of Caring as a Health Care System Framework**
>
> Nurses from a multihospital health care system were educated regarding the five processes of caring based on Swanson's theory and were encouraged to implement actions consistent with the five processes (Higdon & Shirey, 2012). The 15-item Swanson's Caring Professional Scale (CPS) was used to measure patients' perceptions before and after the adoption of the framework. There was a significant difference ($Z = -3.05$, $p = .002$) between pre- and postadaptation scores, and in two subscales: compassionate healer ($Z = -2.34$, $p = .020$) and competent practitioner ($Z = -2.67$, $p = .008$).

Box 5.1 summarizes how nurse leaders from a multihospital organization applied and implemented Swanson's Theory of Caring in Nursing as a framework for patient care delivery.

Kolcaba's Theory of Comfort

Works of multiple nursing theorists inspired the development of Kolcaba's Theory of Comfort. She conceptualized comfort as a noun and describes it as a sense of being strengthened. She reconstructed comfort into three types: relief, ease, and transcendence. Each type is addressed in one of four contexts: physical, psychospiritual, sociocultural, and environmental (Wilson & Kolcaba, 2004). These terms represent the central concepts of her theory and describe the types of comfort provided and the context in which comfort occurs.

The concept of relief, based on Ida Jean Orlando's work, is described as the patient's experience or feelings when the nurse has met the patient's comfort needs. The concept of ease was inspired by Virginia Henderson's 13 basic human needs and refers to the patient's status of being calm and content. For the final type of comfort, Kolcaba originally used the term *renewal*, but reconceptualized it as transcendence to refer to the state where the recipients of nursing care rise above difficulties (Wilson & Kolcaba, 2004).

As mentioned earlier, Kolcaba (1991) speculated that the person experiences comfort in four contexts: physical, psychospiritual, environmental, and sociocultural. The physical context refers to bodily functions and homeostasis. The psychospiritual context focuses on comfort within one's self, such as identity, self-esteem, purpose, and spirituality. The environmental context describes factors outside the person's body or psychospiritual awareness that could affect human experiences, such as temperature, odor, lighting, and noise. Finally, the sociocultural context refers to the person's relationship with other people, his or her family, and society, including situations involving finances, education, and the health care system. The sociocultural context also incorporates one's cultural upbringing.

Comfort needs may arise from each of the four contexts. Usually, one can overcome a comfort need through internal and external support systems. However, a health care need develops when comfort needs cannot be met using the traditional system. The nurse's role is to provide comfort interventions to address the patient's comfort needs. Comfort measures have three components that a nurse should consider: (a) appropriateness and timeliness, (b) a nursing care delivery model that allows for caring and empathy, and (c) the nurse's intent to comfort the patient. Nurses need to know which intervening variables could affect how comfort measures would be delivered and whether the outcomes of comfort care will be met or not. Examples of intervening variables are the patient's support system, socioeconomic status, the prognosis of illness, and health habits (Kolcaba, 2004).

Kolcaba's Theory of Comfort is a middle range theory composed of relatively concrete concepts that can be easily understood and applied by nurses regardless of their specialty or level of expertise. The conceptualization of three types of comfort and four contexts in which comfort occurs provides a comprehensive perspective, making the theory easy to implement for patients with diverse health conditions and comfort needs.

Duffy's Quality-Caring Model

The Quality-Caring Model blends the biomedical and holistic paradigms by integrating psycho-socio-spiritual factors associated with quality health care (Duffy & Hoskins, 2003, p. 80). The model is depicted using a structure–process–outcome format. The structure component refers to the "causal past" or things that are present before the need for health care services. Structure includes the patient, family, providers, health care system, and the descriptive characteristics of each. Patient demographics, such as age and education, past experiences, severity of illness, and the presence of comorbidities, influence the type and frequency of interaction with the nurse.

The interactions or encounters among the participants are depicted in the process component. Development of caring relationships is described as independent (between patient/family and nurse) and collaborative (between the health care team and nurse). These independent and collaborative relationships produce the outcomes constituting quality care. Intermediate outcomes may include the patient or family feeling cared for, reduction in anxiety, early symptom detection, and patient adherence to health care. Terminal outcomes for the patient, providers, and the health care system result from the participant's interaction and relationships. Terminal outcomes for providers include satisfaction and personal growth. Patient outcomes include increased knowledge and satisfaction with care, safety, and enhancing the quality of life (QOL). The health care system outcomes focus on economic factors such as the cost of care, the length of stay, readmission rates, and use of resources.

Several assumptions underlie this model. One is that people are multicontextual beings who are interdependent on others. Therefore, achieving quality health care outcomes relies on interdependence and partnership among the patient, family, nurse, and other care providers. Another assumption is that evidence is continually changing and is sought to validate the application of nursing care for patient outcomes. The Quality-Caring Model values evidence-based practice, yet views caring processes as a key factor in achieving quality health care outcomes.

Locsin's Technological Competency as Caring in Nursing Model

The use of technology is pervasive in the delivery of patient care and nursing education. In health care, technology is used for monitoring the patient's status, collecting data, analyzing trends, and documentation. In nursing education, virtual learning settings and high-fidelity human simulation technologies provide technologically based interaction experiences for nursing students. However, Locsin's definition of *technology* is broader than using mechanical devices. It includes the activities of nursing, or "anything that creates efficiency" (Locsin, 2010, p. 467).

According to Locsin, "Technological knowing is the use of technologies (i.e., activities of nursing) to know persons more fully" (2008, p. 48). As a way of knowing, technology expands on Carper's four fundamental patterns of knowing, which are empirical (factual and scientific), personal (self-knowledge and empathy), ethical, and aesthetic (perceptual) ways of knowing. Therefore, the primary role of the nurse is to know the patient holistically through technology and Carper's four ways of knowing.

Five theoretical assumptions provide a foundation for the Technological Competency as Caring in Nursing (TCCN) model. Three assumptions relate to nursing or the nurse's actions by (a) seeing nursing as a profession, (b) recognizing humanism as the basis for caring, and (c) knowing the patient allows the nurse to appreciate the patient's uniqueness. The fourth assumption is that people are viewed as whole and complete. And the final assumption concerns the use of technology to know people in a holistic sense (Parcells & Locsin, 2011).

> **BOX 5.2 Research Application of the Technological Competency as Caring in Nursing Theory**
>
> Parcells and Locsin (2011) conducted a study of the validity of the 30-item Technological Competency as Caring in Nursing (TCCN) Instrument. Based on the five assumptions that underlie the TCCN model, a combined sample of nurse theorists and practice experts ($n = 13$) provided feedback on the content validity of the instrument. Items with a validity index of less than .70 were eliminated, and items between .70 and .95 were revised based on expert feedback. This resulted in a 25-item instrument with a validity index increased from .63 to .72.

Based on these assumptions, a tool was developed and validated to study technological competency in nursing (Box 5.2).

Using technologies in health care provides a means to recognize, realize, and understand patients as participants in their care. However, in health care, the pervasiveness of technology, especially mechanical technology, has the potential to create the perception of diminished caring by the nurse. The TCCN model values the link between the key concepts of caring, technology, nursing, and positive health outcomes. According to Locsin (2010), "In creating a nursing situation of care, there is a requisite competency to know persons fully, to understand, and to appreciate the important nuances of the person's dreams and desires" (p. 464). The nurse is expected to use multiple ways of knowing the person to achieve technological competence.

Ray's Theory of Bureaucratic Caring

Ray and Turkel (2010) view caring in health care organizations as a complex process that occurs within economic and political contexts. In the Theory of Bureaucratic Caring (TBC), the goal is to achieve quality outcomes that demonstrate humanistic, spiritual–ethical caring. The TBC views caring as part of and a result of the complexity of health care organizations. The complexity is seen in the synthesis of multiple environmental factors that operate in society, the health care system, and the institutional culture of the hospital (Ray & Turkel, 2012). The hospital's complex physical, technical, economic, political, sociocultural, educational, and legal aspects interact within the larger context of the health care system and society to affect spiritual/ethical caring.

The TBC depicts these complex factors as interconnected but recognizes that economic and political factors play a more dominant role in influencing caring and health care change. A shift in emphasis has occurred from reimbursement for the quantity or volume of services provided to reimbursement based on achieving quality outcomes such as patient safety, reduced complications, reduced readmission rates, and increased patient satisfaction. These quality outcomes are a direct reflection of caring within the hospital system depicted by the TBC.

On a deeper level, the TBC blends personal and organizational foci, with Rogers's Science of Unitary Human Beings and complexity sciences. Aspects that denote Rogerian influences are the use of concepts of person–environment interaction, change, and transformation. Complexity science emphasizes interconnectedness, relationships, self-organization, and the interrelatedness between environmental factors and the dynamic practices that occur in the caring process (Ray & Turkel, 2012). The TBC has been described as a grounded, holographic theory, which also reflects Rogers's influence.

TABLE 5.1 Comparison of Caring Frameworks

Framework (Theorist)	Grounding Influences	Key Concepts	Unique Attributes
Cultural Care Diversity and Universality Theory (Leininger)	Anthropology	Culture care accommodation or negotiation and repatterning or restructuring	Broad definition of culture that influences care expressions, patterns, and practices
Core, Care, and Cure (Hall)	Biological and social sciences; basic human needs and functions	Core = human and social science knowledge; Care = nurturing comforting role of nurse; Cure = dealing with disease process	Interconnectedness of core, care, and cure concepts
Prescriptive Theory (Wiedenbach)	Ida Orlando and the nursing process	Central purpose is the nurse's philosophy, prescription (plan and actions), and realities (influencing factors)	Four steps of nursing practice: realization, insight, design, and decision
LIGHT Model (Andersen)	Science of Unitary Human Beings and Aristotle's ethics	LIGHT acronym for identifying nursing care and patient actions	An intervention model with emphasis on unconditional love and well-being as the desired outcome
Carative Factors (Watson)	Science of Unitary Human Beings	10 carative factors and caring processes	Holistic, transpersonal emphasis
Caring in Nursing (Swanson)	Watson's Caring Science	Processes of caring: maintaining belief, knowing, being with, doing for, and enabling.	Focused on the process of caring in nursing
Comfort Theory (Kolcaba)	Orlando, Henderson, and Paterson and Zderad	Types of comfort (relief, ease, and transcendence) occur in the four contexts of comfort	Taxonomy of comfort and physical, sociocultural, psycho-spiritual and environmental contexts of comfort
Quality-Caring Model (Duffy)	Grounded in Donabedian and Watson's work and influenced by King, Mitchell, and Irvine	Uses structure–process–outcomes framework; provider, patient, and system characteristics provide structure and sources for caring relationships (process)	Considers caring outcomes for the provider, patient, and health system

(continued)

TABLE 5.1 Comparison of Caring Frameworks *(continued)*			
Framework (Theorist)	**Grounding Influences**	**Key Concepts**	**Unique Attributes**
Technological Competency as Caring in Nursing (Locsin)	Heidegger Phenomenology; Carper's ways of knowing	Caring, technology, nursing, and health outcomes	Technology (i.e., nursing actions) is used to know people holistically
Theory of Bureaucratic Caring (Ray & Turkel)	Rogers's Science of Unitary Human Beings and complexity sciences	Person–environment interaction, change, transformation, interconnectedness, relationships, and self-organization	Organizational foci; considers the influence of physical, technical, economic, political, socio-cultural, educational, and legal aspects on caring
Caring Effectiveness Model (Smith)	Roy's Adaptation Model	Caregiving concepts and context + adaptive concepts and context = caregiving effectiveness outcome	Explain/predict outcomes of technology-based home caregiving

Smith's Caregiving Effectiveness Model

The Caregiving Effectiveness Model involves "the provision of technical, physical, and emotional care by family members that results in outcomes of optimal patient condition yet maintains caregivers' well-being" (Smith et al., 2002, p. 51). The model is based on Roy's Adaptation Model and has been refined using concept analysis and published research. Assumptions of the model include recognition that home care is stressful and disrupts family activities, and technology-based home care is preferred over institutional care. Finally, theories related to terminally ill caregiving do not provide useful guidance for those requiring long-term technology-based care.

Smith's model combines the influences of the caregiving context, adaptation context, and caregiving effectiveness outcomes (Smith et al., 2002). Caregiving context and concepts include caregiving characteristics, the nature of caregiving and care-receiving interactions, and home care management including education and resource management. These factors interact with the adaptive context and concepts, which include family economic stability, caregiver health, family adaptation (coping), and reactions to caregiving. The model depicts major caregiving outcomes as the effective use of resources, patient health status, technological side effects, and QOL of both the patient and the caregiver.

Relational statements derived from the model were developed to identify and test the effectiveness of interventions on four dependent variables: caregiver QOL, patient QOL, patient physical condition, and technological side effects. Four interventions derived from the model focus on (a) preventing catheter-related infection, (b) preventing caregiver depression, (c) facilitating problem-solving, and (d) effective resource management. The Caregiving Effectiveness Model provides a comprehensive picture of factors that affect caregiving in the home for technology-dependent patients. Unique aspects of the model are the comprehensive consideration of factors affecting outcomes for both the caregiver and the care receiver.

⊙ CONCLUSION

The care and caring frameworks represent a diverse knowledge base that, when combined, provides a comprehensive and holistic frame of reference for nursing practice. The concepts of care and caring have been recognized by many nursing scholars and leaders as essential components of nursing and the nurse–patient relationship. The theories and models of care and caring provide frameworks for nurse–patient relationships, interactions, goal setting, and interventions. A comparison of grounding influences, key concepts, and unique attributes of care and caring frameworks is found in Table 5.1.

⊙ KEY POINTS

- Leininger's Cultural Care Diversity and Universality Theory emphasizes the interrelationship between culture and care. Culture influences how the individual expresses care, care patterns, and care practices for health and wellness.

- The goal of Hall's Core, Care, and Cure Model is to make patients comfortable and support them in performing activities of daily living. Care is integral to the concepts of core and cure, which involve establishing an interpersonal relationship and assisting the patient to work through his or her disease process.

- Wiedenbach's Prescriptive Theory comprises three concepts: (a) central purpose, (b) prescription, and (c) realities. Central purpose refers to the nurse's personal philosophy of caring, and it influences the prescription (actions taken) and realities experienced.

- LIGHT is an intervention model based on Rogers's Science of Unitary Human Beings and Aristotle's Theory of Ethics. The acronym LIGHT identifies attitudes and actions of the nurse and patient that facilitate well-being.

- Watson identified 10 carative factors that constitute the main characteristics of a caring relationship. The nurse's role is to use the carative factors to help patients achieve holistic harmony through human-to-human caring processes and caring transactions.

- Swanson's Theory of Caring in Nursing describes and explains the five processes used in caring as: (a) maintaining belief, (b) knowing, (c) being with, (d) doing for, and (e) enabling.

- Kolcaba's Comfort Theory identifies three types of comfort: relief, ease, and transcendence. Each type is addressed within physical, psychospiritual, sociocultural, and environmental contexts.

- Quality-Caring Model proposed by Duffy uses a structure–process–outcome format and blends aspects of the biomedical and holistic paradigms by integrating psycho-socio-spiritual factors associated with quality health care.

- In Locsin's Theory of Technological Competence as Caring in Nursing, the nurse uses technologies defined as activities of nursing, to fully know the patient and create a nursing situation of care.

- Ray's TBC considers the effects of physical, technical, economic, political, sociocultural, educational, and legal aspects of a hospital; it is interaction with the healthcare system and society on spiritual/ethical caring.

- The Caregiving Effectiveness Model based on Roy's Adaptation Model identifies factors that affect caregiving in the home for technology-dependent patients.

REFERENCES

Andersen, M. D. (1986). Personalized nursing: An intervention model for use with drug dependent women in an emergency room. *International Journal of Addictions, 21*(1), 108–122.

Andersen, M. D., & Smereck, G. A. (1989). Personalized nursing LIGHT model. *Nursing Science Quarterly, 2*(3), 120–130.

Andersen, M. D., Smereck, G. A., & Braunstein, M. S. (1993). LIGHT model: An effective intervention model to change high-risk AIDS behaviors among hard-to-reach urban drug users. *American Journal of Drug and Alcohol Abuse, 19*(3), 309–325.

Clegg, T. (2012, September 24). Nurses see results from caring theory. Retrieved from https://www.watsoncaringscience.org/files/PDF/Nursecomarticle-092412.pdf

Cossette, S., Cara, C., Ricard, N., & Pepin, J. (2005). Assessing nurse-patient interactions from a caring perspective: Report of the development and preliminary psychometric testing of the caring nurse-patient interactions scale. *International Journal of Nursing Studies, 42*, 673–686.

Dalpezzo, N. K. (2009). Nursing care: A concept analysis. *Nursing Forum, 44*(4), 256–264. doi:10.1111/j.1744-6198.2009.00151.x

Duffy, J. R., & Hoskins, L. M. (2003). The quality-caring model: Blending new paradigms. *Advances in Nursing Science, 26*(1), 77–88.

Hall, L. (1959). Nursing: What is it? *Canadian Nurse, 60*(2), 150–154.

Hall, L. (1969). The Loeb Center for Nursing and Rehabilitation at Montefiore Hospital and Medical Center. *International Journal of Nursing Studies, 6*, 81–95.

Higdon, K., & Shirey, M. (2012). Implementation of a caring theoretical framework in a multihospital system. *Journal of Nursing Administration, 42*(4), 190–194.

Hockman, E., Andersen, M., & Smereck, G. (2000). The impact of an intervention program for HIV-positive women on well-being, substance use, physical symptoms, and depression. In G. J. Huba (Ed.), *Evaluating HIV/AIDS treatment programs: Innovative methods and findings* (pp. 145–161). New York, NY: Haworth Press.

Kolcaba, K. Y. (1991). A taxonomic structure for the concept of comfort. *Image: Journal of Nursing Scholarship, 23*(4), 237–240.

Kolcaba, K. Y., & Kolcaba, R. (1991). Analysis of the concept of comfort. *Journal of Advanced Nursing, 16*, 1301–1310.

Leininger, M. (1988). Leininger's theory of nursing: Cultural care diversity and universality. *Nursing Science Quarterly, 1*(4), 152–160.

Leininger, M. (1995). *Transcultural nursing: Concepts, theories, research, and practice.* Columbus, OH: McGraw-Hill.

Leininger, M. (2002). Culture care theory: A major contribution to advance transcultural nursing knowledge and practices. *Journal of Transcultural Nursing, 13*(3), 189–192.

Locsin, R. C. (2008). Caring scholar response to: Grounding nursing simulations in caring: An innovative approach. *International Journal for Human Caring, 12*(2), 47–49.

Locsin, R. C. (2010). Rozzano Locsin's technological competency as caring and the practice of knowing persons in nursing. In M. E. Parker & M. C. Smith (Eds.), *Nursing theories and nursing practice* (pp. 460–471). Philadelphia, PA: F. A. Davis.

Malat, J. (2013). The appeal and problems of a cultural competence approach to reducing racial disparities. *Journal of General Internal Medicine, 28*(5), 605–607.

New nursing model enhances care, reduces stress. (2013, January 9). *Beyond* [forum]. Retrieved from http://www.beyond.com/articles/New-Nursing-Model-Enhances-Care-Reduces-Stress-12040-article.html

Nurse.com. (2010, June 14). Local hospitals embrace Jean Watson's caring theory. Retrieved from https://news.nurse.com/2010/06/14/local-hospitals-embrace-jean-watson%C2%92s-caring-theory

Parcells, D., & Locsin, R. (2011). Development and psychometric testing of the technological competency as caring in nursing instrument. *International Journal for Human Caring, 15*(4), 8–13.

Potter, D. R., & Fogel, J. (2013). Nurse caring: A review of the literature. *International Journal of Advanced Nursing Studies, 2*(1), 40–45.

Ranheim, A., Kärner, A., & Berterö, C. (2012). Caring theory and practice: Entering a simultaneous concept analysis. *Nursing Forum, 47*(2), 78–90. doi:10.1111/j.1744-6198.2012.00263.x

Ray, M., & Turkel, M. (2010). Marilyn Anne Ray's theory of bureaucratic caring. In M. E. Parker & M. C. Smith (Eds.), *Nursing theories & nursing practice* (pp. 472–494). Philadelphia, PA: F. A. Davis.

Ray, M., & Turkel, M. (2012). A transtheoretical evolution of caring science within complex systems. *International Journal for Human Caring, 16*(2), 28–39.

Reich, W. T. (1995). History of the notion of care. In W. T. Reich (Ed.), *Encyclopedia of bioethics* (pp. 319–331). New York, NY: Simon & Schuster Macmillan.

Rosenberg, S. (2006). Utilizing the language of Jean Watson's caring theory within a computerized clinical documentation system. *Computers, Informatics, Nursing, 24*(1), 53–56.

Smith, C. E., Pace, K., Kochinda, C., Kleinbeck S., Koehler, J., & Popkess-Vawter, S. (2002). Caregiving effectiveness model evolution to a midrange theory of home care: A process for critique and replication. *Advances in Nursing Science, 25*(1), 50–64.

Swanson, K. M. (1991). Empirical development of a middle-range theory of caring. *Nursing Research, 40*(3), 161–166.

Swanson, K. M. (1993). Nursing as informed caring for the well-being of others. *Image: The Journal of Nursing Scholarship, 25*(4), 352–357.

Swanson, K. M. (1999). The effects of caring, measurement, and time on miscarriage impact and women's well-being in the first year subsequent to loss. *Nursing Research, 48*(6), 288–298.

Swanson, K. M. (2015). Kristen Swanson's theory of caring. In M. C. Smith & M. E. Parker (Eds.), *Nursing theories and nursing practice* (pp. 521–531). Philadelphia, PA: F. A. Davis.

Watson, J. (1996). Watson's theory of transpersonal caring. In P. H. Walker & B. Neuman (Eds.), *Blueprint for use of nursing models: Education, research, practice, & administration* (pp. 141–184). New York, NY: NLN Press.

Watson, J. (2001). Jean Watson: Theory of human caring. In M. E. Parker (Ed.), *Nursing theories and nursing practice* (pp. 343–354). Philadelphia, PA: F. A. Davis.

Wiedenbach, E. (1963). The helping art of nursing. *American Journal of Nursing, 63*, 54–57.

Wiedenbach, E. (1969). *Meeting the realities in clinical teaching.* New York, NY: Springer Publishing.

Wiedenbach, E. (1977). The nursing process in maternity nursing. In J. P. Clausen, M. H. Flook, & B. Ford (Eds.), *Maternity nursing today* (pp. 39–51). New York, NY: McGraw-Hill.

Wilson, L., & Kolcaba, K. (2004). Practical application of comfort theory in the peri-anesthesia setting. *Journal of PeriAnesthesia Nursing, 19*(3), 164–173.

Human Development Frameworks

Rose Utley

All that is valuable in human society depends upon the opportunity for development accorded the individual.
—Albert Einstein

⬤ KEY TERMS

Activity Theory
Bronfenbrenner's Ecological
   Systems Theory
chronosystem
Continuity Theory
Disengagement Theory
ecosystem
Erikson's Psychosocial
   Theory of Development
Flood's Theory of
   Successful Aging
Gerotranscendence Theory
Gilligan's Theory of Moral
   Development

Kohlberg's conventional
   stage
Kohlberg's Moral
   Reasoning Theory
Kohlberg's
   post-conventional stage
Kohlberg's
   pre-conventional stage
macrosystem
mesosystem
Piaget's concrete
   operational stage
Piaget's formal
   operational stage

Piaget's preoperational
   stage
Piaget's sensorimotor
   stage
Piaget's Theory of Cognitive
   Development
Synactive Theory
Vygotsky's more
   knowledgeable other
Vygotsky's Social
   Development Theory
Vygotsky's zone of proximal
   development

⬤ LEARNING OBJECTIVES

1. Describe developmental frameworks in terms of attributes, assumptions, processes, tasks, and goals that characterize the individual's development.

2. Differentiate developmental processes, tasks, attributes, and goals of developmental frameworks for adults, adolescents, children, and infants.

3. Categorize, compare, and contrast developmental frameworks in terms of perspective, key concepts, and emphasis.

4. Appreciate how developmental frameworks are useful in nursing education, clinical practice, and research.

Developmental frameworks describe, explain, and predict the human development and aging processes from diverse perspectives. These frameworks have focused on psychosocial development (Erikson), cognitive development (Piaget), and moral development (Kohlberg, Gilligan, Eisenberg) of multiple age groups. Other frameworks have focused on understanding the aging process or on understanding the phenomena experienced by a specific age group (Synactive Theory and Gerotranscendence Theory). As a body of knowledge, developmental frameworks help us understand a patient's physical, cognitive, social, and/or emotional abilities, tendencies, perspectives, and attributes. This chapter explores human developmental frameworks and their usefulness in education, clinical nursing, and research.

STAGE THEORIES OF HUMAN DEVELOPMENT

Stage theories of human development are focused on specific functions of the individual over a range of ages. Theories in this section describe and explain the progression of the individual's psychosocial, cognitive, and moral development. Developmental theories focus on the progression of the individual's psychosocial development (Erikson), cognitive development (Piaget), and moral development (Kohlberg, Gilligan, Eisenberg) in multiple age groups.

Erikson's Psychosocial Theory of Development

Erikson, a neo-Freudian psychologist, developed a stage theory to explain and predict the individual's psychosocial development from birth through adulthood (Erikson, 1950, 1968). Erikson's Psychosocial Theory of Development focuses on how the individual develops a sense of identity within a community of people by progressing through stages characterized by specific psychosocial needs or types of stimulation. For healthy development, the needs of each stage must be met, and the developmental tasks associated with each stage must be accomplished.

Each stage is associated with a time of life and a general age span in which the tasks are the focal experience. The stage of trust versus mistrust is the focus from birth to 1 year. During this stage, the infant learns to trust or not trust other people for meeting physical and emotional needs. Consistency in having needs met at this stage supports the establishment of trust. However, when infants receive inconsistent care, are neglected, handled in an erratic manner, or do not receive loving touch, they may experience difficulty in trusting others to support them in later years when needed.

From 1 to 3 years of age, the child's focus or need is for autonomy. During this stage, the child learns how to navigate and explore the environment and as a result experiences opportunities to make choices and decisions. When the environment is supportive and safe for exploration and the child does not feel shame or uncertainty, positive self-esteem and autonomy develop. When a child feels shame and doubt about the actions and decisions made, development of self-confidence is hampered.

In the third stage, from approximately age 3 to 6 years, the emphasis is on developing initiative versus guilt. As the child continues to develop, the desire to try new things increases. Children at this age can move and navigate through different physical environments and try new things. If a safe environment is provided where the child can experiment and is stimulated to learn, the child will continue to find purpose and demonstrate initiative. However, a child who has limited opportunities to explore the environment or experiences an unsafe environment may not have the opportunities to demonstrate initiative and success, resulting in feelings of guilt.

Around school age (6–11 years old) the child begins exploring the world outside of the home. School activities provide a major source of exposure for development. Socialization and academic achievements during this stage challenge the child's coping and provide the opportunity to demonstrate industry and accomplishment of goals. Failure to achieve competency in socialization and academic achievement produces a sense of inferiority.

The adolescent years, ages 12 to 18, are characterized by the challenge of clarifying one's identity. Failure to do so can manifest as role confusion. Socialization with peers through school, after-school activities, and community organizations are primary means of establishing a sense of self and resolving the conflict between identity and role confusion.

Adulthood, age 19 years and older, is characterized by three stages. In the young adult stage, age 19 to 39 years, the individual is faced with resolving the conflict of intimacy versus isolation. The establishment of strong, loving relationships with a spouse, partner, or family members is essential during this stage. In middle adulthood, ages 40 to 65 years, the individual is confronted with the need to nurture and create things through family and work accomplishments. The basic conflict during this stage is generativity versus stagnation. The eighth and final stage for adults, age 65 years and older, involves reflecting on life accomplishments and achieving a sense of purpose for one's life. The process of reflection enables the adult to develop ego integrity if a sense of accomplishment is generated or a sense of loneliness if one's accomplishments fall short. Unlike Freud's psychosexual theory, which addresses only childhood development, Erikson's stage theory contributes to our understanding of psychosocial development throughout the life span.

Piaget's Theory of Cognitive Development

Jean Piaget, a Swedish psychologist, formed the Theory of Cognitive Development to describe how a person's thinking develops through interaction with the world around him or her (Piaget, 1970, 1977). He described four stages of cognitive development from birth through adolescence: (a) sensorimotor, (b) preoperational, (c) concrete operational, and (d) formal operational. During the *sensorimotor stage*, from birth to approximately 2 years of age, the child learns how to learn through the senses. As the child's exposure to the outside world is limited, his or her thinking and perception are egocentric. During this stage, language development begins. Simultaneously, the child's motor skills develop, which facilitates further exploration and learning as the child moves about and interacts with the environment by crawling, walking, pointing, and grasping.

During the *preoperational stage*, from ages 2 to 7 years, the child's learning experiences change from exploring through the senses to understanding and interacting with the world. The child begins to "decenter" and sees things from a different perspective. The child learns to understand language, shows progressive verbal interaction with others, and engages in imaginary play with objects and later with peers.

In the third stage, called *concrete operational*, the child develops the ability to think logically, solve problems, classify, and categorize what has been learned. However, during this stage, from approximately ages 7 to 11 years, the child's thinking and problem solving is limited to concrete ideas versus abstract concepts. Cognitive abilities are further developed during the final stage called the *formal operational* stage, which begins around age 11 to 12 years. This stage is marked by developing the ability to think about abstract ideas, use symbols, and solve problems that are not concrete. Life experiences and cognitive restructuring facilitate the eventual development of abstract thinking. For Piaget, cognitive development involved reorganization of mental processes that children use to build an understanding of their world and their experiences. The goal of his theory is to explain the processes used by the child to develop reasoning and thinking skills.

Vygotsky's Social Development Theory

Around the time Piaget was developing his ideas, Vygotsky, a Russian psychologist, developed a sociocultural theory of cognitive development. However, Vygotsky (1978) stressed the fundamental role of social interaction in developing cognition and the role the community plays as central to ascribing meaning. Social Developmental Theory highlighted the important contributions of social, interpersonal, and linguistic factors in facilitating the child's mental development. Unlike Piaget's notion that development precedes learning, Vygotsky argued that social learning precedes the individual's development. Higher mental processes have their origin in social processes and need to be understood within the individual's social and cultural context.

A term central to Vygotsky's theory of development is "scaffolding." *Scaffolding* is a cognitive process in which experiences create greater understanding and provide a structure for building or constructing knowledge. As the child's mental scaffolding develops, he or she needs less guidance and instruction in the processes of learning and creating knowledge.

The internalization of language is another central concept in the child's cognitive development. The development of thought and language stems from separate systems that merge around 3 years of age to produce verbal thought or inner speech. The child uses language to socialize, get help from others, and solve problems. This internalization of language allows the child to think in new ways, communicate with others, and engage in other forms of language development.

A deeper understanding of Piaget and Vygotsky's theories of development is possible by considering the central concepts, sources, and contributing factors viewed as important to human development (Table 6.1). Vygotsky coined the term "zone of proximal development" to describe the difference between what the child can do alone, without help, and what the child can do with assistance. The child's zone of proximal development initially comprises the immediate family and siblings. As the child ages, the zone expands to include neighbors, classmates, social organizations, and clubs.

An environment that provides a range of experiences within the child's zone of proximal development and involves interactions with "more knowledgeable others" is most likely to foster cognitive development. The concept of *more knowledgeable other* not only includes parents and teachers but anyone who has more knowledge or ability than the learner related to a specific task or process. When these tasks or processes are accompanied by prompting, questioning, and adjustments, they create the optimal environment to facilitate the child's development. According to Vygotsky (1978), cognitive development stems from social interactions and guided learning experiences within the child's zone of proximal development.

Kohlberg's Moral Reasoning Theory

Lawrence Kohlberg, an American psychologist, developed a theory that describes the processes through which people learn to discriminate right from wrong. His theory is based on Piaget's developmental theory and proposes that cognitive developmental level determines moral reasoning ability. The theory was developed by studying young boys' responses to a moral dilemma. The boys, aged 11 to 16 years, were asked to respond to the following question: Should a man steal an overpriced drug that he can't afford, to save his wife from cancer? Analysis of the boys' responses identified three distinct levels of moral reasoning that he termed *pre-conventional*, *conventional*, and *post-conventional*.

Pre-conventional reasoning occurred in the youngest boys and was characterized by actions that were primarily motivated to gain a reward or avoid punishment (Kohlberg & Hersh, 1977). Thus, moral actions in this stage were motivated by self-interest, to avoid punishment, or to do what was in one's immediate interest. Thus, doing what is morally right is to follow the rules.

The *conventional stage* is when a person acts in a certain way because he or she believes that following the rules is the best way to promote good relationships. Following the rules is still valued but not for selfish reasons. For example, a person demonstrating conventional morality would believe it is wrong to steal because of the consequences it may have on others, not because they would risk punishment if discovered. Right actions involve living up to the expectations held by family and friends.

The final stage, called *post-conventional* morality, describes those whose view of moral behavior transcends what rules or laws say. Rather than following societal rules without

TABLE 6.1 Comparison of Human Development Frameworks

Theory (Theorist)	Perspective	Emphasis	Key Concepts
Psychosocial Theory of Development (Erikson)	Psychosocial	Developmental tasks focus on resolving psychosocial crisis or needs	Eight sequential stages; successful resolution of the crisis in each stage is needed for healthy development
Theory of Cognitive Development (Piaget)	Cognitive	Explains the processes used by the child to develop reasoning and thinking skills	Stages of development are sensorimotor, preoperational, concreate operational, and formal operational
Social Development Theory (Vygotsky)	Sociocultural cognitive	Social, interpersonal, and linguistic factors	Scaffolding, internalization of language, zone of proximal development
Theory of Moral Development (Kohlberg)	Moral development stages of boys	Principle of justice governs decision making	Three stages: pre-conventional, conventional, and post-conventional
Theory of Moral Development (Gilligan)	Moral development stages of women	Caring and relationships are key	Socialization of women results in the use of different decision-making factors compared to men
Model of Moral Development (Eisenberg)	Blends Kohlberg and Gilligan's theories	Justification for actions based on partially and fully internalized values	Six levels of moral reasoning: self-centered, needs-oriented, approval-oriented, empathic, partially internalized, and fully internalized
Ecological Systems Theory (Bronfenbrenner)	Ecological environment	Conflict between ecosystem levels impedes development	Four levels of environment: micro-, meso-, eco-, and macrosystems
Synactive Theory (Als)	Neuro-behavioral	Infants communicate stress and functional abilities through behaviors	Five interdependent subsystems: motor, autonomic, attention/interaction, states of consciousness, and self-regulation
Gerotranscendence Theory (Tornstam)	Older adult	A positive shift from materialistic, rational to a cosmic, transcendent perspective	Involves a change in perception of time and personal relationship boundaries
Theory of Successful Aging (Flood)	Adapted from Roy and Tornstam	Adapting to change is essential	Three coping mechanisms: functional, intrapsychic, and spiritual

(continued)

TABLE 6.1 Comparison of Human Development Frameworks (*continued*)

Theory (Theorist)	Perspective	Emphasis	Key Concepts
Disengagement Theory (Cumming and Henry)	Social science	Disengagement from societal roles is normal and expected	See the nine postulates in Table 6.2
Activity Theory of Aging (Havighurst)	Social science functionalist perspective	Successful aging requires maintenance of social interactions	Activity is physical and intellectual
Continuity Theory of Aging (Maddox and Atchley)	Adaptation to maintain equilibrium	Use of strategies that have worked in the past	Internal structures (personality, ideas, beliefs) and external structures (relationships and roles)

questioning them, those in the post-conventional stage use their personal values or beliefs to determine what constitutes moral and immoral behavior. The post-conventional thinker may choose actions guided by other ethical principles such as human rights, or respect for the dignity of human beings.

Kohlberg viewed the stages of moral development as cumulative with each building on the previous stage. He saw moral development as a lifelong task and acknowledged many people fail to develop more advanced stages of moral understanding. His theory spurred the formation of other theories of moral–ethical development by Gilligan and Eisenberg.

Gilligan's Theory of Moral Development

Carol Gilligan, a Harvard-educated psychologist, worked alongside Lawrence Kohlberg in 1969 as a research assistant. Her contribution to psychology stems from her criticism of Kohlberg's theory as biased because of sampling that was limited to White males. In her classic publication *In a Different Voice*, she presents her argument and describes the differences in women's moral development (Gilligan, 1982). Using Kohlberg's stages framework, she described female moral development not as inferior to that of males but simply different. Instead of focusing on the concept of justice for making moral decisions as Kohlberg did, Gilligan found that women made moral choices based on caring and relationships.

Gilligan's Theory of Moral Development parallels the structure used in Kohlberg's theory, with the pre-conventional stage being characterized as a concern with self-interest and practicality. Transition to the conventional stage involves a shift from self-interest to responsibility and caring for others and a focus on goodness as self-sacrifice. Moral decisions are greatly influenced by society or things external to the person. The child wants to be an upstanding citizen and therefore wants to obey the rules and laws of society. In the post-conventional stage, women see morality as nonviolence, doing no harm to self or others.

Although Gilligan used the same three stages as Kohlberg to describe the development process, she found that the motivation for moral decision making differed across gender. The underlying principle guiding moral decision making in females was not justice as Kohlberg advocated, but caring. Thus, in Gilligan's stages of moral development, the pre-conventional stage is concerned with self-care, self-interest, and self-survival. In the conventional stage, one internalizes and prioritizes caring for others and the need for self-care. In the post-conventional stage, one becomes critical of the ideas adopted in the conventional stage and learns to balance caring for self with caring for others. She argued that the differences in male and female moral development were likely a product of social influences and gender conditioning. Morality in women was influenced more by interpersonal connections and relationships compared with men whose morality was influenced by the principle of justice.

Eisenberg's Prosocial Model of Moral Development

American psychologist, Nancy Eisenberg, developed the Prosocial Model of Moral Development, which views the child's moral reasoning as less predictable but more advanced than Kohlberg proposed. She noted that the scenario Kohlberg presented to young boys may have been too complex to allow an accurate response. The levels of moral reasoning are viewed as evolving from egocentric to concern for others to being focused on values. This evolution occurs owing to our increased ability to empathize, sympathize, and to see others' points of view.

A unique characteristic of her theory is that children are capable of reasoning from several levels rather than using one level. Eisenberg's theory also gives equal importance to Kohlberg's justice-oriented and Gilligan's caring-oriented moral reasoning. She identified six levels of moral reasoning based on (a) self-centered, (b) needs-oriented, (c) approval-oriented, (d) empathic, (e) partially internalized, and (f) fully internalized principles (Eisenberg, Reykowski, & Staub, 1989).

According to Eisenberg et al. (1989), when using self-centered reasoning, the individual is most concerned with the consequences to oneself; the benefit or loss; the expectation of reciprocity; and his or her likes, dislikes, or needs. With needs-oriented reasoning, there is a concern for meeting needs even though there may be a conflict with one's needs or interests. Using approval-oriented reasoning relies on stereotyped ideas of good/bad people, good/bad behavior, and the desire for approval. With empathetic reasoning, the individual shifts to a perspective that recognizes another's humanness. The individual knows of and experiences the emotional consequences of helping or not helping others and learns to recognize how his or her behavior affects others.

Justification of a person's actions involves partially and fully internalized values. Once a person reaches adulthood, he or she begins to use partially internalized values. Partially internalized values are not thought out or strongly stated. In contrast, fully internalized values are based on strongly felt values and principles that are abstract, such as wanting to improve society or the belief in equality. According to Eisenberg's theory, few adults reach the fully internalized stage, in which the person is motivated by the need to live up to personal expectations.

◉ NON-STAGE-RELATED DEVELOPMENTAL THEORIES

Most of the developmental frameworks discussed so far have focused on different aspects of human development such as psychosocial, cognitive, or moral development. Many have been organized around progressive, developmental tasks that focused on the movement from one stage of development to the next. These developmental theories originated primarily from psychology and depicted progressive changes through the life span. In this section, we introduce developmental theories from a variety of disciplines. They share the commonality that they do not depict development as occurring in stages. For example, Bronfenbrenner's Ecological Systems Theory emphasizes environmental development, while age-specific theories, such as Als Synactive Theory, focuses on the neurological development of neonates, and Gerotranscendence and Flood's Theory of Successful Aging address positive, nonphysical aspects of development in older adults. Each offers a unique perspective that adds to our understanding and sensitivity to the processes and results of human development.

Bronfenbrenner's Ecological Systems Theory

American psychologist and cofounder of the Head Start program, Urie Bronfenbrenner developed the Ecological Systems Theory to explain how the environment affects the child's growth and development. He identified four levels of the environment that influence child development: the microsystem, the mesosystem, the ecosystem, and the macrosystem (Bronfenbrenner, 1990). The *microsystem* is a child's immediate environment, including parents, siblings, caregivers, and teachers. Nurturing the microsystem relationships facilitates growth and development. The interactions between the child and people within the microsystem are influenced by the child's temperament, which is genetically determined and biologically influenced.

The *mesosystem* describes the interaction between the people in the child's microsystem, for example, the parent's interaction with the child's school, sports, or church activities. The *ecosystem* level describes environments with which the child interacts less frequently or ones that exhibit less impact on the child and the child's microsystem and ecosystems. Examples of ecosystems include the family workplace, community service organizations, media, and the neighborhood.

The *macrosystem* is composed of the largest and most abstract set of environmental conditions that influence the child's development. It includes attitudes and ideologies expressed by the government, culture, national economy, laws, and the overall stability and volatility of the environment. These factors affect the child's development either positively or negatively. Conflict between these four ecosystem levels impedes the child's development, whereas positive interactions facilitate the child's development. An application of Bronfenbrenner's Ecological Systems Theory is presented in Box 6.1, which elaborates the development of policy and programs to facilitate healthy aging.

According to Bronfenbrenner, a fifth system develops from the person's life history and experiences, referred to as the *chronosystem*. The chronosystem is composed of the person's life experiences, including interactions between the micro-, meso-, eco-, and macro-environmental systems. The five systems denoted in the Ecological Theory produced a shift in developmental theory that emphasized microsystems and broader social, cultural, political, and economic influences on development (Figure 6.1).

BOX 6.1 Research Application of Bronfenbrenner's Ecological Systems Theory

Using Bronfenbrenner's Ecological Systems Theory and Powell Lawton's General Ecological Model of Aging, Greenfield (2011) conceptualized a range of aging-in-place initiatives. Similarities and differences in factors that promoted aging-in-place were identified. The theoretically derived dimensions of aging-in-place initiatives were classified as being environment or person-focused. Environment-focused initiatives were concerned with the types of social systems and structures that the initiatives target for change, whereas the person-focused initiatives were concerned with the extent to which the initiatives target particular subgroups of older adults. Program leaders will be able to use these findings to select initiatives that best meet the needs of the population. Awareness of the theoretically derived dimensions can be used to advance program research, further program development, and advocate for health care policy. The findings can be used to support and expand aging-in-place initiatives that are most appropriate for individuals within specific environments.

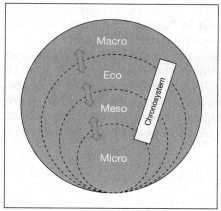

FIGURE 6.1 Bronfenbrenner's Ecological Systems Theory.

Synactive Theory of Neurobehavioral Infant Development

Als's Synactive Theory of Neurobehavioral Infant Development provides a framework for assessing an infant's biological and neurobehavioral functioning. It also offers a basis for providing care and support to enhance the development of preterm infants. A major premise of the theory is that the neonate communicates his or her stress tolerance and functional abilities through assessable behaviors (Als, 1982/2006). Als categorized these abilities as within five interrelated, interdependent subsystems that simultaneously mature. These systems are: (a) motor, (b) autonomic, (c) attention/interaction, (d) states of consciousness, and (e) self-regulatory subsystems. Instability in one subsystem affects other subsystems and subsequently affects the neonate's behavior.

Nursing care using Synactive Theory involves assessing the infant's behaviors related to each subsystem and providing interventions. The motor system assessment includes noting the infant's motor tone, movement, activity, and posture. Observation of skin color, tremors/startle response, heart rate, and respiratory rate evaluates the autonomic system. The state of consciousness subsystem refers to the infant's level of central nervous system arousal such as crying or sleeping. The attention and interaction subsystem describes the ability and strength the infant displays in interacting with things in the environment. Finally, the self-regulatory subsystem is concerned with synaction, which is the process of subsystems interacting with each other. Therefore, the self-regulatory subsystem is concerned with the infant's ability to maintain a balance with the other subsystems. Interventions involve controlling the environment, providing aids to promote flexion and self-regulation, clustering care to reduce the frequency of stimuli and stress, and encouraging parental involvement in caring for the child.

In healthy, full-term infants, these subsystems work together smoothly and support each other. However, in the preterm infant, these subsystems are not fully developed, and function is more erratic. Therefore, a major premise of the Synactive Theory is that when the subsystems are not fully developed, the preterm infant is more dependent than the full-term infant on environmental interventions to support and maintain a balanced equilibrium. Interestingly, in today's neonatal intensive care units (NICUs), the technology focuses on assessment and interventions for the autonomic system such as heart rate, breathing, regulation of body temperature, and digestive functions, with little attention given to other subsystems. Support for and regulation of the autonomic subsystem may come at the expense of the motor, state, intention/attention, and self-regulatory systems, which are interdependent and responsive to an adaptive environment.

Based on the Synactive Theory, an assessment tool and training program have been developed for implementation in NICUs. The Infant Behavioral Assessment tool can be used by nurses to assess theory-based needs and interventions. It has been studied and used extensively in NICUs to assess the six subsystems of physiology: motor, state, attention/ interaction, regulatory functions, and examiner facilitation. In the 1980s, the Newborn Individualized Developmental Care and Assessment Program (NIDCAP) was developed. The NIDCAP is used to assess the infant's subsystems and provide nursing care that reduces stress and promotes physiological stability (Ohlsson & Jacobs, 2013). This program provides training for caregivers to enable them to assess the neonate in each of the areas identified by the theory.

Gerotranscendence Theory

According to Lars Tornstam, a Swedish sociology professor, human aging is characterized by moving toward gerotranscendence (1994). In contrast to other geriatric-based theories, gerotranscendence represents a positive shift in perspective from a materialistic and rational view of the world to a more cosmic and transcendent view. Gerotranscendence acknowledges changes in the way older adults perceive and value their experiences in the world. The change in perception involves a change in the perception of time, so the boundaries among past, present, and future become less distinct. The boundaries between one's self and others may also become diffused and superfluous as we age (Tornstam, 1994). This results in a sense of affinity with others and a sense of being part of a whole (Tornstam, 2011).

The individual with a transcendent perspective values and turns to spirituality and experiences greater life satisfaction. A person who has experienced gerotranscendence may view the younger generations as more concerned with materialistic endeavors and superficial relationships. In gerotranscendence, there is less self-preoccupation and a more altruistic focus. Individuals experiencing gerotranscendence express the need for contemplation time, referred to as *positive solitude*. As people age, they tend to become more selective in their choices of social and other activities, and may avoid social interactions that are judged to be unnecessary. Gerotranscendent individuals accept the mysteries of life and acknowledge that they cannot understand everything. They view death as a natural part of the life process, and they fear death less than those who are younger. It is important to view the hallmarks of gerotranscendence as a natural part of aging and not indicative of a pathological process. Health care providers are exploring how gerotranscendence can be recognized and supported in a variety of communities and health care settings. Research is beginning to focus on understanding and support for gerotranscendence as a normal developmental process.

Flood's Theory of Successful Aging

Flood's Theory of Successful Aging represents the first middle range nursing theory of aging adapted from Tornstam's Theory of Gerotranscendence and Roy's Adaptation Theory (see Chapter 9). Flood defined *successful aging* as "an individual's perception of a favorable outcome when adapting to the cumulative physiologic and functional alterations associated with the passage of time while experiencing spiritual connectedness, and a sense of meaning and purpose in life" (Flood, 2005, p. 36). Successful aging is viewed as the ability of the individual to adapt to alterations that occur over time. Adaptation to aging relies on three coping mechanisms: (a) functional performance mechanisms, (b) intrapsychic factors, and (c) spirituality. Functional performance mechanisms refer to our use of conscious choice to adapt to physical changes and losses. Positive adaptation is indicated through physical health, mobility, and engagement in health promotion activities. Intrapsychic coping mechanisms are engaged when character traits such as creativity, optimism, and personal control are activated. Spiritual coping strategies involve prayer and processes that enhance awareness of a connection with a greater power. These coping mechanisms are interdependent, with each influencing the others. Successful integration of these coping mechanisms is believed to facilitate achievement of gerotranscendence and promote successful aging (Figure 6.2).

To facilitate functional coping and achievement of gerotranscendence, physical interventions might include maintenance of mobility through exercise programs, healthy eating, health education for management of health problems, or completing routine physical examinations. Intrapsychic interventions include counseling and activities that increase one's sense of personal control and decrease negative affectivity. These may include creative problem solving and facilitating inner peace through listening to music, painting, or writing. Interventions to enhance spiritual coping include expressing one's religiosity through attending church, being part of a prayer group, reading inspirational literature, or journaling. Interventions for promoting gerotranscendence include reminiscence, listening, facilitating quiet environments, and allowing time for contemplation.

With a growing population of older adults, understanding successful aging and ways to promote it has become paramount. Researchers have explored the Theory of Successful Aging in diverse populations, including older adults living independently, those in assisted-living settings, and those of low socioeconomic status. A study that used the Theory of Successful Aging in older adults from a low-income retirement community is featured in Box 6.2.

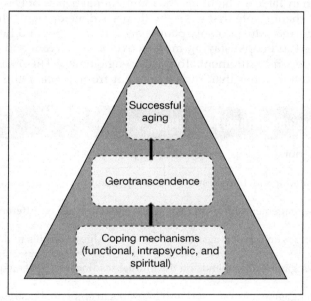

FIGURE 6.2 Flood's Theory of Successful Aging.

BOX 6.2 Research Application of Flood's Theory of Successful Aging

McCarthy (2011) explored successful aging in older adults with chronic disease, physical limitations, and racial or socioeconomic disadvantages. Three key concepts of Flood's Theory of Successful Aging were measured: (a) adaptation, using the Proactive Coping Inventory Subscale; (b) transcendence, using the Self-Transcendence Scale; and (c) successful aging, using the Successful Aging Inventory. Both adaptation and transcendence were found to be significant predictors of successful aging for this diverse and disadvantaged sample.

◉ SOCIAL SCIENCE THEORIES OF AGING

In this section, three social science theories of aging are presented: Disengagement, Activity, and Continuity Theories. Each takes a distinct perspective on psychosocial processes and factors that influence normal and successful aging.

Disengagement Theory

The Disengagement Theory is a descriptive and explanatory theory that views aging as an expected, acceptable, mutual withdrawal or release of the older adult from earlier societal roles. Withdrawal is evident in decreased interaction between the aging person and others within society such as the shift from work/career to retirement and the shift from actively raising children to having raised children into adulthood. Disengagement Theory was the first theory of aging developed by social scientists and was popularized by Cumming and Henry in the 1961 book titled *Growing Old*.

Three key assumptions of Disengagement Theory are: (a) the disengagement process is modal for the aging population, (b) it is inherent and inevitable; and (c) it is a normal and natural process. Proponents believe that the process of disengagement between society and the aging individual is mutual and beneficial as it enables the individual to engage in self-reflection. The postulates shown in Table 6.2 highlight the foundational beliefs of Disengagement Theory.

Opponents of the theory note that since the theory's development, changes in the aging population have occurred. Most notably people are living longer and healthier lives. These changes have resulted in people staying more active in later years and often remaining in the workforce well beyond retirement. Today, Disengagement Theory is viewed as a shift from one role to another rather than disengagement from a role. Others have abandoned

TABLE 6.2 Disengagement Theory Postulates	
Postulate 1	Deterioration, loss, and death are expected over time
Postulate 2	Limited interactions result in disengagement that becomes self-perpetuating
Postulate 3	Disengagement differs in men and women because of different social roles
Postulate 4	Aging is an ego change that causes knowledge and skills to deteriorate
Postulate 5	Disengagement depends on the mutual readiness for disengagement
Postulate 6	Disengagement from central roles results in emotional distress unless new roles are assumed
Postulate 7	Readiness for disengagement occurs when the individual is aware of the shortness of life, scarcity of time, perceives life space as decreasing, and experiences a loss of ego energy Societal readiness occurs because of requirements in the legal, occupational system, characteristics of the nuclear family, and differential death rates
Postulate 8	Changes in the degree of involvement in key roles affect the individual's functioning in noncentral roles
Postulate 9	Disengagement occurs across cultures, but the way it manifests is culturally determined

Sources: Cole (2017); Cumming and Henry (1961).

the theory in favor of other perspectives, while some, such as Tornstam, have suggested a reformulation of the theory to incorporate gerotranscendence.

Activity Theory

Developed by Havighurst in 1961, Activity Theory focuses on what constitutes successful aging. It proposes that when older adults stay active and maintain social interactions, successful aging occurs. In contrast to Disengagement Theory, Activity Theory values the connection between the older adult and the community and the roles assumed by older adults. Proponents of the Activity Theory emphasize that satisfaction in old age depends on the active maintenance of personal relationships and other endeavors and views activity as both physical and intellectual in nature.

  While Activity Theory acknowledges role losses in old age, the theory predicts that older adults who experience role loss will choose to engage in other roles and activities to maintain life satisfaction. Operating from a functionalist perspective, activity theory values the interaction and involvement developed during middle age and supports maintaining a similar level of activity in later years. Intellectual and physical activities are viewed as essential for maintaining a positive self-image and well-being as people age. New interests, hobbies, roles, and relationships are developed to replace those that are diminished or lost as one ages. Activity Theory has been validated in research studies in the United States and England (Knapp, 1977).

Continuity Theory

Continuity Theory describes an adaptive strategy that stems from the individual's preferences and societal approval. According to the theory, many older adults display consistency in activity, personality, and relationships with age, despite changes in physical, mental, and social statuses that are common with aging. Thus, behaviors and actions in old age are considered a continuation of the patterns developed throughout the person's life. Successful adaptation methods used in early adulthood will likely continue to be used in old age. According to Continuity Theory, older adults try to maintain continuity of lifestyle by adapting strategies they have successfully used in past experiences.

  Maddox (1968) and Atchley (1971, 1989, 1999) developed the Continuity Theory. The key concepts influencing the need for adaptation and equilibrium include internal and external structures. Internal structures such as the personality, ideas, and beliefs of the individual remain relatively constant with aging. However, external structures such as the person's relationships and roles change with advanced age. Through continuity, the individual strives to maintain equilibrium.

◉ CONCLUSION

Human development is an ongoing process achieved through life experiences and the passage of time. Each developmental theory presents a unique perspective and emphasis regarding the process. Most developmental stage theories view specific age ranges only as a guide for determining when a person would typically progress to a different stage of development. However, some developmental theories, such as syntactic and gerotranscendence, focus on a limited age range but explore a variety of dimensions relevant to the age group. As a body of knowledge, developmental and aging theories provide perspectives that enlighten, inform, and enhance our understanding of the processes of change on an individual level.

  Many theories have attempted to explain the aging process. They describe the adaptation that occurs as related to changes in human biology or changes due to an adverse outcome of conditions that act on the person. Table 6.1 compares the perspectives, emphases, and key concepts of psychosocial developmental and aging frameworks.

⊙ KEY POINTS

- Erikson's Psychosocial Development Theory depicts seven needs or task-focused stages of development. Successful development requires meeting the developmental tasks associated with each stage.

- Piaget's Cognitive Development Theory describes how thinking develops as we interact with the world. Cognitive development occurs from infancy through adolescence in four stages: sensorimotor, preoperational, concrete, and formal operational.

- Vygotsky's Social Development Theory emphasizes the role of social, interpersonal, and linguistic factors in the child's mental development.

- Bronfenbrenner's Ecological Systems Theory explains how the environment affects the child's growth and development. Four levels of environmental influence are identified: the micro-, meso-, eco-, and macrosystem levels.

- Kohlberg's Theory of Moral Development describes three progressive stages of moral development: the pre-conventional, conventional, and post-conventional.

- Gilligan's Theory of Moral Development emphasizes moral development in women, which is characterized by valuing relationships and caring.

- Eisenberg's Prosocial Theory of Moral Development blends aspects of Kohlberg's justice-oriented and Gilligan's caring-oriented moral reasoning. Eisenberg differentiated six levels of moral reasoning concerned with self, needs, approval, empathy, and partially and fully internalized values and principles.

- The Synactive Theory provides a framework for assessing an infant's biological and neurobehavioral development and providing care that supports further development.

- Gerotranscendence represents a positive shift in older adults from materialistic self-interests to more altruistic endeavors.

- Disengagement Theory is a descriptive, explanatory theory of normal aging that acknowledges the change in roles for older adults.

- Activity Theory values the connection between the older adult and the community and sees successful aging as depending on maintaining social roles.

- Continuity Theory is based on the observations that older adults display consistency in activity, personality, and relationships as they age.

REFERENCES

Als, H. (1982/2006). Toward a synactive theory of development: Promise for the assessment and support of infant individuality. *Infant Mental Health Journal, 3*(4), 229–243.

Atchley, R. C. (1971). Retirement and leisure participation: Continuity or crisis? *The Gerontologist, 11*(1), 13–17. doi:10.1093/geront/11.1_part_1.13

Atchley, R. C. (1989). A continuity theory of normal aging. *The Gerontologist, 29*(2), 183–190. doi:10.1093/geront/29.2.183

Atchley, R. C. (1999). *Continuity and adaptation in aging: Creating positive experiences.* Baltimore, MD: Johns Hopkins University Press.

Bronfenbrenner, U. (1990). Discovering what families do. In D. Blankenhorn, S. Bayme, & J. Elshtain (Eds.), *Rebuilding the nest: A new commitment to the American family.* Milwaukee, WI: Family Service America Publishers.

Cole, N. L. (2017). Disengagement theory. Retrieved from http://sociology.about.com/od/D_Index/g/Disengagement-Theory.htm

Cumming, E., & Henry, W. (1961). *Growing old. The process of disengagement.* New York, NY: Basic Books.

Eisenberg, N., Reykowski, J., & Staub, N. (1989). *Social and moral values: Individual and social perspectives.* Hillsdale, NJ: Erlbaum.

Erikson, E. (1950). *Childhood and society.* New York, NY: W. W. Norton.

Erikson, E. (1968). *Identity, youth, and crisis.* New York, NY: W. W. Norton.

Flood, M. (2005). A mid-range nursing theory of successful aging. *Journal of Theory Construction & Testing, 9*(2), 35–39.

Gilligan, C. (1982). *In a different voice: Psychological theory and women's development.* Cambridge, MA: Harvard University.

Greenfield, E. A. (2011). Using ecological frameworks to advance a field of research, practice, and policy on aging-in-place initiatives. *The Gerontologist, 52*(1), 1–12. doi:10.1093/geront/gnr108

Havighurst, R. J. (1961). Successful aging. *The Gerontologist, 1*(1), 8–13.

Knapp, M. R. (1977). The activity theory of aging: An examination in the English context. *The Gerontologist, 17*(6), 553–559.

Kohlberg, L., & Hersh, R. (1977). Moral development: A review of the theory. *Theory Into Practice, 16*(2), 53–59.

Maddox, G. L. (1968). Persistence of lifestyle among the elderly: A longitudinal study of patterns of social activity in relation to life satisfaction. In B. L. Neugarten (Ed.), *Middle age and aging: A reader in social psychology* (pp. 181–183). Chicago, IL: University of Chicago Press.

McCarthy, V. L. (2011). A new look at successful aging: Exploring a mid-range nursing theory among older adults in a low-income retirement community. *Journal of Theory Construction and Testing, 15*(1), 17–23.

Ohlsson, A., & Jacobs, S. E. (2013). NIDCAP: A systematic review and meta-analyses of randomized controlled trial. *Pediatrics, 131*(3), e881–e893. doi:10.1542/peds.2012-2121

Piaget, J. (1970). Piaget's theory. In P. Mussen (Ed.), *Carmichael's handbook of child psychology* (pp. 703–732). New York, NY: Wiley.

Piaget, J. (1977). The role of action in the development of thinking. In W. F. Overton & J. M. Gallagher (Eds.), *Knowledge & development* (pp. 17–42). New York, NY: Springer Publishing.

Tornstam, L. (1994). Gerotranscendence: A theoretical and empirical exploration. In L. E. Thomas & S. A. Eisenhandler (Eds.), *Aging and the religious dimension* (pp. 203–225). Westport, CT: Greenwood Publishing.

Tornstam, L. (2011). Maturing into gerotranscendence. *The Journal of Transpersonal Psychology, 43*(2), 166–180.

Vygotsky, L. S. (1978). *Mind in society: The development of higher psychological processes.* Cambridge, MA: Harvard University Press.

Frameworks for Teaching and Learning

Rose Utley

Tell me and I forget. Teach me and I remember. Involve me and I learn.
—Benjamin Franklin

affective domain
andragogy
behaviorism paradigm
Bloom's taxonomies
classical conditioning
cognitive developmental
   frameworks
cognitive domain taxonomy
Cognitive Social Theory
cognitivism
connectionism

constructivism paradigm
discriminant learning
desensitization
field theory
gestaltism
humanism paradigm
Information
   Processing Theory
Kolb's Experiential
   Learning Theory
learning styles

locus of control
Multiple Intelligences
   Theory
operant conditioning
pedagogy
psychomotor domain
schema
Social Cognitive Theory
Social Learning Theory
Visual, Auditory, Kinesthetic
   Learning Channels

⬤ **LEARNING OBJECTIVES**

1. Describe the key concepts, assumptions, and perspectives of classical educational frameworks related to teaching and learning.

2. Differentiate behaviorism, cognitivism, social cognitivism, andragogy, information processing, social learning theory, constructivism, gestalt, and humanism in terms of assumptions, key concepts, and perspectives.

3. Describe learning domain taxonomies, including Bloom's original cognitive domain taxonomy, Bloom's revised cognitive taxonomy, Bloom's affective domain taxonomy, and psychomotor learning taxonomies.

4. Explain how frameworks related to teaching and learning are used in nursing education, clinical practice, leadership, and research.

Teaching is the core intervention for nurses in faculty roles and staff development. For clinicians, patient education is an essential skill and intervention for health promotion, preoperative and postoperative care, disease management, and discharge care. Knowing the theoretical rationale behind teaching and learning frameworks helps educators and clinicians plan and implement effective teaching strategies for individuals and groups. This chapter looks at classical learning frameworks from a historical perspective followed by learning processes and styles; teaching styles; and taxonomies for cognitive, affective, and psychomotor learning.

Regardless of the nursing role, whether teaching others or conducting research on teaching and learning, the nurse will likely use one or more of the frameworks described in this chapter. As with most categories of theory, each takes a slightly new perspective and emphasizes different concepts and relationships. With close inspection, the reader will find that aspects of many of the earlier frameworks are still used today in academic and clinical education.

CLASSIC LEARNING FRAMEWORKS

In this section, classic learning frameworks and schools of thought are presented. Over the years, the assumptions, key concepts, relationships between concepts, and the underlying perspectives of the dominant frameworks have shifted. Nonetheless, aspects of earlier frameworks are still observable in educational practices today. Awareness of the diversity and spectrum of learning frameworks will broaden the educator and clinician's perspective and facilitate the expansion of the educational approaches used with our learning audiences.

Behaviorism Paradigm

Behaviorist frameworks of learning were developed from psychology in the early 1900s. Before the development of behaviorism, the field of psychology was focused on the study of consciousness, which was difficult to observe and measure. To bring greater objectivity to the discipline of psychology, a shift to the study of events and stimuli occurred. Behaviorists viewed learning as a change in behavior and studied the relationship between observable stimuli and response. The works of four behaviorists are described in the following sections, beginning with Thorndike's Theory of Connectionism, followed by Pavlov's classical conditioning in animals, Watson's classical conditioning in humans, and Skinner's operant conditioning.

Connectionism

Perhaps the earliest and most fundamental idea in behaviorism was the notion of trial and error learning, often referred to as "connectionism" or stimulus–response. Thorndike, an American psychologist, believed that learning involved forming associations or connections between sensory impulses and neural responses. He studied the ability of dogs, cats, and baby chickens to learn by placing them in a box with a mechanism that would open a door and release the animal when activated by the animal (Thorndike, 1898a, 1898b). Eventually, through trial and error, the animals learned to trigger the mechanism and open the door. The animals performed this act with less and less delay on subsequent attempts. This connection between sensory input and neural responses is known as the Law of Effect. It explains that behavior immediately followed by pleasant consequences will likely be repeated but behavior followed by unpleasant conditions is not likely to be repeated or the response will be weakened. For people, the connections also develop gradually over time by trial and error as a person makes the connections, experiences the results, and decides if the event will be repeated.

The Law of Effect is the first of three laws that Thorndike specified within Connectionism. The second, the Law of Exercise, accounts for the need for frequent repetition of the stimulus–response connection for the behavior to be learned and the need for periodic reinforcement to maintain the learned behavior. The third, the Law of Readiness, is applied when stimulus–response connections are chained together. Several principles have been deduced from these laws, including (a) learning requires repetitive behaviors and rewards; (b) positive outcomes establish the stimulus–response connection, and (c) the connection between stimulus and response becomes weaker if the stimulus and reward are not repeated frequently. These associations between the stimulus and the effect lead the way for developing classical conditioning and operant conditioning.

Classical Conditioning

In his well-known study of salivation of dogs, Ivan Pavlov, a Russian physiologist, observed that dogs salivated in response to the attendants feeding them meat powder (Pavlov, 1932, 1949). Later, he noticed that salivation also occurred in response to hearing the attendant's footsteps. This spontaneous salivation prompted Pavlov to study whether another stimulus coupled with the sound of footsteps could also trigger the dogs to salivate in anticipation of receiving food. He paired the sound of a metronome with giving the dogs meat powder. Soon the dogs salivated at the sound of a metronome whether or not it was accompanied by meat powder. The dogs had learned to pair the unconditioned stimulus (metronome) with the conditioned stimulus (meat powder) and produced a conditioned response (salivation), even when the meat powder was not present. The new piece Pavlov added to the behaviorist paradigm was that learning was a conditioned response and did not require the real conditioned stimuli to be present.

Pavlov established two laws or generalizations about learned behavior. First, the conditioned reflex could become extinct by repeated administration without the unconditioned stimulus. The effects of extinction could be reversed, and the original conditioned response could be restored with repeated exposure to the stimulus. Second, the response could be generalized to stimuli that are similar to the conditioned stimuli. This generalization process helped to clarify a mechanism for developing phobias and also provided a mechanism for facilitating change in human behavior.

Watson and Rayner (1920) conducted what is now known as the Little Albert experiment to determine if classical conditioning could occur in people. They exposed a 9-month-old boy, named Albert, to various stimuli, including an image of a white rat. They noted that Albert showed no fear of any of the images. When the appearance of the white rat was repeatedly paired with a loud noise, Albert cried. Eventually, the image of the white rat alone would elicit crying and fear. Besides establishing that classical conditioning occurred in humans, they determined that a generalization response could occur in which fear was elicited by objects associated with the unpleasant stimuli. Thus, crying and a fear response were eventually elicited by anyone wearing a white lab coat because the attendants associated with the white rat stimuli wore white lab coats.

Although the Little Albert experiment is not considered ethical, nor well designed by today's standards, it helped explain the origin of phobias and provided a means of treating phobias and anxiety through discriminant learning and desensitization. The concept of *discriminant learning* involves helping the learner see and appreciate differences between seemingly similar stimuli and is useful for weakening a conditioned response. *Desensitization* involves progressive exposure to the stimuli to form a new conditioned response, which does not elicit anxiety.

Operant Conditioning

B. F. Skinner added to our understanding of behaviorism by focusing on the importance of valued internal processes, rewards, and expectations in the learning process (Skinner, 1932, 1985). Skinner's focus represented the beginning of a shift in behavioral psychology, in which the internal processes of the person were explored instead of studying only external stimuli and responses. Today, evidence of Skinner's behaviorism, called *operant conditioning*, is seen when providing motivation or rewards to reinforce behavior. Reinforcement can be supplied through rewards to either increase or decrease a response. Positive reinforcement involves applying a pleasant stimulus or removing a negative or unpleasant stimulus. Nonreinforcement or no positive reenforcement can be administered, or a negative stimulus can be applied to decrease a response.

In contrast to Thorndike's trial-and-error learning, in operant conditioning, the connection is made rather quickly by incorporating stimuli that would motivate or demotivate behavior. Operant conditioning techniques have been used to promote desirable behavior and discourage undesirable behavior in the classroom and other group settings. In health care, we see behaviorism as the basis for behavioral modification. Aversion therapy is used to promote habit change. Educational approaches derived from Skinner's perspective include the use of learning contracts, behavioral modification, positive and negative reinforcement, and decreasing the association between stimulus and response to produce extinction of behaviors.

Behaviorists view all behavior as learned. Thus, learning can be confirmed by observation of a change in behavior. Learning occurs through the individual's actions, which may include Thorndike's trial-and-error learning or connectionism, Pavlov's classical conditioning, or Skinner's operant conditioning. Experiencing the consequences of one's behavior is key to learning. Behaviorism emphasizes the outcomes of learning and the external conditions that occur to facilitate learning.

Application of behaviorism is especially evident in the fields of psychology and education. In psychology, both positive and negative reinforcement are often used to manage habits, shape behavior, or eliminate undesirable responses. Positive reinforcement is accomplished by providing a positive reward or removing a negative stimulus after a desirable behavior is performed. In contrast, negative reinforcement involves applying negative or undesirable stimuli or removing a positive reward when an undesirable behavior is displayed.

Teaching approaches based on behaviorism involve providing repetition, reinforcement, reward, and promoting incremental achievement of tasks. Programmed instruction is an educational approach developed by Skinner and Holland in 1954, which incorporates all four activities while completing self-paced instruction. In print form, programmed instruction content is repeatedly presented in logical incremental sequences, interspersed with self-assessment questions. Progression through the program is dependent on successfully answering the self-assessment questions. Reinforcement and reward are provided through written feedback built into the document. Similarly, computer technology can deliver programmed instruction and provide repetition, reinforcement, reward, and incremental instruction.

Cognitivism Paradigm

The behaviorists' emphasis on environmental and external stimuli opened the way for a shift in perspective that emphasizes the learner's cognitive or mental processes referred to as *cognitivism*. Cognitivism grew out of the need to recognize and understand the internal factors related to the learning process. Therefore, cognitivism represented a dramatic shift from the passive role of the learner as seen in behaviorism, to more active involvement of the learner.

Cognitivism encompasses a large family of frameworks, including Gestaltism, Information Processing Theory, cognitive developmental, social constructivism, and social cognitive frameworks. Gestalt psychology, which is the basis for Gestalt Learning Theory, emphasizes perception and seeing the whole versus the parts. According to Gestalt Learning Theory, it is natural to want to understand the big picture before understanding details. Information Processing Theory is concerned with cognitive processes used when information is processed and stored in short- and long-term memory. *Cognitive developmental frameworks* look at how our thinking, perceiving, and reasoning develop with age. Social constructivism views the social context, which had been ignored by the other cognitive perspectives, as important in learning. Social constructivists see learning as influenced by developmental status and the cultural context of the person. They believe that learning occurs through interaction and collaboration, wherein the individual constructs knowledge. They see motivation to learn as strongly influenced by the person's values and beliefs. We create explanations of how and why the world is the way it is based on those values and beliefs. Social cognitivism empha-sizes the importance of social factors on influencing what we perceive and think. These cog-nitive theoretical perspectives are explored further in the following sections.

Gestalt Learning Theory

The term *gestalt* is rooted in German, meaning *shape* and *form*. Gestalt psychology origi-nated in 1912 from the works of Max Wertheimer from the Berlin School of Experimental Psychology. *Gestaltism* refers to a theory of the mind that emphasizes perception and how our mind organizes and perceives visual data. Although gestaltism applies to all aspects of learning, it is especially pertinent for visual learning and successful problem solving, as it considers the overall picture or structure of a problem. Grouping visual information is rel-evant for perceptual interpretation, problem solving, and detecting patterns.

Gestalt psychologist Kurt Koffka is credited with the often-quoted statement, "The whole is other than the sum of its parts" meaning the whole is independent of the parts. Unlike behaviorists, gestaltists do not believe you can take apart a complex phenomenon and examine the parts to understand it; the meaning will be lost (Ellis, 1938). The idea of whole-ness and the Law of Organization are fundamental to gestaltism. According to the Law of Organization, the attributes of proximity, similarity, closure, and simplicity determine the grouping of visual information.

Each of the four attributes described within the Law of Organization provides the foun-dation for an additional law. Thus, the Law of Proximity proposes that we tend to group things together that are near each other. The Law of Similarity explains nonspatial factors that influence our ability to group items together. Therefore, when items are similar in shape, color, texture, or size, we tend to group them together. The Law of Closure is in operation when we perceive incomplete shapes, letters, and pictures as being complete and the Law of Simplicity refers to grouping items together based on shared symmetry or regularity. These four laws are easily applied when interpreting visual data and when developing visual educational material. Applying these laws will facilitate classification, organization, seeing things in a different way, and seeing the complete picture.

Psychologist and well-known change theorist Kurt Lewin endorsed gestaltism in educa-tion. For Lewin, learning was determined by the totality (gestalt) of an experience; influ-enced by motivating and demotivating factors; and included social influences, motivation, and meeting human needs. Lewin's Field Theory may seem obvious now, but at the time, it represented a shift in thinking from behaviorism, which did not acknowledge internal cognitive processes to the recognition of internal processes such as motivation. Lewin saw motives as goal-directed forces. He believed that behavior was purposeful and determined by the totality of the individual's situation. He coined the term "field theory" to describe the motivational forces behind our behavior (Lewin, 1951). Field Theory considers restraining and driving forces as influencing the performance of behavior, including learning.

Gestalt Theory also emphasizes the importance of perception and the selective nature of perception. The gestalt approach is used in psychological therapy and education. A gestalt-based therapist tends to view the whole person and not just particular signs, symptoms, or problems. From a gestalt perspective, an educator operates from the assumption that it is easier and more desirable for the learners to see the big picture first versus the details. Thus, when learners perceive the whole of the situation, learning is facilitated.

Information Processing Theory

Information Processing Theory focuses on the operation of memory and recall and how both can be enhanced. Information processing theory also examines how information is most easily retrieved by the learner. The mental organization or *schema* used by the individual is of key importance. According to Gagné, Wagner, Golas, and Keller (2005), learning moves through four stages: (a) attention, (b) processing, (c) memory storage, and (d) action or response. The attention stage is initiated by the instructor or the educational material and requires the learner attend to the stimuli so the information may be processed and encoded into short-term memory. The final stage involves validation and reinforcement of learning through action or the response of the learner.

Within the four stages of learning, nine events of information processing are used to guide instruction. Each event or principle involves an internal cognitive process and suggests instructional practices to enhance learning (Table 7.1). The first four events of instruction depict things that occur during the early stage of learning. The first event depicts that learning is facilitated by attention, which involves the internal process called *reception*. Reception is facilitated by using teaching techniques that heighten awareness. These teaching techniques often provide a shift in physical or mental stimuli or a change in the pace of instruction. The second event explains that memory processing and retrieval are enhanced by making the information meaningful. Clarifying the objectives or expected outcomes from a learning activity sets up the cognitive process of expectancy and makes the information more meaningful. Integrating the mental organization of the information into the learner's cognitive structure by associating new information with old enhances memory processing. The third event of instruction acknowledges that recalling prior knowledge facilitates learning. Recall of prior knowledge is accomplished by creating cognitive connections or associations with

TABLE 7.1 Principles of Information Processing Theory and Teaching Strategies

Principle	Description	Teaching Strategies
Reception	Get learner's attention	Novelty, questioning, storytelling
Expectancy	Set objectives/expectations	Inform learners of benefits, specify what they will learn
Retrieval	Stimulate recall of prior learning	Explain how new information builds on previous knowledge
Selective perception	Present information	Present selected content with visual cues and verbal instructions appropriate for objectives and type of learning
Semantic encoding	Guide learner to understand	Explain, give examples
Responding	Have learner engage in new learning	Ask questions about new information.
Reinforcement	Give feedback to learner	Verbal feedback, written feedback, test results
Retrieval	Assess learner's performance	Give feedback and provide varied opportunities to apply information to new situations
Generalization	Apply and practice in diverse situations	Present multiple scenarios, apply new learning to diverse case studies

Sources: Gagné (1985); Gagné, Wager, Golas, and Keller (2005).

previous learning. Establishing associations facilitates the retrieval of information into working memory. The fifth process involves providing guidance to facilitate selective perception. To accomplish this, the instruction or learning stimulus must relate to the learning objectives and to the type of learning such as intellectual, cognitive, affective, motor, or verbal.

The remaining events of instruction occur after the content or information has been presented. The fifth event involves guiding the process of semantic encoding, which involves creating a cognitive structure for memory storage and retrieval of knowledge. Instructor guidance, explanations, chunking information, and using mnemonic devices can assist in the encoding process. Performance or practice is the basis of the sixth event of instruction. Based on the type of learning expected, the learner may be asked to verbalize, demonstrate, or solve a problem. The seventh principle is that learning is reinforced by informative feedback. This is an instructor-focused principle in which observations related to the student's learning or performance are conveyed verbally, nonverbally, or in writing to the learner. The goal of feedback is to inform the learner about the achievement of learning outcomes. The final two instructional events are concerned with the retrieval of information and involve the assessment of new learning and generalization of learning. Assessment of learning helps consolidate the learning and provides feedback for the learner. Retrieval and generalization of learning help to enhance learning and can be accomplished by providing varied opportunities for application of information to new situations. These principles describe the cognitive processes used in learning and identify useful instructional methods and teaching approaches to facilitate learning (Table 7.1).

According to Gagné (1985), cognitive learning from an information-processing perspective involves hierarchical skills that vary in complexity. These are: (a) recognition of the stimulus, (b) generation of a response, (c) following a procedure, (d) use of terminology, (e) discrimination, (f) formation of concepts, (g) application of rules, and (h) solving problems. The hierarchy is useful for identifying tasks that should be completed before each intellectual skill to facilitate learning at each level of the hierarchy.

First in the hierarchy is recognition of a stimulus. This is the most basic form of learning and corresponds to behaviorism's classical conditioning (see the earlier discussion of Pavlov's Classical Conditioning Theory). The second level of learning is the generation of a response, which corresponds to operant conditioning, in which a reward or punishment is presented after a response. This type of conditioning is characteristic of programmed instruction where the learner is presented with information, quizzed on the information, and then given immediate positive or negative feedback. The third level involves following a procedure by connecting two or more previously learned items such as when learning psychomotor skills to perform a procedure. In the fourth level, the use of terminology requires verbal association, which is necessary for language development. These processes involve qualitative changes in perception, thinking, and reasoning that progress with age or experience.

As a group, cognitive developmental frameworks represent a shift in theoretical thinking by valuing the importance of aging, development, and experience in the individual's cognitive processes. In this section, Adult Learning Theory developed by Malcolm Knowles is described. The works of other developmental theorists such as Piaget (cognitive development), and Kohlberg and Gilligan (moral development and decision making) were discussed in Chapter 6.

Andragogy

Malcolm Knowles, an adult educator, is credited with the development of andragogy, known as the science and methods of teaching adults (1984). Before Knowles, learning had been conceptualized as a childhood phenomenon, and the focus of education was on *pedagogy* or the methods used to teach children. Today the term *pedagogy* refers to teaching approaches used in general, regardless of age group, whereas the term *andragogy* refers to teaching approaches for adults based on Knowles's theory.

Knowles views teaching adults as a learner-centered process in which the adult has an active role in the phases of assessment, planning, implementation, and evaluation. The theoretical teaching approach used would, therefore, vary depending on the complexity of the task. Behavioristic approaches would work best for simple tasks. Cognitive approaches would work best for medium complex tasks, whereas humanistic and adult education models would work best for highly complex learning.

Based on the unique characteristics and experiences of adult learners, Knowles (1984) identified concepts relevant to adult learning. These are: (a) self-concept, (b) experience, (c) needs-based readiness to learn, (d) problem-focused learning, (e) internal or intrinsic motivation, and (f) relevance/importance of learning. Development of one's self-concept leads to self-directed and independent learning, where the adult learner chooses the what, when, and how of learning. Using this concept in teaching and curriculum development allows the learner to tailor learning activities to meet personal interests and goals.

Unlike children, adult learners bring diverse life experiences to the learning situation. The adult learner's life experiences and educational history provide context, previous knowledge, skills, and opportunities for sharing and learning from others' experiences. Past experiences, however, may also bias the learner or create barriers to learning that must be addressed by the teacher. Readiness to learn is based on the adult's self-perceived need to learn. If the subject matter is perceived as helping the learner deal with life or career, then readiness is facilitated. A related concept involves using a problem-centered focus. Adults must see the immediate application of learning. Therefore, they seek learning opportunities that will enable them to solve problems.

Adults are also more internally motivated to learn than children. Although adults will seek learning opportunities that are externally motivated, self-esteem, better quality of life, and self-actualization are potent internal motivators. For adults, learning is no longer focused on memorization of foundational reading and writing. Instead, they use those foundational skills to achieve deeper learning. However, adults who are busy with career and family must know how this new knowledge can be immediately applied to their lives or careers. Adults need to know why they need to learn the subject matter or how it will benefit them or their family.

Social Cognitive Theory

The development of Social Cognitive Theory (SCT) represents another significant shift in thinking about learning processes. Previous learning frameworks had emphasized the person's responses to environmental stimuli (behaviorism) or the mental processes used in learning (cognitivism). Building on behaviorism and cognitivism, SCT recognizes the importance of the social environment or the social context in which learning occurs. Central to this paradigm is the belief that social factors influence learning by influencing what we perceive, how we think, and our sources of motivation to learn. In SCT, much of what is learned is gained through observation and is filtered through the individual's values and beliefs. Therefore, SCT focuses on identifying the learner's values and beliefs and understanding how these factors contribute to explaining events in our world.

As a subtype of social cognitivism, Social Learning Theory (SLT) represents a synthesis of behaviorism, Information Processing Theory, SCT, and psychodynamic perspectives. However, in SLT, the learning experiences do not need to be directly experienced by the learner for learning to occur. Learning can occur simply by observing another. The person whose behavior is being observed and emulated is referred to as a *role model*. When the learner observes and internalizes a meaning for an observed or role-modeled behavior, whether positive or negative, learning occurs. According to SLT, the observer can learn both positive behaviors that should be performed as well as negative behaviors that should not be repeated.

Rotter's SLT

When psychologist Julian Rotter published his theory of social learning in the 1950s, behaviorism was the dominant school of thought. However, unlike behaviorism, which emphasized motivation from one's instinctual drives, Rotter's SLT viewed behavior as stemming from the individual's interaction with the environment, which shapes the individual's personality. Personality is viewed as a relatively stable but changeable aspect of the individual, a set of potential ways one is inclined to respond to situations. Cognitive aspects of personality such as internal and external locus of control are key concepts.

Locus of control is a term popularized by Rotter that refers to the origin of expectancies as being reinforced by either internal or external factors (Rotter, 1982). Locus of control exists on a continuum of internal to external. Those with an internal locus of control believe reinforcement comes from within. Those with an external locus of control believe their actions have little impact on reinforcement and factors outside of their control are dominant. Therefore, individuals with an internal locus of control feel responsible for what happens in their lives. Those with an external locus of control perceive life events as the result of external forces or factors outside of their direct control.

Four components of Rotter's theory are: (a) behavior potential, (b) expectancy, (c) reinforcement value, and (d) psychological situation (Rotter, 1982). Behavior potential is related to one's personality. An individual will engage in a behavior that has the highest potential for a successful outcome. Expectancy is a subjective attribute that influences learned behavior. It answers the question: How likely is it that a behavior will lead to the desired outcome or receive reinforcement? Having a high expectancy depends on the person's belief in his or her capacity to perform the behavior and the belief that the behavior will be positively reinforced. Interestingly, expectancy can be influenced directly by our past experiences and indirectly through observing others' behaviors and the reinforcement they received.

The next concept in Rotter's theory includes the idea that reinforcement is based on the desirability of the outcome and desirability depends on one's life experiences. A high reinforcement value exists for things we want to happen, whereas a low reinforcement value exists for things we do not want to happen. A person will demonstrate the behavior that has the higher reinforcement value provided the expectancies of the choices are equal. The combination of expectancy, reinforcement value, and behavior potential provides a predictive model in which the effects of expectancy and reinforcement value result in a behavioral potential. Thus, a person's tendency to demonstrate a behavior is based on the probability that the behavior will lead to an outcome (expectancy) and on the desirability of that outcome (value reinforcement).

The fourth component of Rotter's SLT is the psychological situation, which is subjective and unique to each person. The psychological situation accounts for the unique interpretation and meaning that each person gives to life experiences. It is how the person interprets the environment and the stimuli that give meaning and significance to the behavior.

Bandura's SLT

According to Albert Bandura, an American-trained psychologist, human functioning is explained using *reciprocal determinism*. In this theory, the concepts of behavior, environment, and the person are interrelated, with each concept influencing the other (Bandura, 1986). Learning through role modeling is a central idea in SLT that explains how learners can change or learn through observing the behavior of others. However, Bandura differentiated role modeling from simple imitation. Role modeling is not just repeating an observed behavior, but it is also a means for acquiring values and attitudes. Role modeling requires cognitive skills and impacts psychological aspects of the learner. The learner models a behavior based largely on his or her values and beliefs about the behavior and about the person who performed the behavior.

Four processes necessary for observational learning to occur, are: (a) attention, (b) retention, (c) motor reproduction, and (d) motivation. For attention to occur, the observer must have sufficient sensory capacity to observe the modeled behavior. The observer must also demonstrate a level of arousal and establish a perceptual set or readiness to perceive certain aspects of the situation. And the final requirement for ensuring learner attention is to have received positive reinforcement for modeling the behavior in the past. The process of attention involves self-directed exploration and can be encouraged by behaviorist incentives such as praise and positive recognition. The modeled event must demonstrate functional value and a level of distinctiveness. Retention of observed behavior relies on information processing concepts such as "coding" the behavior using words, labels, or images. Another aspect of retention involves metacognitive thinking, such as self-reflection, to facilitate cognitive organization and mental rehearsal of the behavior. Motor reproduction of the observed behavior requires physical abilities, self-observation of the motor reproduction, and the receipt of accurate feedback. Drawing from behaviorism, the motivation to perform a behavior involves positive or negative vicarious reinforcement, internal self-reinforcement, and/or external reinforcement. Vicarious reinforcement is achieved by observing the effect of the behavior or noting others' responses to the modeled behavior. Internal self-reinforcement occurs when the individual evaluates the qualities of the behavior using his or her internal standards and expectations. External reinforcement is achieved by receiving external rewards or negative feedback.

Bandura later modified his SLT, giving more emphasis to the internal processes of intentionality, self-regulation, and self-efficacy in the learning process. He extrapolated several principles of SLT. One principle is that adoption of an observed behavior is more likely when the behavior is perceived as valued or results in outcomes perceived as valued. Another principle notes that when behavior is cognitively coded into words or images, greater retention results. Finally, internal processes of intentionality, self-regulation, and self-efficacy facilitate learning through modeling. Emphasizing these concepts and principles strengthens the application of SLT to interventions that support the person's internal capabilities.

SLT is important for learning psychomotor skills, communication techniques, and attitudes and values. In nursing education, SLT can explain how and why a student learns from clinical observation and clinical simulation scenarios in which the student plays only an observational role. In clinical practice, SLT is useful for understanding how nurses are socialized into the profession, including learning negative social behaviors such as aggression and addiction. An example of a study of addiction-quitting interventions using Bandura's SLT is explored in Box 7.1.

Constructivism Paradigm

Constructivists believe that we construct our understanding and knowledge of the world through experience and by reflecting on those experiences. Constructivism values the cultural environment in which learning occurs and views the processes of interaction and collaboration as essential for learning to occur. Culture, social interaction, and construction of knowledge through interaction with the content and with the learning environment are important considerations. In constructivism, the learner takes an active role in developing, learning, and creating knowledge.

The foundation for constructivism was laid by developmental psychologist Jean Piaget and educational reformist, philosopher, and psychologist, John Dewey. Piaget's Theory of Human Development (see Chapter 6) emphasized the child's cognitive processes that rely on the child's growth, development, and interaction with people and things in the environment. Dewey's work in education was grounded in experiential learning, which was

> ### BOX 7.1 Research Application of Bandura's Social Learning Theory
>
> In this study by Heydari, Dashtgard, and Moghadam (2014), Bandura's theory was used to guide the measurement of self-efficacy and to develop interventions that would address self-efficacy. The researchers conducted an experimental study of 60 patients enrolled in an addiction-quitting clinic, with 30 in the intervention group and 30 in the control group. All patients completed a self-efficacy questionnaire before the intervention, with no significant differences noted between groups. The intervention groups then received addiction education to increase knowledge and participated in four sessions designed using concepts relevant to Bandura's Social Learning Theory. Information was provided to increase knowledge of the addiction process, complications, and treatment. Small groups were conducted to facilitate change in attitude and to develop self-regulatory skills. Four sessions were conducted to enhance self-efficacy, one session each for learning problem solving, decision making, self-projection, and communication skills. The final component of the intervention included two group sessions dealing with family support and self-governing groups. The control and intervention groups were reevaluated 1 month postintervention to determine morphine use and measure self-efficacy. Only 4% in the theory-based intervention group experienced a relapse compared to 40% in the control group. In addition, significant differences in the self-efficacy scores were noted postintervention.

articulated through the classic text *Experience and Education* published in 1938. Later, Dewey's conceptualization of experiential learning was implemented at the University of Chicago's Laboratory School.

The common attributes of constructivist approaches include learning that is constructed, active, reflective, collaborative, and inquiry based. Constructed learning stems from the student's prior knowledge, which provides the foundation for exploring and building new understandings. Learners are encouraged to take an approach to problem solving that is self-determined, meaning the learners find their own ways of solving problems or studying issues. Active learning involves using mental or physical activity to promote learning such as asking questions, application of concepts learned to real situations, and hands-on problem-solving activities. Constructed learning also requires reflection on the learning experience by engaging in processes such as thinking about what was learned, journaling, or discussion.

Collaboration is also crucial for constructed learning as it enables the individual to learn from interactions with others. Activities that rely on collaboration include small-group problem solving, working through case studies, group projects, and presentations. Inquiry-based methods, such as asking questions, exploring a topic, or using resources to solve problems, can be used to facilitate collaboration. Inquiry is a cyclical process in which exploring a topic leads to questions, which leads to further exploration and new questions.

The final aspect of constructivism is its evolving nature. The learning experience is both a process and an outcome. However, in constructivism, the process includes temporary, evolving steps, and personal realizations, which are key to achieving the learning outcomes. Proponents of constructivism report that its use encourages critical thinking, and fosters teamwork, communication, and development of social skills. In constructivism, learning is derived from students' questions, explorations, and reflections. Emphasis is placed on learning how to think and understand which are the processes readily transferable to situations outside of a classroom.

Humanism Paradigm

Humanism is a teaching paradigm that values personal growth, curiosity, and the uniqueness of individuals. It represents a shift away from a behaviorist's and a cognitivist's aspects to personal growth and affective aspects of learning. Development of the learner's positive self-concept, self-esteem, and self-regard are important considerations for learning. Humanists do not accept that behavior is predetermined by the environment or one's subconscious state as in behaviorism and psychoanalytical approaches. Instead, they believe that the individual controls his or her destiny and possesses unlimited potential for growth and development.

Two well-known proponents of humanism are discussed in this section. Abraham Maslow, the father of humanistic psychology, offers a perspective that focuses on the sources of personal motivation that influence learning. Psychologist and educational reformist Carl Rogers emphasized experiential learning that occurs when the focus shifts from teacher-centered to learner-centered approaches. Although each offers distinctive features not emphasized by the other, each also values personal growth and development of the learner.

Maslow's Hierarchy of Needs

Abraham Maslow's Hierarchy of Human Needs outlines a motivational framework for human behavior (1954, 1987). The hierarchy is typically depicted as a triangle with the physiological needs positioned at the base of the triangle followed by safety needs, then higher order needs, culminating in self-actualization. The physiological needs for air, water, food, and safety are deprivation needs, which must be met before the individual can focus on higher order needs. Once deprivation needs are met, the individual can focus on social needs of love and belonging and personal growth needs of self-esteem and self-actualization.

Three assumptions underlie Maslow's Hierarchy of Human Needs. First, the motivation to learn is intrinsic to the learner. It is an internal process that depends on the individual's past and present experiences and circumstances. Second, learning contributes to psychological health by facilitating the individual's progress toward self-actualization. This movement toward goal achievement or self-actualization facilitates psychological well-being. Finally, self-actualization is the primary goal of learning.

Maslow's theory has been used extensively in nursing education programs and in clinical practice for prioritizing nursing care and developing care plans. Nurses can use the hierarchy as a framework for assessing the patient's needs, prioritizing interventions, and determining the patient's readiness to learn. Once the patient's deprivation needs have been addressed, the nurse can focus on higher order needs and on facilitating learning.

Rogers's Experiential Learning

In 1969, Carl Rogers popularized his learning perspective in the text, *Freedom to Learn*. His ideas of humanistic education correlated closely with his ideas regarding psychology. He believed that learning was (a) self-initiated; (b) required learner involvement; (c) influenced the behavior, attitudes, and personality of the learner; and (d) was best evaluated by the learner. He acknowledged two types of learning: the academic or cognitive type for mastery of subject matter content and experiential or applied learning. A key difference between the two types of learning is that experiential learning is learner centered and focuses on the individual's engagement with the learning experience, whereas cognitive learning focuses on internal processes of learning and the subject matter. Also, experiential learning addresses the learner's needs and wants, and promotes personal growth through active involvement and application of knowledge.

Rogers viewed learning as a natural process the teacher facilitates by (a) developing a positive learning environment, (b) clarifying the purpose of learning activities, (c) providing

TABLE 7.2 Comparison of Teaching and Learning Frameworks		
Theory	**Key Concepts**	**Assumptions**
Connectionism	Stimulus–response, association	Learning involves an association between sensory impulses and neural responses.
Classical Conditioning	Unconditioned stimulus, conditioned response, generalization response, discriminant learning, desensitization	Learning is a conditioned response to a stimulus. The response to a stimulus can be generalized.
Operant Conditioning	Motivation, rewards, positive reinforcement, negative reinforcement	Internal cognitive processes, rewards, and expectations are important in the learning process.
Gestalt	Pattern recognition based on proximity, similarity, closure, and simplicity	Learning is facilitated when learners perceive the whole of the situation. The whole is other than the sum of the parts.
Information Processing	Memory storage, short- and long-term memory, recall, schema	Learning occurs in four stages: (a) attention, (b) processing, (c) memory storage, and (d) action or response.
Adult Learning Theory (Andragogy)	Self-concept, experience, readiness, problem focused, motivation, and relevance	Internal motivators are important to adult learners.
Social Cognitivism	Social environment, social context, observation, perception, values, and beliefs	The social environment and social context for learning are important. Social factors influence our perceptions, thinking, and motivation.
Rotter's Social Learning Theory	Environment, personality, internal and external locus of control, behavior potential, expectancy, reinforcement value, and psychological situation	Behavior stems from interaction with the environment which shapes personality. Personality is a set of potential ways a person is inclined to respond.
Bandura's Social Learning Theory	Reciprocal determinism, behavior, environment, person, and role modeling	Learners model behavior based on values and beliefs about the behavior and the person performing the behavior.

(continued)

TABLE 7.2 Comparison of Teaching and Learning Frameworks *(continued)*		
Theory	**Key Concepts**	**Assumptions**
Maslow's Hierarchy of Needs	Hierarchy of needs, deprivation needs, higher order needs, personal growth needs	Sources of personal motivation can influence learning. Learning contributes to psychological health.
Rogers's Experiential Learning	Intellectual learning, experiential learning, learner-centered approach	Experiential learning occurs when the focus shifts from teacher-centered to learner-centered approaches.

resources, (d) organizing the learning experience, and (e) incorporating a balanced emphasis on intellectual and experiential learning. Learners participate actively and have control over the learning experiences that involve applying knowledge to understand or solve practical problems. According to Rogers and Freiberg (1994), learning occurs more quickly and easily when the threat to the learner's self-perception is low. Reducing the learner's perceived threat is a key component of creating a positive learning environment. Learning is more significant and long-lasting when it is self-initiated and when the individual has a personal interest in the subject.

The learning frameworks discussed in this section build on previous theoretical knowledge, and each shares some attributes of his or her theoretical predecessors. Each framework also adds a unique perspective and understanding of how learning occurs, which sometimes manifests as a subtle shift and at other times a dramatic shift in perspective. The key concepts and assumptions of these frameworks are compared in Table 7.2.

○ LEARNING STYLES

Learning styles refer to "characteristic cognitive, affective, and psychosocial behaviors that serve as relatively stable indicators of how learners perceive, interact with, and respond to the learning environment" (Curry, 1981, p. 535). Other terms used to describe this group of frameworks are *learning channels* and *learning preferences*. Learning styles stem from diverse perspectives. Some are personality based, such as the Myers–Briggs Personality Types and the Kolb Learning Model, while others look at preferred modes of processing information such as the Visual, Auditory, and Kinesthetic Theory and Multiple Intelligences. These frameworks are useful in understanding and appreciating personal differences in learning and planning and implementing teaching interventions that will maintain the interest, focus, and arousal of the learners.

Using teaching approaches that are congruent with specific learning styles is helpful when teaching patients one on one. However, when teaching groups composed of individuals with diverse learning styles, knowing and using a range of strategies that address individual differences may be more valuable. In addition, a fit between the learning style approach used and the nature of the content is important. Some types of content and topics are more amendable to certain approaches than others. For example, learning CPR emphasizes kinesthetic and visual learning approaches, whereas music appreciation would involve auditory learning approaches. Regardless of the learning style framework used, all are based on the assumptions that maintaining arousal, attention, and focus are enhanced when the teaching methods match the learner's preference and match the nature of the content to be learned.

Visual, Auditory, Kinesthetic Learning Channels

Learning channels are perhaps the most widely known and widely used category of learning style theory. One of the most well known is referred to as the Visual, Auditory, and Kinesthetic Theory or VAK (Barbe, Swassing, & Milone, 1979). It is simple, easy to use, and people tend to have an intuitive sense of their preferred learning channel. Ask adults whether they prefer learning through visual, auditory, or kinesthetic strategies, and many can tell you their preference. According to the VAK Theory, people have preferred ways or channels for receiving, processing, and applying information. However, an individual will display some degree of preference for each channel.

Understanding learning channels is valuable for the teacher and the learner. Learners may learn more easily or be more satisfied with the learning experience if teaching methods address their preferred style. Teachers will find that using a range of teaching strategies will appeal to more learners, and will help provide novelty, stimulate arousal, and enhance the student's engagement in the learning process. Strategies for teaching that address visual, auditory, and kinesthetic learners are outlined in Table 7.3.

Multiple Intelligences Theory

Multiple intelligences (MI) refer to an individual's abilities and learning potential using one or more learning modes. The concept of multiple intelligences was popularized by Gardner in his 1983 book titled *Frames of Mind*. In 2011, he presented an updated version that identified the nine types of intelligences as linguistic, logical-mathematical, musical-rhythmic, bodily kinesthetic, spatial, naturalist, interpersonal, intrapersonal, and existential intelligence. Individuals have varying degrees of skill and comfort with each of the nine types of intelligences represented in Table 7.4.

MI represents preferred modes of receiving, processing, and learning information. Each intelligence is also appropriate for learning specific types of information or skills (Table 7.4). All types of MI are believed to exist in varying degrees in each individual. The person's level of comfort with diverse intelligences can be enhanced or facilitated through individual effort. In addition, some types of intelligence are more relevant for certain content areas than others, so a balance between the use of content-appropriate intelligences with the personal strengths of the learner may be needed.

Myers–Briggs Personality Types

Although the Myers–Briggs is a personality classification system, it has been valuable in understanding how aspects of personality affect learning by understanding the driving forces in the person's approach to the world and others. The theory is based in part on the

TABLE 7.3 Visual, Auditory, and Kinesthetic Teaching Strategies	
Learning Channel	**Teaching Strategies**
Visual	Seeing, reading, graphics, videos, models, watching a demonstration
Auditory	Hearing, speaking, lecture, discussion, podcasts, teaching classmates
Kinesthetic	Touching, doing, moving, experiments, demonstrating a skill, role-playing, field trips, mind mapping

Sources: Barbe, Swassing, and Milone (1979); About Education (2017).

TABLE 7.4 Characteristics of Gardner's Multiple Intelligences and Teaching Approaches

Intelligence	Characteristics	Teaching–Learning Approaches
Linguistic	Sensitive to the meaning and order of words	Listening, speaking, humor, reading (oral or silent), writing, or journaling
Logical-mathematical	Handle chains of reasoning, recognize patterns, and order	Use of abstract symbols, formulas, outlining, organizing, sequencing, calculating, and problem solving
Spatial ability	To perceive the world accurately and recreate it	Use of photos, graphics, mind mapping, visual patterns, color schemes, or imagery
Musical	Sensitive to pitch, melody, rhythm, and tone	Music, singing, whistling, humming, environmental sounds, litening to rhythmic and tonal patterns in heart, lung, and bowel sounds
Kinesthetic	Skillful use and movement of the body	Role-playing, drama, physical exercise, body language, technical skill performance
Interpersonal	Understand people and relationships	Group projects with assigned roles, giving and receiving feedback
Intrapersonal	Accurate self-awareness and self-understanding	Emotional processing, reflection, thinking strategies, higher order reasoning, centering, metacognitive strategies

Sources: Gardner (1983, 2011).

work of Carl Jung who introduced the ideas on introversion and extroversion as a major personality dimension. The Myers–Briggs Inventory classifies people according to four personality dimensions: (a) introversion–extroversion, (b) sensing–intuiting, (c) thinking–feeling, and (d) judging–perceiving. The pairing of these four dimensions results in 16 personality types (Myers & Briggs Foundation, n.d.).

Each of the four personality dimensions represents a dichotomous continuum of behaviors, preferences, or cognitive activities. Each dimension has value and is viewed in a nonjudgmental fashion. Thus, the tendency to behave or perceive more strongly in one direction is not considered superior to another. Introversion and extroversion describe what energizes a person: the inner world of ideas and abstractions (introversion) or the outer world of people and things (extroversion). Individuals leaning toward introversion will feel more at ease and energized working on projects alone or engaging in solo, cognitive-based learning activities. Those who relate to extroversion are more energized by connecting with others and engaging in group learning activities. The sensing or intuiting dimension refers to how individuals perceive the world, either by directly observing the surrounding reality (sensing) or by using impressions and imagining possibilities (intuiting). This dimension is important to teaching as it reflects how the person prefers to receive information. The third dimension is thinking–feeling, which is concerned with how the person makes decisions. Thinkers make decisions impersonally by analyzing the situation, and their decisions are rooted in the value of fairness. Feelers value empathy and harmony and consider a person's needs as they make decisions. The final dimension is judging–perceiving, which refers to how a person views the world. Judgers are decisive, self-starters who focus on completing tasks. Perceivers are curious and spontaneous and may find it difficult to meet deadlines. They are process oriented and tend to focus on how the task is completed. Each of these dichotomous dimensions has the potential to influence the individual's observations, perspectives, perceptions, and interactions in the world. As a result, each dichotomous dimension influences learning behaviors and processes.

Kolb's Experiential Learning Theory

American psychologist, David Kolb, defined experiential learning as "the process whereby knowledge is created through the transformation of experience. Knowledge results from the combination of grasping and transforming experience" (Kolb, 1984, p. 41). Experiential Learning Theory (ELT) describes two ways of grasping experience: through concrete experience and abstract conceptualization. The learner transforms the experience by engaging in reflective observation and active experimentation.

The four phases in ELT are typically linked to form a four-quadrant cycle, with the learner able to enter the cycle at any point and progress through the phases for optimal learning. Based on ELT, which focuses on ways of acquiring and transforming learning experiences, Kolb developed a learning style theory that describes four learning styles: diverging, assimilating, converging, and accommodating, with each corresponding to respective quadrants of the ELT. Each learning style represents a merging of the ways of grasping information (i.e., concrete experience and abstract conceptualization) and ways of transforming knowledge (i.e., reflective observation and active experimentation). The diverging style, referred to as *divergers*, represent the merging of concrete experience and reflective observation. Therefore, divergers do well with brainstorming and gathering information. Learners with an assimilating style (i.e., *assimilators*) understand information best using abstract conceptualization, and they transform knowledge through reflective observation. As a result, assimilators do well with grouping and compiling information. Individuals with a converging style (i.e., *convergers*) use the processes of abstract conceptualization and active experimentation and are therefore good at finding practical uses for theory. The fourth learning style is accommodating, which relies on active experimentation and concrete experience. Therefore, *accommodators* are hands-on learners who like to carry out plans and solve problems.

Kolb's Learning Style Theory

Kolb's ELT identifies learning styles that identify personality, education, and work experience factors that shape learning styles. The types of learners described earlier (i.e., divergers, assimilators, convergers, and accommodators) represent personality types and their preferred ways of interacting with and adapting to the world as well as preferred ways of working with information. Previous educational experiences influence the person's learning style by reinforcing attitudes toward particular learning skills. Experiences in the work world provide exposure to others with shared values and beliefs, similar professional expectations, and career training. The person's job performance also necessitates adaptive competence in which the demands of the task are matched with the required skills. Thus, each learning style and corresponding tasks require certain skills for effective performance. For the accommodative learning style, taking the initiative and other action skills in leadership are needed. The diverging learning style is associated with valuing skills such as interpersonal relationships and helping others. Thinking skills, including information gathering and analysis, are needed for the assimilating learning style. Finally, the converging learning style is associated with decision skills that rely on the use of technology and goal-setting.

ELT and Kolb's Learning Style Theory are useful in understanding learning and the flexibility that is inherent in the process. These theories provide deep and comprehensive frameworks for understanding the learning process and learners. Educators can use these theories to guide learners to improve their learning and to design effective processes in education.

DOMAINS OF LEARNING

Bloom's taxonomies have been used to generate learning objectives in the cognitive and affective domains for individual learning sessions and entire courses and curriculums. Each domain of learning depicts a hierarchy of progressively higher learning processes. Other authors have developed taxonomies for the *psychomotor domain*, which describe the stages of psychomotor skill acquisition and refinement. The learning taxonomies for cognitive, affective, and psychomotor learning are reviewed next.

Cognitive Domain Taxonomy

In 1956, Bloom et al. developed a taxonomy for the cognitive learning domain, comprising six progressively higher levels of learning labeled knowledge, comprehension, application, analysis, evaluation, and synthesis. In 2001, Anderson, one of Bloom's students and Krathwohl, one of the original authors of the 1956 cognitive taxonomy, along with others, published a revision of the cognitive taxonomy (Anderson et al., 2001). Major differences in the 2001 version are: (a) renaming and reordering of several taxonomies levels, (b) using verbs instead of nouns for each level, and (c) differentiating four types of knowledge (i.e., factual, conceptual, procedural, and metacognitive) within each of the six cognitive levels. See Table 7.5 for a comparison of the original and revised taxonomies.

TABLE 7.5 Comparison of Bloom's Original and Revised Cognitive Taxonomies		
Domain Levels	**Bloom's Original Taxonomy**	**Revised Taxonomy**
1	Knowledge	Remember
2	Comprehension	Understand
3	Application	Apply
4	Analysis	Analyze
5	Evaluation	Synthesize
6	Synthesis	Create
Knowledge types	Not emphasized	Integrated into each taxonomy level
1	—	Factual
2	—	Conceptual
3	—	Procedural
4	—	Metacognitive

Sources: Anderson et al. (2001); Bloom (1956).

In level 1 of the revised taxonomy, the noun *knowledge* has been replaced by the verb *remembering*. The second taxonomy level, originally called *comprehension*, was replaced by the verb *understanding*. The term *synthesize* was changed to *creating* and moved to the sixth level. All other levels were renamed to the verb form resulting in the new taxonomy of "remembering, understanding, applying, analyzing, evaluating, and creating."

In the revised taxonomy, each cognitive level is characterized and differentiated further using four levels of knowledge. *Factual knowledge* refers to basic elements and terms a student must know to solve problems in the content area. *Conceptual knowledge* involves knowing the relationships between basic elements and the functioning of those elements. It involves classifying, making generalizations, and identifying principles and frameworks relevant to the discipline. *Procedural knowledge* includes using the information, skills, techniques, or methods appropriate for the content area. The final level, *metacognition*, involves the ability to think about one's thinking and regulate and guide one's cognitive processes. It includes understanding how to solve problems and perform cognitive tasks.

The cognitive domain taxonomy is useful for developing leveled objectives to guide educational content and guide the development of ways to evaluate learning. Educators use the taxonomy to level learning objectives in nursing curriculums for undergraduate and graduate nursing programs. Nurse administrators may apply the taxonomy to clinical ladder programs and use the verbs identified for each level to describe clinical evaluation outcomes for novice through expert nurses. The four levels of knowledge delineate the knowledge outcomes expected with each domain level.

Affective Domain Taxonomy

The *affective domain* delineated by Krathwohl, Bloom, and Masia (1964) consists of five hierarchical levels that depict a person's progressive development of values, beliefs, attitudes, and their expression. The affective domain describes the inner processes involved in reorganizing our thoughts, feelings, and ultimately changing our actions. Thus, the affective domain is linked to both the cognitive (thinking) and psychomotor (action) domains.

The first affective level involves receiving information that is new to our experience, and it has three aspects: (a) awareness, (b) willingness to receive, and (c) acquiescence. At the receiving level, the learner is relatively passive. But with each successive level, the degree of active involvement, the initiative assumed by the learner, and the degree of internal change experienced increases. Willingness to receive information that is new or to challenge our values requires some degree of initiative and depicts internal change beyond the passive awareness level. Acquiescence represents even more active involvement and internal change as the learner accepts new attitudes, values, and beliefs.

Responding describes the second affective level, where the learner demonstrates a willingness to respond and satisfaction in that response. Willingness may be demonstrated by the learner taking action to become familiar with a specific issue, whereas satisfaction is a subjective feeling experienced by the learner as a result of responding.

At the third and fourth levels, the learner experiences further internal changes. The valuing level has three aspects: (a) acceptance of other's values or situation; (b) preference, which involves examining viewpoints and forming an opinion; and (c) making a commitment to act in a manner that respects the patient. Once valuing behaviors have been demonstrated, the learner can engage in metacognitive processes that characterize the organization domain level. Thus, the fourth level, organization, refers to the cognitive process involved in the acquisition of an affective change. The learner is involved in conceptualizing a value and using evaluation processes to organize and create a value system.

The final level is referred to as "characterization by a value or value complex." This level is where the learner actively responds to an ethical situation. It can be achieved in two ways: first, by responding to an ethical dilemma using ethical principles, referred to as *generalized set* or by characterization, which involves using internalized values to respond to an ethical dilemma. Affective learning is often difficult to quantify in learning objectives, yet it is essential for social integration of students and novice nurses into professional nursing practice.

Psychomotor Learning Domain

Several educators have developed taxonomies for psychomotor learning. Dave (1970) outlined a five-level taxonomy that focuses on skill refinement over time. Similarly, Simpson (1972) developed a five-level taxonomy, later revised to have seven levels. Simpson depicts the learner's movement from awareness of the components involved in performing a skill and culminates in the learner adapting his or her performance of the skill to new situations. The taxonomies discussed subsequently are useful in creating objectives that level the learner's skill performance. Each taxonomy adds to our understanding of how people learn and how skill performance improves over time.

Dave's Psychomotor Taxonomy

Dave's psychomotor taxonomy focuses on the processes that occur during performance of a skill. The five-level taxonomy includes the processes of (a) imitation, (b) manipulation, (c) precision, (d) articulation, and (e) naturalization. The first level, imitation, relies on observing and copying the performance of a skill. In the manipulation process, the learner focuses on manipulation of the environment, equipment, and supplies used to perform the skill. The precision level focuses on developing greater accuracy and the ability to perform the skill without guidance. In the fourth level, articulation, the learner combines several skills and performs them in a consistent manner. At the naturalization level, the learner has integrated two or more skills and can perform them sequentially and automatically with little mental effort.

Dave's taxonomy can be used to determine the level of a student's skill performance and identify teaching strategies useful at each level. The taxonomy also provides verbs to delineate progressively higher ordered learning objectives. At the imitation or copying level of performance, repeated demonstrations followed by practice are the main teaching strategies. Verbs used in learning objectives of this first level are the most basic and include *identify, copy, follow,* or *repeat*. The next level of skill performance called manipulation involves a higher level of performance in that the learner can perform the skill with only verbal or written guidance. Learning objectives may specify that the person can perform the skill with only written or verbal instructions or may incorporate verbs such as *implement, perform,* or *execute*. At the precision level, the performance of the skill should demonstrate increased independence. Accuracy of performance is enhanced with additional practice and feedback. Skill performance is evaluated using learning objectives that denote consistent demonstration or completion of the skill without additional instruction or feedback.

The remaining levels of Dave's taxonomy denote refinement of the skill performance. At the articulation level, the learner performs the skill efficiently in diverse settings or situations. Effective performance is evaluated using objectives denoting constructing, developing, or adapting the skill to novel situations. The naturalization level is the habituation level in which the skill is easily performed or taught to others. The learner is able to create an individualized version of the skill and teach others. Verbs such as *design, manage,* and *invent* are commonly used in psychomotor learning objectives at this level.

Simpson's Psychomotor Taxonomy

Simpson's psychomotor taxonomy published in 1972 describes the process of skill learning and refinement. The first domain level is *perception*, or awareness of the objects, qualities, and characteristics that are needed to perform the skill. The individual uses his or her senses to determine what is required to perform the skill. Perception is necessary for effective implementation of the next level referred to as "set." Performing a skill at the set level involves achieving physical and mental readiness to perform the skill. The third level referred to as *guided response* occurs during the earliest attempts to perform the skill with guidance from the teacher or from written or visual instructions. After the learner has repeatedly practiced using guided response, the next level called *mechanism* is achieved. The mechanism level is characterized by performing the skill with less reliance on direct guidance. The fifth taxonomy level is called *complex overt response*, which is characterized by smooth and efficient performance.

Later modifications to Simpson's taxonomy have focused on the refinement of skill performance that occurs after the complex overt stage is mastered. *Adaptation* is the sixth level, which occurs when the learner is able to change the skill to meet the needs of unique situations. The seventh and final level is *origination*. The learner who demonstrates origination goes beyond adaptation by actually creating new movements within the procedure to meet the unique needs of the situation. Each skill level from guided response through origination is achieved through repeated practice over time.

In each psychomotor taxonomy, the learner progresses from an initial state of dependency and lack of proficiency. The lower levels of performance require high mental effort until smooth, efficient, adaptable, and automatic performance is eventually achieved. Both Dave's and Simpson's taxonomies share the perspective that the progression of skill refinement improves with practice over time. They also agree that achieving the highest psychomotor taxonomy level enables the learner to exert less mental effort when performing the skill and focus instead on interacting with and observing others while performing the skill.

◉ CONCLUSION

Each theoretical perspective discussed contributes a slightly different understanding or perspective on education, teaching, and learning. With learning frameworks we have seen progressive development that expands our understanding and builds an increasingly comprehensive explanation of learning and knowledge acquisition.

Models, theories, and taxonomies are used throughout the teaching/learning process. More than one theory or model may be useful in a teaching and learning situation. You may discover that you prefer the use of certain frameworks as a teacher and learner. However, diversity is the key to adaptability in learning and teaching. For one-on-one teaching, each learner will have unique preferences and strengths; so identifying and using them to enhance the learning experience are essential. When teaching groups, the use of a variety of strategies will appeal to the majority of learners and will enhance the learner's focus, engagement, and satisfaction with the learning experience.

◉ KEY POINTS

- Classic learning frameworks are categorized as behaviorism, cognitivism, cognitive developmental, social cognitive, constructivism, and humanism.
- Behaviorism sees learning as a change in behavior. Three behaviorist frameworks are connectionism, classical conditioning, and operant conditioning.
- Gestaltism is a cognitive framework that is concerned with how we perceive and organize information, especially visual information.
- Four stages of learning involved in Information Processing Theory are attention, processing, memory storage, and action or response.

- Gagné describes a cognitive learning process that involves (a) recognition of the stimulus, (b) response, (c) following a procedure, (d) use of terminology, (e) discrimination, (f) formation of concepts, (g) application of rules, and (h) solving problems.

- Cognitive Developmental Theory, such as andragogy, focuses on changes in perception, thinking, and reasoning that occur with age and experience.

- Social cognitivist frameworks, such as Rotter's SLT, emphasize the cognitive aspects of personality and the individual's internal and external locus of control.

- Bandura's SLT sees the person, environment, and behavior as reciprocal concepts that influence learning.

- Constructivism values the cultural environment and the processes of interaction and collaboration in learning.

- Humanists value teaching approaches that emphasize personal growth, curiosity, and utilize experiential learning. Humanism values objectives from within the affective domain.

- Learning style frameworks describe preferred ways of perceiving and/or processing information.

- Three domains of learning are cognitive, affective, and psychomotor. The process of learning in each domain is described using hierarchical taxonomies.

REFERENCES

About Education. (2017). The three different learning styles. Retrieved from http://testprep.about.com/od/tipsfortesting/a/Different_Learning_Styles.htm

Anderson, L. W., Krathwohl, D. R., Airasian , P., Cruikshank , K., Mayer, R., Pintrich, P., & Wittrock, M. C. (2001). *A taxonomy for learning, teaching, and assessing: A revision of Bloom's taxonomy of educational objectives.* New York, NY: Addison Wesley Longman.

Bandura, A. (1986). *Social foundations of thought and action: A social cognitive theory.* Englewood Cliffs, NJ: Prentice Hall.

Barbe, W. B., Swassing, R. H., & Milone, M. N. (1979). *Teaching through modality strengths: Concepts and practices.* Columbus, OH: Zaner-Bloser.

Bloom, B. S. (Ed.). (1956). *Taxonomy of educational objectives: The classification of educational goals. Handbook I: Cognitive domain.* New York, NY: David McKay.

Curry, L. (1981). Learning preferences in continuing medical education. *Canadian Medical Association Journal, 124,* 535–536.

Dave, R. H. (1970). Psychomotor levels. In R. J. Armstrong (Ed.), *Developing and writing behavioral objectives* (pp. 20–21). Tucson, AZ: Educational Innovators Press.

Dewey, J. (1938). *Experience and education.* Toronto, ON, Canada: Collier-MacMillan.

Ellis, W. D. (1938). *A source book for gestalt psychology.* New York, NY: Harcourt, Brace & World.

Gagné, R. M. (1985). *The conditions of learning and the theory of instruction.* New York, NY: Holt, Rinehart & Winston.

Gagné, R. M., Wager, W. W., Golas, K. C., & Keller, J. M. (2005). *Principles of instructional design.* Belmont, CA: Thomson/Wadsworth.

Gardner, H. (1983). *Frames of mind: The theory of multiple intelligences.* New York, NY: Basic Books.

Gardner, H. (2011). *Frames of mind: The theory of multiple intelligences* (3rd ed.). New York, NY: Basic Books.

Heydari, A., Dashtgard, A., & Moghadam, Z. E. (2014). The effect of Bandura's social cognitive theory implementation on addiction quitting of clients referred to addiction quitting clinics. *Iranian Journal of Nursing and Midwifery Research, 19*(1), 9–23.

Knowles, M. (1984). *The adult learner: A neglected species.* Houston, TX: Gulf Publishing.

Kolb, D. A. (1984). *Experiential learning: Experience as the source of learning and development.* New Jersey, NJ: Prentice Hall.

Krathwohl, D. R., Bloom, B. S., & Masia, B. B. (1964). *Taxonomy of educational objectives: Handbook II: Affective domain.* New York, NY: David McKay.

Lewin, K. (1951). *Field theory in social science: Selected theoretical papers.* New York, NY: Harper & Row.

Maslow, A. (1954). *Motivation and personality.* New York, NY: Harper & Row.

Maslow, A. (1987). *Motivation and personality* (3rd ed.). New York, NY: Harper & Row.

Myers & Briggs Foundation. (n.d.). MBTI basics. Retrieved from http://www.myersbriggs.org

Pavlov, I. P. (1932). The reply of a physiologist to psychologists. *The Psychological Review, 39*(2), 91–127.

Pavlov, I. P. (1949). Conditioned responses. In W. Dennis (Ed.), *Readings in general psychology.* New York, NY: Prentice Hall.

Rogers, C. R. (1969). *Freedom to learn.* Columbus, OH: Merrill.

Rogers, C. R., & Freiberg, H. J. (1994). *Freedom to learn* (3rd ed.). Columbus, OH: Merrill/Macmillan.

Rotter, J. B. (1982). *The development and applications of social learning theory.* New York, NY: Praeger.

Simpson, E. (1972). *The classification of educational objectives in the psychomotor domain: The psychomotor domain.* Washington, DC: Gryphon House.

Skinner, B. F. (1932). On the rate of formation of a conditioned reflex. *Journal of General Psychology, 7,* 274–286.

Skinner, B. F. (1985). Cognitive science and behaviourism. *British Journal of Psychology, 76,* 291–301.

Thorndike, E. (1898a, January/June). Some experiments on animal intelligence. *Science, 7,* 818–824.

Thorndike, E. (1898b). Animal intelligence: An experimental study of the associative processes in animals. *Psychological Monographs: General and Applied, 2*(4), i–109.

Watson , J. B., & Rayner, R. (1920). Conditioned emotional responses. *Journal of Experimental Psychology, 3,* 1–14.

Moral and Ethical Perspectives

Rose Utley

One's philosophy is not best expressed in words; it is expressed in the choices one makes....And the choices we make are ultimately our responsibility.
—Eleanor Roosevelt

Whatever you are, be a good one.
—Abraham Lincoln

KEY TERMS

ANA *Code of Ethics*
autonomy
beneficence
care-based ethics
consequentialism
Crisham's MORAL
 Decision-Making Model
DECIDE Model
deontological
duty-based ethics
ethics
eudemonia

intellectual virtues
International Council of
 Nurses *Code of Ethics*
Jonsen's Four Box Method
justice
Kidder's Shared Values
moral exclusion
Moral Exclusion Theory
moral virtues
morality
morals
nonmaleficence

Nurses Ethical Reasoning
 Skills Model
principle-based ethics
principlism
Symphonological
 Bioethical Theory
symphonology
teleological
utilitarianism
values
veracity
virtue ethics

LEARNING OBJECTIVES

1. Define principles and terms used to describe ethical perspectives and ethical decision making.
2. Explain and compare ethical concepts, frameworks, and perspectives.
3. Explore the role of morals and ethics in nursing education, clinical practice, administration, and research.

Values, morals, and ethics are interconnected and pervasive in nursing, health care, and all aspects of life. *Values*, defined as qualities that are important to individuals and communities, are the foundation for *morals* (i.e., values demonstrated by behaviors). *Morality* is the expression of our ethics through human behavior or adhering to accepted standards of behavior. The terms ethics and morals are distinct but interrelated and often used interchangeably. *Ethics* is a branch of knowledge that deals with principles that underlie moral behaviors, as well as a branch of philosophy concerned with establishing criteria for evaluating the goodness or desirability of behavior (Robb, 1989). Ethics also refers to the study of ideal human behavior and ways of being in the world, which is based on theories of moral values and principles. As a system of moral principles or rules of conduct for individuals, groups, and cultures, ethics relies on nontangible beliefs and values. When expressed through behavior, ethics becomes a study of morals or behaviors of individuals, groups, and cultures. To distinguish between morals and ethics, it may be helpful to think of ethics as the science of morals and morals as one's practice of ethics.

Our interconnectedness with each other necessitates that we understand and explore our values, morals, and ethical judgments when attempting to resolve ethical dilemmas. Ethical dilemmas occur when a person is forced to choose between two or more actions, each with its own rationale that justifies its goodness. The goal of ethical inquiry is to distinguish between right and wrong, good and not good, and facilitate decision making in the face of ethical dilemmas.

Our values, beliefs, decision making, and behavior are described, influenced, and guided by ethical principles including justice, beneficence, and nonmaleficence. Values, morals, and ethics play a key part in all nursing roles including nursing educator, clinician, leader, and researcher. In this chapter, ethical concepts, principles, philosophies, and frameworks used in nursing are explored. Application of these concepts and perspective to the roles of the nurse educator, clinician, leader, and researcher are highlighted.

◉ ETHICAL PRINCIPLES

Ethical principles are used in all nursing roles. In the clinician and nurse leadership roles, the issues of health care costs, access to treatment, limited resources, end-of-life care, genetics, and technological advances in medical interventions have resulted in numerous ethical issues that require our attention. In the researcher role, evidence-based health care practices require ethically conducted research. Therefore, attention to human subjects' concerns and participants' rights to autonomy, justice, beneficence, nonmaleficence, and veracity are emphasized. Nurse educators are charged with teaching students about moral and ethical principles and frameworks, and they often facilitate students' clinical decision making. Additionally, nurse educators determine and enforce academic integrity policies and evaluate student behaviors based on ethical principles. Thus, the use of ethics is pervasive in all nursing roles. Ethical principles are discussed in the following sections to provide a basis for personal understanding, reflection, and decision making.

Autonomy underlies human and patient rights and supports the person's right to decide based on personal values and beliefs. Autonomy values the individual's right to participate or not in decisions and actions without undue influence. It involves the freedom to act independently to achieve self-determined goals. In health care, autonomy refers to the patient's right to decide the type, timing, and continuation of treatment. In research, autonomy protects the person's freedom to choose to participate in a research study without coercion or to withdraw from a study without the fear of repercussions. Informed consent whether for medical treatments or participation in a research study helps ensure the individual has the information needed for autonomous decision making. Providing informed consent supplies needed information for decision making such as risks, benefits, and a description of procedures conducted. Interference with autonomy may be subtle such as offering incentives to participate in research that could motivate disadvantaged individuals to participate when they would not do so otherwise.

The principle of *justice* is based on equality, equity, and fairness. It is foundational for dealing with vulnerable populations that experience health disparities and social injustice, and for addressing health policy issues. With the emphasis on treating others equitably, justice seeks to distribute both benefits and burdens equitably. Application of the principle of justice often involves advocacy for the patient's rights to treatment.

The actions of health care professionals are typically guided by *beneficence* which is the obligation to do good for others and contribute to their welfare. Beneficence typically involves three components: (a) to prevent harm, (b) remove harm, and (c) do good. A related principle, *nonmaleficence*, is often cited in the guiding maxim, "First, do no harm." This maxim is concerned with the obligation not to inflict harm intentionally on another. This principle is important in clinical practice, administrative policy making, and in nursing research.

Veracity is honesty and truth telling, or one's duty to tell the truth. It is based on the respect for human dignity and autonomy. It incorporates related concepts such as avoiding deceit and misrepresentation. It is integral to the process of informed consent, which mandates that issues affecting decision making, such as full disclosure of risks, be identified.

ETHICAL PERSPECTIVES

Ethical perspectives can be described regarding ethical principles, which serve as the basis for ethical rules. These ethical principles and rules can then be used for decision making. Ethical perspectives provide a rationale that explains and justifies our ethical stance and provides structure for our reasoning. The use of ethical principles enables the nurse to make decisions in a comprehensive and well-reasoned fashion as opposed to relying on personal opinion and intuition. Knowledge of ethical frameworks can be used to clarify the underlying argument and reasoning for decision making and to help identify ethical aspects of a situation that should be considered.

Duty-Based Ethics

Before moral/ethical frameworks are explored, it is important to understand the foundations and underlying principles of major schools of ethical thought. German philosopher Immanuel Kant (1724–1804) was a proponent of the *deontological* perspective, which is based on the study of duties and rules (Gibson, 1993). Kant believed that people are ethically required to take action from their sense of duty regardless of the consequences. In a deontological perspective, the focus is on the act itself, which is judged right or wrong independent of the consequences. Acting as a good samaritan is an example of acting from duty-based ethics.

Deontologists live according to a set of moral rules to do the right thing, even if it produces a bad result. If an action is a right action, then it should be carried out; if it is a wrong action, it should not be carried out. Duty-based ethical practices give equal respect to all human beings. They require that the interests of a single person be considered even when those interests oppose those of a larger group. According to duty-based ethics, some actions are inherently right or wrong, and people have a duty to act accordingly, regardless of the good or bad consequences that may be produced (Chowning & Fraser, 2007).

Consequentialism

When compared to duty-based ethics, consequentialism introduces greater uncertainty because it is concerned with the consequences of an action. It is also known as a *teleological* perspective or *utilitarianism*, and it values the achievement of good results regardless of the methods. Consequentialists support actions that produce the greatest overall benefit for the majority (Chowning & Fraser, 2007). An example of consequentialism is seen in mass casualty triage where patient care is prioritized by the severity of the illness or injury yet tempered by the caveat "do the greatest good for the greatest number."

Consequentialism is based on two principles. First, the result of an action determines whether it is right or wrong. Second, the degree of goodness or rightness is determined by a number of good consequences that result. Therefore, consequentialists believe people should choose actions that produce the greatest amount of good for the greatest number.

Virtue Ethics

Virtue ethics fall outside of the deontological/teleological dichotomy of duty and consequentialism and instead values the individual's character traits. Virtue ethics is concerned with striving to be the best that one can be and emulate positive character traits (Chowning & Fraser, 2007). An individual's traits such as honesty, trustworthiness, wisdom, justice, courage, integrity, and temperament are what make an action right or wrong. Virtue ethics is not concerned with outcomes or processes but encourages the cultivation of human excellence by asking: What kind of person do I want to be?

Andorno (2012) stressed that both understanding and action are necessary components for applying virtue ethics. "The idea that knowing moral theories is enough for making sound moral decisions is as naïve as expecting that just by reading a book about how to swim one will be able to swim" (Andorno, 2012, p. 459). For proponents of virtue ethics, the goal of human life is *eudemonia* meaning *happiness* or *well-being*. Virtue, as a character trait, is needed for people to flourish and live well.

Virtues are categorized into two types; moral and intellectual. *Moral virtues* include prudence, justice, fortitude, and temperance; and *intellectual virtues* incorporate theoretical and practical knowledge. Aristotle proposed that each moral virtue represents a desirable middle ground between two undesirable extremes. For example, courage represents a concept midway between the two extremes of cowardice and foolhardiness. According to virtue ethics, evaluating actions and consequences as either positive or negative depends on the ethical judgments we make about the traits of those who perform the actions.

Principle-Based Ethics

Principlism, or principle-based ethics, integrates the principles of personal autonomy, justice, beneficence, and nonmaleficence, and upholds these principles according to the situation (Chowning & Fraser, 2007). Principle-based ethics considers the actions emphasized in duty-based ethics, the outcomes emphasized in consequentialist-based ethics, and the individual's character as emphasized in virtue-based ethics.

Elements of principlism are found in the Constitution of the United States which acknowledges the individual's right to justice and in the autonomy of action. Principlism was formally articulated in the Belmont Report developed by the National Commission for the Protection of Human Subjects of Biomedical Research (1979). In the report, adherence to the principles of autonomy, justice, and beneficence were identified as essential for research conducted on human subjects.

Wide agreement exists on the importance and acceptance of the values of autonomy, nonmaleficence, beneficence, and justice. The universality of these principles across cultures and situations is a strength, as is the ease of application of these principles to ethical scenarios. Principlism describes how people make moral decisions and how they ought to act based on society's intersubjective agreements. Proponents of principlism contend that from the beginning of recorded history, decision makers have used moral principles and they are compatible with most intellectual, religious, and cultural beliefs.

Care-Based Ethics

Care-based ethics emphasizes that the development of morals relies on learning behaviors in specific social-cultural contexts and is not the result of learning and applying principles. In contrast to principle-based ethics, care-based ethics are less guided by rules and instead focus on the needs of others and on one's responsibility to meet those needs. The ethics of care emerged from the work of American psychologist and ethicist, Carol Gilligan, who studied ethical decision making in women. She differentiates decision making by women, which is based predominantly on caring, from that of men who rely on the principle of justice (see Chapter 6).

Care-based ethics has continued to develop through the works of Toronto (1993, 2005). He identified four components of care as (a) attentiveness, (b) responsibility, (c) competence, and (d) responsiveness. To provide care, one must demonstrate actions consistent with these components. First, one must recognize or be attentive to other's needs. If an individual is not aware of the need, there is no basis for caring. The second component, responsibility, is more ambiguous than an obligation, and it is often tied to preestablished social norms, roles, or legal obligations. Responsibility is not mandated but is something the individual decides to do. The action part of care is denoted by providing care that is competent and accurate. Responsiveness refers to the care receiver's reaction to the care. According to Toronto, the nature of caring is concerned with addressing needs related to vulnerability and inequality.

ETHICAL FRAMEWORKS

Ethical concepts and principles have been combined to form theories and models that describe and explain codes of ethics and ethical decision-making processes. In this section, the American Nurses Association (ANA) *Code of Ethics, International Code of Ethics for Nurses*, Moral Exclusion Theory, and Kidder's Shared Values Theory are explored. Then, several frameworks useful for ethical decision making are reviewed including Jonsen's Four Box Method, Nurse's Ethical Reasoning Skills Model, Crisham's MORAL Decision-Making Model, and the DECIDE Model.

ANA *Code of Ethics for Nurses*

The ANA *Code of Ethics for Nurses* was initially developed in 1950 as a guide for nursing practice. The purpose was to delineate the ethical obligations of nurses and nursing's commitment to society as a whole. The code addresses several categories of ethical relationships (see Table 8.1) including the nurse to patient, nurse to self, nurse to nurse, nurse to others, nurse to society, nurse to the profession, and the nursing profession to society (ANA, 2015; see Table 8.1).

The code is organized into nine provisions that describe the nurse's relationships, responsibilities, and obligations to self and others. Interpretive statements explain the application of each provision. The first three provisions focus on the nurse's responsibilities in dealing with others. The first provision addresses the nature of the nurse's relationships with others, addressing the need to practice with compassion and respect regardless of the situation. Second is the importance of the nurse's commitment to the patient, which is defined broadly as an individual, family, group, or community. The third provision describes the nurse's actions to promote and advocate for the patient's health, safety, and rights.

Provisions four and five address the nurse's responsibilities to self. Provision four delineates the nurse's accountability for his or her nursing practice including decisions about delegation of tasks. The nurse's responsibility to maintain integrity and safety in practice through personal and professional growth is emphasized in provision five.

The final four provisions address the nurse's responsibility to others such as employers, other professionals, the community, and the nursing profession. Provision six is concerned with taking individual and collective actions to establish, maintain, and improve the health care environment. The nurse's responsibility for the advancement of the profession through nursing education, clinical practice, leadership, and research is described in provision seven. Provision eight explains the importance of collaborating with other professionals and the general public to address local to global health needs. The final provision emphasizes the

TABLE 8.1 Provisions of the ANA *Code of Ethics for Nurses*

Provision #	Description
1	Provide compassionate, respectful care
2	Demonstrate commitment to the patient
3	Promote, advocate, and protect the rights, health, and safety of patients
4	Demonstrate authority, accountability, and responsibility
5	Promote personal health, safety, integrity, and competence
6	Facilitate an ethical work environment
7	Take actions to advance the profession
8	Collaborate to protect human rights, promote health, and reduce health care inequities
9	Articulate nursing values and incorporate principles of social justice into practice

ANA, American Nurses Association.

Source: American Nurses Association (2015).

role of professional nursing organizations in maintaining practice integrity and shaping health care practices.

International Council of Nurses *Code of Ethics*

In 1953, the first *International Code of Ethics for Nurses* was developed and adopted by the International Council of Nurses (ICN). The 2012 version of ICN *Code of Ethics* is organized around four elements that encompass the scope of nursing practice regarding (a) nurses and people needing nursing care, (b) nurses and practice, (c) nurses and the profession, and (d) nurses and coworkers. In each element, standards of conduct are identified.

The first element, "nurses and people needing nursing care," outlines standards that value responsibility, confidentiality, cultural sensitivity, and advocacy. The importance of demonstrating professional values of respectfulness, responsiveness, compassion, trustworthiness, and integrity is incorporated in this element. The second element is "nurses and practice," which contains six standards. These standards revolve around responsibility for one's practice, including competence, personal health, personal conduct, acceptance and delegation of responsibilities, and ensuring a safe, respectful practice culture. The third element delineates the roles and responsibilities of the nurse and the profession. Six standards describe the expectations of nurses to create an ethical professional environment, which includes sustaining and protecting the natural environment and ensuring an equitable and safe working environment. Practices that sustain professional values, research-based knowledge, and implement standards for clinical, educational, administrative and research practice are valued. The final element concerns the nurse and the coworkers and consists of three standards. These standards revolve around the need for collaboration and respect when interacting with coworkers. They serve as a safeguard when coworkers endanger the patient's health and guide and support nurses to engage in ethical behavior.

The ICN *Code of Ethics* offers a comprehensive framework for nursing practice. It empha-sizes social, cultural, and professional competence as well as individual's actions, and the impact of those actions on ethical behaviors. It reflects universal values and beliefs about nursing, among which is: "Nursing care is respectful of and unrestricted by considerations of age, color, creed, culture, disability or illness, gender, sexual orientation, nationality, pol-itics, race, or social status" (ICN, 2012, p. 1). The code provides a usable document that can serve as a framework for nursing practice, regardless of geographical boundaries.

Moral Exclusion Theory

Moral Exclusion Theory is relevant when dealing with subtle, individual-focused forms of moral exclusion such as discrimination, bullying, sexual harassment, and blatant forms of persecution such as hate crimes and ethnic cleansing (Opotow, Gerson, & Woodside, 2005). The theory explains "the thinking of individuals or groups towards other individuals or groups on difficult social problems and the underlying conflicts that may occur between groups" (Brinson, 2011, p. 6).

Moral exclusion occurs when the application of justice is limited in certain contexts. It emphasizes fairness, resource sharing, and concern for the well-being of others (Opotow et al., 2005). Moral exclusion varies in scope from narrow to broad and ranges from subtle to blatant in the intensity of manifestation. Moral exclusion behaviors that are narrow in scope and subtle include double standards, condescension, and derogation. Blatant manifes-tations that are narrow in scope include violence and persecution in the form of hate crimes. Behaviors that are broad in scope but subtle include oppression and structural violence man-ifesting as racism, poverty, and some cases of domestic violence. Examples of moral exclu-sion that are broad in scope and blatant include direct violence and infringement of human rights on a massive scale such as ethnic cleansing and mass murder.

Conflict and a sense of disconnectedness are antecedents for moral exclusion. How we communicate with or about others may demonstrate disconnectedness. According to Leets (2001), "Communication is one of the primary means by which people affect and are affected by others" (p. 1859). Therefore, communication plays a pivotal role in the exclusion process through deprecating speech and may play an equally important role in reversing the cycle of moral exclusion.

Kidder's Shared Values

Kidder, a writer, ethicist, and founder of the Institute for Global Ethics, sees the development of a values-driven culture as essential in today's world (Kidder, 1994, 1995). A values-driven culture requires four factors: (a) shared core values, (b) shared language, (c) commitment by the leadership, and (d) moral courage. To identify shared values, Kidder questioned 24 men and women who had been identified by others from their country, religion, or cultural group as having a strong ethical conscience. The following questions were posed: "Is there a set of values that wise, ethical people from around the world use to make decisions? And if so can those values be identified?" (Curtain, 2000, p. 9). The values were identified and ranked in order of importance as love, truthfulness, fairness, freedom, unity, tolerance, and respon-sibility. A values-based culture sees these core values as the driving force behind decision making. "A culture of ethics is what links people to those above, below, and beside them, connections which, although invisible, make the whole organization immeasurably stron-ger" (Institute for Global Ethics, 2016, para. 2).

Subsequently, a common language is needed to facilitate communication, discussion, and ethical decision making and the common language is based on an understanding of the core values. These values provide a critical foundation for problem solving, consensus building, and organizational leadership. Commitment by the leadership to foster a culture of ethics and connection is also necessary. These shared connections, although nontangible, make the

---

BOX 8.1 Application of Kidder's Shared Values in Administration

Using the values identified by Kidder and the principles of beneficence, nonmaleficence, and honesty, Curtain (2000) outlined 10 principles to guide nurse administrators. These principles reflect the nurse administrator's dual roles in facilitating patient
care and functioning as a steward of the organization's resources. Curtain notes that
the nurse administrator must align with the ethics of professional nursing, which focus
on doing no harm, protecting, and maintaining confidentiality. These professional ethical perspectives are duty oriented or deontological. However, the nurse administrator
also operates from a set of business ethics focused on resource allocation and being a
steward of patient resources including nursing staff.

---

organization cohesive and strong. In addition, moral courage by decision makers is needed.
There will be times when a decision is not popular, or a decision must be made quickly
before all influencing factors are known. In these cases, moral courage of the leadership is
needed to take action that is believed to be the best ethical decision. An example that builds
upon Kidder's Shared Values is presented in Box 8.1.

FRAMEWORKS FOR MORAL DECISION MAKING

In Chapter 6 several theories were discussed that describe developmental stages in the person's ethical decision-making skills. Among them is Kohlberg's Moral Reasoning Theory
which describes the cognitive processes in the moral development of children. Kohlberg
characterized the person's moral reasoning ability as developing in sequential stages from
birth to adulthood and saw moral decision making as being influenced by the principle of
justice. Similarly, developmental theorist Carol Gilligan developed a theory of moral reasoning using Kohlberg's sequential stages. However, she found that women develop moral
reasoning in the context of caring and relationships, rather than from the principles of justice or fairness as did men. Eisenberg's Prosocial Theory of Moral Reasoning represents a
synthesis of some of Kohlberg's and Gilligan's main points. However, depending on the
situation, Eisenberg sees the child as able to engage in moral reasoning from more than one
developmental level (see Chapter 6). The remainder of this section focuses on decision-making frameworks used specifically in nursing practice.

Jonsen's Four Box Method

Jonsen's Four Box Method is useful for analyzing individual cases that involve medical treatment dilemmas (Jonsen, Siegler, & Winslade, 2010). Each case is examined for the following
factors: (a) medical indications, (b) patient preferences, (c) quality of life, and (d) contextual
features. Medical indications are concerned with factual data about the efficacy of specific
treatments or nontreatments and with the congruence with the principles of beneficence and
nonmaleficence. Patient preference is based on the principle of respect for autonomy. When
examining patient preference, biases related to age, race, culture, class, or other personal
attributes are acknowledged. Inherent in the third factor, quality of life, are the principles of
beneficence, nonmaleficence, and personal autonomy. Each of these principles is important
to maintain the quality of life. For example, respect for patient autonomy acknowledges that
the patient is most qualified to judge his or her quality of life. The principles of beneficence
and nonmaleficence are applied to determine the appropriateness of accepting or rejecting
potential therapeutic options. As the individual defines the quality of life, the perceptions of

what constitutes quality may vary significantly from one person to the other. Beliefs about the importance of the individual's mental, physical, and social capacities are considered. Subsequently, contextual features based on the principles of justice and fairness are considered. Potential issues such as resources, family dynamics, provider issues, costs, and legal and religious concerns are captured in this model.

The central issue needing intervention is determined by examining information about the situation and sorting it into each of the four categories or boxes. Answering the question, In what box does the issue seem to lie? helps guide the practitioner to the area that needs additional assessment data and to identify potential areas to intervene.

Symphonological Bioethical Theory

Husted and Husted (2008) outlined an ethical decision-making model for nurses that uses the principles of autonomy, freedom, objectivity, self-assertion, beneficence, and fidelity. Named "symphonology" (after the Greek word *symphonia* meaning *agreement*), the theory holds that all interactions between the nurse and patient are ethically bound by agreements based on bioethical principles. Agreements are universal and exist between all rational beings.

In health care situations, there are agreements between patients and care providers, administrators, and employees, and health care institutions and the community, to not act opposed to each other. In each instance of agreement, the professional assumes the greater burden of the agreement. For example, the care provider agrees to do for the patient what the patient would do, if able. The patient agrees to be the patient, to fulfill his or her responsibilities in the treatment plan and not place any unreasonable demands on the health care professional. The administration agrees to treat employees fairly, and the employees agree to perform their specified functions in the organization. Agreements may not be made if we think the person with whom we are agreeing would not demonstrate fidelity or be faithful to the agreement. To enter into any agreement, each party must perceive some good will be achieved. Also, agreements require consent, which entails objectivity or truthful sharing of information. Self-assertiveness operates in the person's ability to control the time and effort needed to participate in the situation. Finally, agreements are valid when and if the parties have the freedom to choose and to make agreements that maintain their autonomy.

Using the Symphonological Bioethical Theory, knowledge about agreements is combined with an appreciation of the context of the situation and is used to guide ethical decision making. "In ethics everything is contextual, and the context of every action is unique and unduplicable with the result that even a small difference between two situations may yield a difference in our moral verdict" (Hospers, 1972, p. 63). The principles of autonomy, freedom, objectivity, self-assertion, beneficence, and fidelity are used to analyze and better understand ethical situations from the constituents' perspectives and resolve ethical dilemmas.

Nurses Ethical Reasoning Skills Model

The Nurses Ethical Reasoning Skills Model (NERS) was developed by Fairchild (2010) using three metacognitive processes: reflection, reasoning, and review. NERS uses these strategies, called *the 3Rs*, before engaging in ethical decision making.

Reflection refers to being self-aware of interactions with the environment. It involves self-monitoring, analyzing, and evaluating situations. The reflection process is foundational to nursing practice and allows the nurse to manage and reconcile ethical dilemmas. Reasoning involves a dialectical or backward and forward thinking process in which the thinker recognizes that concepts exist on a continuum, and as a continuum, these concepts reflect an interrelated whole. This reasoning process allows the nurse to see the big picture and analyze oppositional aspects. The reflection and reasoning process culminates in a review of competing values. Competing values are sources of moral and ethical conflict. For example, competing values may be seen in the concept of caring and technology, or when comparing the patient's wishes to the recommended treatment options. Negotiation and seeking a balance between competing demands reduce conflict or dissonance and facilitates ethical decision making.

As an experienced nurse working in the emergency department, Fairchild (2010) used intuition, reflection on ethics literature, and personal nursing experiences to develop the NERS model. The model acknowledges the complexity of the health care system and the need to maintain a caring focus in decision making. The processes of reflection, reasoning, and review of competing values combine to provide a synergistic framework for decision making in real time. The 3Rs can be used to support the maintenance of a caring, ethical stance while managing clinical practice within today's complex health care system.

According to Fairchild (2010), "being reflectively mindful of self, and of our individual or collective actions in the context of professional practice, is proposed to be the cornerstone skill for nurses engaged in caring, ethical practice" (p. 359). To facilitate understanding and application of the NERS model, Fairchild presents a case study of a pregnant teenager found unconscious in the emergency department (Box 8.2). Through a case study, NERS is applied to demonstrate the thinking and problem-solving processes used to resolve a complex ethical issue.

Crisham's MORAL Decision-Making Model

Crisham (1985) developed a decision-making model using the acronym MORAL to define the cognitive and action processes used in decision making. The first step is to "Massage" the ethical dilemma, which means to contemplate and reflect on the different sides of the issue. Next, look at the issue from multiple perspectives. Then "Outline the Options," "Review criteria and Resolve," "Affirm a position and Act," and finally, "Look back."

The model arose from the request of nurses who participated in a study on ethical decision making. They wanted a model that could be easily used in clinical practice to guide ethical decision making about nursing interventions. The first step, massaging the dilemma, involves creating an image of the ethical conflict, determining whose interests are involved, and defining the dilemma from the individual perspectives of those involved. Patient, staff, and family, as well as legal interests, are examined. Kurt Lewin's force field analysis technique is used to analyze the various factors that influence the nurse's choice of action. This process helps the nurse recognize the issues and conflicts inherent in the situation from a broad perspective and recognize the underlying goals of a situation.

BOX 8.2 Use of Nurse's Ethical Reasoning Skills Model in a Clinical Situation

Fairchild (2010) describes the application of the Nurse's Ethical Reasoning Skills Model using a scenario where an unconscious woman collapsed in the hall near the emergency department. The nurses begin providing aid, and in the process, the victim awakens and states she does not want to have this baby. She asks that her parents not be informed of her pregnancy. The complexities of care become known, and the nurse's internal dialogue involving reflection and reasoning is explored. As the story progresses, it becomes known that the victim is a minor who had accompanied her boyfriend who is a patient in the emergency department. She requests that he not be informed of the pregnancy. As the victim stabilizes, questions of the legality of continuing care without parental consent and the question of her status as either a minor or emancipated minor are explored. The internal dialog of the nurses as they engage in reflective reasoning, review competing values, and compare their perspective with those of the patient, hospital, boyfriend, and parents is explored.

The process of outlining the options is a natural result of massaging the dilemma. Using the factors identified in the force field analysis, the nurse brainstorms on strategies that strengthen the driving forces and weaken the restraining forces. Three questions are addressed for each factor identified: (a) What can be done to control the force? (b) What can be done to influence the force? and (c) What effect is the force anticipated to have on the dilemma? From these questions, strategies emerge that are then examined more closely in the following step.

The process of reviewing criteria and resolving the dilemma involves the nurse deciding on an approach that is in line with ethical principles. Two approaches can be used to identify moral criteria. In the first approach, the nurse identifies principles involved by looking at the options identified in the earlier step and answering the question, "Should I (or should I not) take this action because . . .?" The nurse then examines the answer from various theoretical or philosophical perspectives. The second approach is to adopt principles from specific ethical perspectives and use them to filter which actions to take. Based on the previous steps, a foundation is laid for decision making.

The subsequent step involves taking action. "The nurse has shifted from not knowing which alternative is best, to making a judgment about which alternative is best according to moral principles" (Crisham, 1985, p. 36). In this step of the process, a distinction is made between knowing what is best and making a commitment to take action. The nurse makes the transition from deciding that one position is best and choosing that position.

At the affirm and take an action step, several tools are used. One tool is a decision-making grid in which the ethical criteria and alternative actions are evaluated regarding moral and practical considerations. The results of the decision-making grid are then used to guide the nurse's decision. Therefore, the nurse affirms a specific position and the accompanying set of actions. To complete the process, the nurse shifts from affirming a position to choosing to take action congruent with that position. Crisham (1985) recommends using the acronym ACT to facilitate the action part of the process. 'A' stands for anticipating objections and obstacles to taking action. 'C' consists of clarifying the chosen position and clarifying a plan to address the objections and obstacles, and 'T' involves testing the choice by taking action.

The final step of the MORAL Model involves looking back or evaluating the 'MOR' steps of the process which preceded taking action. Looking back at the Massage process, the nurse can identify the types of ethical dilemmas that reoccur in clinical practice. By focusing on the "O" part of the model, the adequacy of options is explored, followed by reviewing the processes used to explore alternatives and arrive at a decision. Using the MORAL model facilitates ethical decision making by identifying moral principles and connecting the nurse's thinking with those ethical principles.

DECIDE Model

The DECIDE Model was developed by Guo (2008) to guide decision making for health care managers. The acronym DECIDE, describes six sequential steps: (a) define the problem, (b) establish the criteria, (c) consider alternatives, (d) identify the best alternative, (e) develop and implement a plan of action, and (f) evaluate and monitor the outcomes. The first step is to define the problem by answering the questions What is happening? and Why does anything need to be done differently? Defining the problem is essential for identifying barriers that must be addressed in the solution. The second step is to establish criteria concerning the desired outcomes. During this step, the absolute requirements are distinguished from nonessential or desirable ones. Common questions to ask include: What is desired regarding achievement? What aspects of the situation should be preserved? and What problems should be avoided? An important consideration is that the established criteria should be consistent with the values, mission, philosophy, and culture of the institution. In the third step, all alternatives are considered by engaging in brainstorming. The importance of congruence with organizational values is emphasized during this process. During the fourth step, the best alternative is identified. This involves maximizing or developing one best solution by ranking each alternative against the criteria identified earlier. Alternatively, when decisions must be made under extreme time pressure, a set of minimum criteria is developed. Any alternative that meets the minimum criteria is deemed acceptable. This simplified approach is referred to as "satisficing." The decision maker recognizes that there may be better solutions in the long run, but that because of the time urgency of the situation a solution that meets the minimum criteria is needed.

TABLE 8.2 Comparison of Ethical Frameworks

Framework	Key Concepts	Unique Attributes
ANA *Code of Ethics*	Describe the nurse's relationships, responsibilities, and obligations to self and others	Nine provisions with interpretive statements describe applications to practice
ICN *Code of Ethics*	Four elements describe the scope of practice and standards of conduct	Cross-cultural applications Values the nurse's social, cultural, and professional competence
Moral Exclusion Theory	Moral exclusion of individuals or groups requires conflict and a sense of disconnectedness	Categorizes exclusion behaviors as subtle-blatant and broad-narrow in scope
Kidder's Shared Values	Love, truthfulness, fairness, freedom, unity, tolerance, and responsibility	Identifies cross-cultural, universal values
Four Box Methods	Considers medical indications, patient preferences, quality of life, and context	Medical ethics decision-making tool
Symphonology	Values autonomy, freedom, objectivity, self-assertion, benevolence, and fidelity	Focuses on nurse-patient interactions
Nurses Ethical Reasoning Skills Model	Uses three metacognitive processes, reflection, reasoning, and review	Emphasizes metacognitive and dialectical reasoning processes
MORAL Model	Outlines a five-step decision-making process for staff nurses	M = massage dilemma; O = outline options; R = review criteria and resolve; A = affirm and act; and L = look back.
DECIDE Model	Uses a six-step acronym developed for nurse managers	D = define problem; E = establish criteria; C = consider alternatives; I = identify best alternative; D = develop and implement plan of action; E = evaluate and monitor

ANA, American Nurses Association; ICN, International Council of Nurses.

In the fifth step, a plan of action is developed and implemented. Two questions are addressed: How is the action plan going to be implemented? and What resources will be needed? During this step, the decision maker focuses on communication and coordination. Contextual factors such as stakeholders, urgency, and preferences are considered in developing goals and objectives and implementing the plan. Developing a detailed plan for implementation involves addressing what will be done and how it will be done. The final step, "evaluate and monitor," follows the actual implementation of the plan. Obtaining feedback is essential to determine how well the solution is working, and to monitor for potential problems. Feedback should be obtained from all constituents involved in the plan. Monitoring feedback is useful in troubleshooting problems and in anticipating potential problems.

The DECIDE Model identifies a systematic, step-by-step process to facilitate making quality decisions. The model recognizes that decision making is a skill that can be facilitated and learned by a structured process. Quality decisions need to reflect the values, mission, and culture of the institution and the individual stakeholders as decisions made ultimately impact the success of the health care organization.

◉ CONCLUSION

In today's complex health care environment, the need for ethical decision-making tools is pervasive regardless of work setting or nursing role. Nurse educators, clinicians, leaders, and researchers all use ethical knowledge and principles in their nursing practices. The ethical principles and frameworks described in this chapter can provide guidance in the decision-making process and facilitate understanding of diverse ethical perspectives. Table 8.2 provides a comparison of key concepts and unique attributes of these frameworks.

Ethics is a critical component of clinical judgment and reasoning that involves reflection and analysis from multiple perspectives. Steps common to the process of ethical decision making include identifying the dilemma, identifying alternative responses to the dilemma, and evaluating the potential outcomes for each response. Then, the nurse takes action, evaluates the effectiveness of the action, and determines whether the action was congruent with one's values. When choosing between alternative actions, recognition of the underlying values is an important determinant. Consideration of the values of the decision maker, patient, family, the profession, and the sociocultural values of the community at large is key.

◉ KEY POINTS

- Ethics deals with the principles that underlie moral behaviors. It is a branch of knowledge and philosophy that is concerned with establishing criteria for evaluating behavior.

- Morals are behaviors that express a person's ethics.

- Ethical principles include autonomy, beneficence, nonmaleficence, veracity, and justice.

- Autonomy underlies the person's right to make decisions and is required for informed consent.

- Beneficence and nonmaleficence are focused on doing good and avoiding harm. Beneficence has three components: (a) doing good, (b) preventing harm, and (c) removing harm.

- Veracity or truthfulness is required for obtaining informed consent.

- Duty-based ethics or deontology focuses on the rightness of an action versus the consequences of the action.

- Consequentialism is the opposite of duty-based ethics and is concerned with the goodness or rightness of the outcome achieved, regardless of the actions taken.

- Virtue ethics values the personality traits or intentions of the individual who takes action.

- Principlism considers aspects of duty-based ethics, consequentialist-based ethics, and virtue-based ethics.

- Proponents of care-based ethics emphasize the way morals are developed. Learning moral behaviors is not the result of applying principles but instead, focuses on meeting the needs of others.

- The ANA *Code of Ethics* emphasizes the nurse's responsibilities, relationships, and obligations to self and others.

- The ICN *Code of Ethics* emphasizes the nurse's social, cultural, and professional competence, individual actions, and the impact of those actions.

- Moral Exclusion Theory describes moral issues that range on a continuum of narrow to broad in scope and subtle to blatant in manifestation.

- Kidder's Shared Values Theory identifies values common across cultures that include love, truthfulness, fairness, freedom, unity, tolerance, and responsibility.

- Frameworks of moral decision making used in nursing include (a) the Four Box Method, (b) Symphonological Bioethical Theory, (c) Nurses Ethical Reasoning Skills Model, (d) the MORAL Decision-Making Model, and (e) the DECIDE Model.

- Ethics is a component of clinical judgment and reasoning. Moral actions can be guided by analysis of the issue from multiple perspectives and the use of decision-making frameworks.

REFERENCES

American Nurses Association. (2015). *Code of ethics for nurses with interpretive statements*. Silver Spring, MD: Nursesbooks.org.

Andorno, R. (2012). Do our moral judgments need to be guided by principles? *Cambridge Quarterly of Healthcare Ethics, 21*(4), 457–465.

Brinson, A. (2011). Using moral exclusion as a framework for redefining of racism in counselor education. *The Journal of Theory Construction and Testing, 15*(1), 4–9.

Chowning, J. T., & Fraser, P. (2007). *An ethics primer*. Seattle, WA: Northwest Association of Biomedical Research.

Curtain, L. (2000). The first ten principles for the ethical administration of nursing services. *Nursing Administration Quarterly, 25*(1), 7–13.

Crisham, P. (1985). Resolving ethical and moral dilemmas. In M. Snyder (Ed.), *Independent nursing interventions* (pp. 25–43). New York, NY: Wiley.

Fairchild, R. (2010). Practical and ethical theory for nurses responding to complexity in care. *Nursing Ethics, 7*(3), 353–362.

Gibson, C. H. (1993). Underpinnings of ethical reasoning in nursing. *Journal of Advanced Nursing, 18*(12), 2003–2007. doi:10.1046/j.1365-2648.1993.18122003.x

Gilligan, C. (1982). *In a different voice: Psychological theory and women's development*. Cambridge, MA: Harvard University Press.

Guo, K. L. (2008). DECIDE: A decision-making model for more effective decision-making by health care managers. *The Health Care Manager, 27*(2), 118–127.

Hospers, J. (1972). *Human conduct: Problems of ethics*. New York, NY: Harcourt Brace Jovanich.

Husted, G., & Husted, J. (2008). *Ethical decision making in nursing and healthcare: The symphonological approach*. New York, NY: Springer Publishing.

Institute for Global Ethics. (2016). Why ethics matters. Retrieved from https://www.globalethics.org

International Council of Nurses. (2012). ICN code of ethics for nurses. Retrieved from http://www .icn.ch/images/stories/documents/about/icncode_english.pdf.

Jonsen, A. R., Siegler, M., & Winslade, W. (2010). *Clinical ethics*. New York, NY: McGraw-Hill.

Kidder, R. (1994). *Shared values for a troubled world: Conversations with men and women of conscience*. San Francisco, CA: Jossey-Bass.

Kidder, R. (1995). *How good people make tough choices*. New York, NY: W. Morrow.

Leets, L. (2001). Interrupting the cycle of normal exclusion: A communication contribution to social justice research. *Journal of Applied Social Psychology, 31*(9), 1859–1891.

National Commission for the Protection of Human Subjects of Biomedical and Behavioral Research. (1979). *The Belmont report: Ethical principles and guidelines for the protection of human subjects of research*. Retrieved from http://www.hhs.gov/ohrp/regulations-and-policy/belmont-report/#xbasic

Opotow, S., Gerson, J., & Woodside, S. (2005). From moral exclusion to moral inclusion: Theory for teaching peace. *Theory Into Practice, 44*(4), 303–318. doi:10.1207/s15430421tip4404_4

Robb, J. W. (1989). A medical ethics primer. *Institute for Laboratory Animal Research News, 31*(4), 21–29.

Toronto, J. C. (1993). *Moral boundaries: A political argument for an ethic of care*. New York, NY: Routledge.

Toronto, J. C. (2005). An ethic of care. In A. E. Cudd & R. O. Andreasen (Eds.), *Feminist theory: A philosophical anthology* (pp. 251–263), Malden, MA: Blackwell.

Health and Illness Frameworks

Lucretia Smith

A wise man ought to realize that health is his most valuable possession.
—Hippocrates

⬤ KEY TERMS

cognator
energy fields
focal stimulus
King's Conceptual
  Framework
King's Theory of Goal
  Attainment
Levine's Conservation
  Model
Levine's conservation
  of energy
Levine's conservation of
  personal integrity
Levine's conservation of
  social integrity
Levine's conservation of
  structural integrity

Life Perspective
  Rhythm Model
Neuman's Systems Model
Newman's Theory of
  Health as Expanding
  Consciousness
openness
pandimensionality
Parse's concept of meaning
Parse's concept of
  rhythmicity
Parse's concept of
  transcendence
Parse's Humanbecoming
  School of Thought
pattern
person–environment
  interaction

regulator
residual stimuli
Rogers's Accelerating
  Change Theory
Rogers's Emergence
  of Paranormal
  Phenomena Theory
Rogers's Manifestations of
  Field Patterning Theory
Rogers's Science of Unitary
  Human Beings
Roy's Adaptation Model
Roy's interdependence mode
Roy's physiologic mode
Roy's role function mode
Roy's self-concept mode

⬤ LEARNING OBJECTIVES

1. Identify the origins, perspectives, and major concepts used in frameworks relevant to health and illness.
2. Describe the application health and illness frameworks in nursing education, clinical practice, and nursing research.
3. Compare and contrast the origin and focus of health and illness frameworks.

It has been noted in nearly every walk of life, that people are motivated to change by forces unseen by the casual observer. The health behaviors of people are no exception. Much theorizing and research have identified and clarified barriers to health as well as factors that motivate, influence, and support health. This chapter focuses on frameworks useful for understanding an individual's health status and appreciating a wide range of factors that contribute to health and illness.

HEALTH AND ILLNESS PERSPECTIVES

Nursing is one of the many professions that conduct research, theorize, and use concepts related to health and illness. The frameworks presented here, although frequently used by nurses, have been influenced by fields of study as diverse as physics, humanistic psychology, and physiology. In theory development, the integration of knowledge from diverse fields is important for capturing the complex aspects of health and illness. In research and clinical practice, the nurse needs to consider the individual's environment and the barriers and facilitators to achieve health and take healthy actions. The frameworks in this chapter provide an understanding of the concepts of health and illness and provide guidance and structure needed for engaging in healthy actions and interventions.

King's Conceptual Framework

In 1968, King introduced a conceptual framework for nursing that was grounded in General Systems Theory (see Chapter 17). She then identified the major concepts important to nursing as social systems, health, interpersonal relationships, and perceptions. Further refinement of the framework included the addition of the concepts of environment, illness, adaptation, and man (Evans, 1991). Later, the concept of adaptation was changed to adjustment, and the concept of man was changed to human being or individual (Evans, 1991). At the core of King's framework is the idea that human beings are open systems constantly interacting with the environment (King, 1997). According to her framework, health is viewed as the goal of nursing and illness as an imbalance in the dynamic state of the person.

King's conceptual framework incorporates three systems, the personal, interpersonal, and social systems. The concept of the personal system is concerned with the individual who is in continual interaction with other individuals (i.e., personal systems) and the environment. The personal system is characterized by the concepts of perception, self, growth and development, body image, time, personal space, and learning. The interpersonal system is formed by the interaction of two or more personal systems, with a focus on interpersonal relationships. The concepts of communication, interaction, roles, stress, coping, and transaction characterize the interpersonal system. The nurse and patient form an interpersonal system that engages in interactions and transactions to achieve the patient's health-related goals. Personal and interpersonal systems interact with and in social systems, which King defined as a structured "system of social roles, behaviors, and practices" (King, 1981, p. 115).

These personal and interpersonal system concepts form the basis for several propositions. These are: (a) congruent nurse and client perceptions and expectations result in transactions, (b) stress in nurse–client interaction occurs when role conflict is experienced, and (c) communication of appropriate information and mutual goal setting facilitates goal attainment. When multiple interpersonal systems interact, social systems are formed that reflect the needs of individuals and smaller groups. Social systems emphasize the concepts of authority, decision making, organization, power, and status.

King's Theory of Goal Attainment

The Theory of Goal Attainment draws directly on King's conceptual framework described earlier. In the Theory of Goal Attainment, King identifies the goal of nursing "is to help individuals maintain or regain health" (King, Sieloff, Killeen, & Frey, 2010, p. 150). Thus, goal attainment is focused on achieving health-related goals with the assistance of interactions and transactions between the nurse and client (Evans, 1991; King, 1997).

The process of goal attainment focuses on assumptions related to King's key concepts and propositions. She describes the individual and the individual's transactions from a holistic perspective. The main concepts are communication, growth and development, interaction, perception, role, space, stress, time, and transaction (King, 1997). Eight propositions about the way individuals, including nurses, interact with their environment, given their rights and responsibilities are identified. The propositions outlined in Box 9.1 reflect a synthesis of the main concepts of her theory.

Both King's Conceptual System and the Theory of Goal Attainment can be applied to the practice roles of nurse educators, clinicians, leaders, and researchers. As these nursing roles involve interaction and goal setting of some kind, King's concepts can provide a solid framework in which to practice, analyze, and transform nursing. This review of her conceptual framework and Theory of Goal Attainment has highlighted the emphasis on health and illness. For a review of her work with an emphasis on interpersonal relationships, see Chapter 10.

Levine's Conservation Model

Myra Levine created the Conservation Model to organize nursing knowledge in a way that nursing students could understand (Levine, 1969). She also sought to change the focus of nursing students' education from a procedural emphasis to a problem-solving approach (George, 2002). Levine's text, *An Introduction to Clinical Nursing*, traces the history of the theory as the editions progressed from 1969 to 1973. The central idea of the theory is that when a person is in a state of conservation, he or she adapts with the least effort while maintaining optimal function and identity. Adaptation is successful when adaptive pathways and behaviors needed for human function have been activated.

BOX 9.1 Propositions of King's Theory of Goal Attainment

Propositions

1. When the nurse and client's role expectations and role performance expectations are congruent, transaction occurs.

2. When there is perceptual accuracy, transaction occurs.

3. When expectations are congruent, transaction occurs.

4. Conflict produces stress that interferes with transactions.

5. Transactions are necessary for goal attainment.

6. Mutual goal setting and goal attainment occur when the nurse communicates appropriate information to the client.

7. Goal attainment results in satisfaction of the nurse and the patient.

8. Growth and development are enhanced when goals are achieved.

Source: Adapted from Alligood and Tomey (2002). Retrieved from http://imogenekingtheory .blogspot.com/p/propositions.html

According to Levine (1973), nursing is concerned with four areas of conservation. The first is the *conservation of energy*, which is the principle of attaining personal energy balance and avoiding fatigue. Conservation of energy includes health behaviors such as rest, exercise, and nutrition. Second is the *conservation of structural integrity*, which involves maintaining and restoring the physical structure of the patient. Third is *conservation of personal integrity*, which is essentially respect and recognition, on the part of the nurse, of the selfhood of others. The fourth principle is the *conservation of social integrity*. This principle recognizes the patient as a part of progressively larger systems of family, community, and eventually global citizenship.

According to Levine, the goal of nursing is to promote adaptation and wholeness by attending to the patient's structural, personal, and social integrity needs (Levine, 1969, 1973). Health is defined as more than the healing of an affected part of a person; it is the holistic, successful adaptation and the ability to pursue interests (Meleis, 1997). Therefore, the nurse's goal is to support wholeness by promoting personalized activities for the patient. Nursing care incorporates qualities of perception, compassion, commitment, devotion to humanity, and self-respect of the patient; while providing patient advocacy and support for the patient's needs.

Five concepts define the relationships among Levine's principles. First, the patient is described as constantly striving for holistic integrity. Second is the idea that the environment of a person completes the person and exists both internally and externally. A third concept is that health and disease are both patterns of adaptive change. Fourth, the nurse is part of a partnership that, consciously or unconsciously, remains part of the patient forever. Finally, the environment becomes congruent with, or part of, a person over time.

The Conservation Model was first proposed and used as a guide to nursing education and continues to be useful when teaching students about health and illness. Researchers have used this model as a framework for studying wound management (Leach, 2006), fatigue (Mock et al., 2001; Schaefer & Potylycki, 1993; St. Ours, Bositis, Hall, & Mock, 2005), as well as staffing patterns (Mefford & Alligood, 2011). Specific practice models continue to use Levine's work as a basis for both evidence and construction (Fawcett, 2014).

The Neuman's Systems Model

Betty Neuman's theoretical ideas began to take shape in the late 1960s with her work in community mental health nursing. By 1970, her work had led to the development of the original Neuman's Systems Model (Neuman & Young, 1972), which was intended to guide nursing education and practice. The model was refined in 1974 and again in 1982. The current model focuses on the response of the client system to actual or potential stressors and the use of three types of prevention (primary, secondary, and tertiary) by the nurse (Neuman, 1996). The goal in Neuman's model is optimal wellness of the client system by attaining and maintaining health. Neuman considers her model to be a metaparadigm of wellness and views wellness as a concept that is defined and negotiated between the client and the nurse. Wellness is a concept that belongs to neither the client nor the nurse. Instead, it is based on the interrelationships between the client and environmental systems and the nurses' perceptions of client system wellness (Neuman, 1995).

The four overarching concepts of the Neuman Systems Model are human beings, environment, health, and nursing. The processes in the model are stress and system feedback. According to Neuman, knowing something about one part of a system clarifies something about another part. As systems become more complex, the internal regulation, and therefore the responses to stress, become more complex. The nurse assists the client to stabilize the system or the system's response to stressors. This stabilization process is based on understanding the positive and negative reciprocal relationships between the client and the environmental systems (Neuman 2002).

The client is an open system, consisting of the usual system components (input, processing, output, and feedback). The characteristics of the client system are physiological, psychological, sociocultural, developmental, and spiritual aspects. The client's interaction with the environment affects the person's well-being and likewise, the individual influences the environment. In addition to the physical and external environment, there is an unconscious and symbolic environment created and progressively developed by the person. This internal symbolic environment is also influential to the person's state of wellness and wholeness. The concept of health, or wellness, is mutually defined by the patient and the nurse and involves assisting the client to stabilize physiological, psychological, sociocultural, developmental, and spiritual aspects to achieve health and wellness.

The combination of all characteristics of the client system interacts with both internal and external environments. This interaction is in the form of matter, energy, and information. Neuman's model depicts lines of defense that are used to maintain homeostasis or decrease energy demands when the internal and external environment stresses the system. The first line of defense is the "flexible line of defense," which can be quickly altered for short periods. The "normal line of defense" is activated when the flexible line fails. It is a protective buffer for maintaining the homeostasis of the system. The normal line of defense is dynamic, rather than static, and is usually the baseline from which deviation from a healthy state is measured. When both lines of defense have failed, and the system is using more energy than available, the lines of defense are activated in an attempt to return the system to homeostasis.

Nursing interventions in Neuman's model are focused on prevention. In primary preventive care, the nurse begins the relationship with the client before the reaction to stress occurs and takes action to increase the available energy to reduce real and potential stresses. Secondary prevention includes actions that enhance the baseline defenses and possibly strengthen the lines of resistance. Tertiary prevention includes actions that rebuild the lines of resistance and enhance the homeostasis at whatever line of functioning the nurse and client have determined are optimal (Neuman, 1995).

Using this model in nursing practice involves creating an environment where nurses view patients as whole systems and work collaboratively with those systems. According to Neuman (2002), the purpose of the model in research is to focus on optimal client stability and the outcomes of specific preventative interventions on client systems and client health.

Roy's Adaptation Model

Sr. Callista Roy began her theoretical work on the Roy Adaptation Model (RAM) while pursuing her master's degree in pediatric and maternity nursing. She developed a systems model of adaptation that views the person as a bio-psycho-social being in continual interaction with the environment (Roy, 1970, 2009). The model was influenced by Bertalanffy's General Systems Theory, Helson's Adaptation Theory, Selye's General Adaptation Syndrome, and Maslow's Humanism and Hierarchy of Human Needs Theory.

The model views that the person is an adaptive system that responds to environmental change using four modes of adaptation: the physiologic, self-concept, role function, and interdependence. Each mode is associated with a need that drives adaptive behaviors. The *physiologic mode* is concerned with the need for wholeness or integrity and consists of physical needs (i.e., oxygen, food, elimination, activity, rest, and protection) that are similar to Maslow's deficit needs. The remaining modes are psychosocial in nature. The *self-concept mode* is the sum of the person's feelings and beliefs about the self, and this mode is concerned with the need for integrity of one's self-concept. *Role function mode* is concerned with the need for social integrity. The need for social integrity is met when the person knows who he or she is in relation to others and can take needed actions to function in specific roles. The need to feel secure in relationships characterizes the *interdependence mode*. Health reflects positive adaptive responses and the integration of these four adaptive modes to achieve wholeness.

In addition to the four adaptive modes, the RAM incorporates concepts relevant to the types of stimuli, coping mechanisms, and adaptation level (Roy 1970, 2009). Types of stimuli include focal, contextual, and residual, which originate from either internal or external environmental sources. A *focal stimulus* is the major concern, event, or situation that confronts the person. *Contextual stimuli* are the contextual factors that surround the event and contribute to the focal stimuli's effect. The *residual stimuli* are nonspecific factors that may have an uncertain influence on the person. Two types of coping mechanisms, the cognator and regulator, characterize the person's response to stimuli. The *cognator* uses mental or cognitive processes to adapt to psychosocial stimuli whereas the *regulator* uses physiological mechanisms to adapt to internal and external stimuli. Drawing on Helson's Adaptation Theory, Roy defined *adaptation level* as a dynamic point that reflects the person's ability to cope. The person's adaptation level along with the types of stimuli provide input into the system. The person adapts to stimuli using coping mechanisms and produces behaviors or responses in one or more of the adaptive modes. The output is either adaptation or an ineffective response that completes the system's feedback loop by providing input into the adaptive system.

Roy's model also incorporates nursing activities that help the person achieve the goal of adaptation and ultimately health. Nursing actions include a six-step nursing process that begins with an assessment of the person's behavior relative to each adaptive mode and assessment of the focal, contextual, and residual stimuli. Then a nursing diagnosis is determined by combining the behavior or response with the focal stimuli (e.g., pain [behavioral response] from surgical procedure [focal stimuli]). The subsequent step in the process is mutual goal setting, with the goal to achieve the desired patient outcome. Nursing interventions are directed to changing the focal, contextual, and residual stimuli that affect adaptation, and by enhancing the patient's coping mechanisms. Evaluation determines if the goals or outcomes have been achieved. The use of a nursing process based on the major concepts of the model makes RAM useful in clinical practice for all phases of care from initial assessment to evaluation of outcomes.

Rogers's Science of Unitary Human Beings

Martha Rogers is known for her futuristic view of nursing and the conceptualization of the person and environment as interacting energy fields. In 1970, she published the first version of her theory titled an *Introduction to the Theoretical Basis for Nursing*. Then in 1994, the final version of the theory was published (Rogers, 1994a, 1994b). Currently, Rogers's theory reflects the belief in a single, infinite, energy field that is the foundation of all life. The flow of energy is unbroken, yet the waves of the energy field are expressed in patterns that are unique to the individual and the environment. These patterns of person–environment interaction are manifestations of health.

Although the concept of health is not given explicit emphasis in the Science of Unitary Human Beings (SUHB), Rogers noted that "health and sickness, however defined, are expressions of the process of life" (1970, p. 85). The life process of the person is depicted in the *person–environment interaction*, which is characterized by openness, energy fields, pattern, and pandimensionality. *Openness* refers to the nature of the environment and person energy fields that freely exchange energy. Conceptualizing the person and environment as open *energy fields* retains the wholeness of each field. *Pattern* is a characteristic or manifestation of an energy field interaction. *Pandimensionality* refers to the idea of a reality outside the usual norm of space and time. In this reality, the boundaries perceived are not the same as the tangible boundaries. Pandimensionality is "a non-linear domain without spacial or temporal attributes" (Rogers, 1992, p. 29). The SUHB perspective sees the person's health as a manifestation of the patterns of person–environment energy field interactions, which are expressions of the process of life.

The SUHB is based on several postulates that incorporate Rogers's main concepts. First, the universe consists of open fields of energy that are distinct, but not separate. These are the person and the environment energy fields. Second, all energy fields, including humans and their environment, are irreducible and pandimensional (i.e., extend across dimensions).

Third, energy fields are continually interacting with each other producing change that is simultaneous in all fields. Fourth, the interaction between energy fields results in energy that flows in an unbroken wave that is characterized by patterning. Finally, the pattern of person–environment interaction, which Rogers defined as health, is observable through rhythms, diversity, and visual awareness.

Rogers further defined the patterns of energy field interaction as exhibiting resonance, which describes the way change occurs, and helicy, which describes the nature of the change (ongoing, creative, and diverse). She described the basis of nursing research and practice as concerned with the continuously fluctuating and unpredictable patterning of person–environment interaction (i.e., health).

Based on these concepts and postulates, Rogers articulated several practice level theories including the Accelerating Change Theory, Emergence of Paranormal Phenomena Theory, and Manifestations of Field Patterning Theory. The *Accelerating Change Theory* views human and environmental field rhythms as speeding up. Aging, when combined with the principle of helicy, is viewed as a creative process that manifests in increased diversity. Therefore, aging is not a process of decline or "running down" but the manifestation of increasing diversity in patterning (Whitbourne, & Whitbourne 2010).

The *Emergence of Paranormal Phenomena Theory* explains that experiences commonly labeled "paranormal" are manifestations of the changing and innovative patterning of the interaction between human and environmental energy fields (Rogers, 1986). These experiences include pandimensional forms of awareness, such as transcendence, visionary insight, and tactic knowing. The effects of distance healing therapies, energy therapies such as therapeutic touch, prayer, and meditation are some of the nursing interventions explained by the Emergence of Paranormal Phenomena Theory.

Originally called the Rhythmical Correlates of Change Theory, the *Manifestations of Field Patterning Theory* is concerned with changes in pattern manifestation. The theory suggests that phenomena of interest to understand the evolutionary changes include the rhythms of motion, time experience, and sleeping-waking cycles. Leddy (1995) described the manifestation of field patterning as "the experience of expansiveness and ease of continuous human-environment mutual process" (p. 21). She developed the Person–Environment Participation Scale to measure the manifestations of field patterning (Leddy, 1995) and has articulated a practice theory that classifies healing interventions into six categories that facilitate energy exchange and patterning (Leddy, 2003).

Although research that explicitly uses Rogers's theories is limited, her conceptual framework and the concepts in the framework have provided a foundation for the development of many other health-related frameworks. Her ideas have been integrated into the works of Parse (Theory of Humanbecoming), Fitzpatrick (Life Perspective Rhythm Model), and Newman (Health as Expanding Consciousness Theory), which are all discussed in this chapter. Additionally, several theorists have used Rogers's concepts to develop frameworks in the area of caring in nursing including Watson's Science of Caring and 10 Carative Factors, and Andersen's LIGHT Model (see Chapter 5).

According to Rogers, the SUHB illuminates the unique position of nursing and the importance of autonomous nursing actions, which fulfills nursing's social contract. Nursing's social contract necessitates the use of all available science to better human life. The person's self-direction, and the use of nursing skills and interventions such as touch, massage, and community-based health resources are valued.

Newman's Theory of Health as Expanding Consciousness

Newman believed that theory was not used by the nurse to practice. Instead, the theory is a way of being with a patient. The development of the Theory of Health as Expanding Consciousness (THEC) grew from her experiences of caring for her terminally ill mother, diagnosed with amyotrophic lateral sclerosis. Her perspective was also influenced by nurse theorist Martha Rogers, chemist Ilya Prigogine, and scientist Itzhak Bentov (Newman, 1994). In regard to Rogers's influence, Newman shared the view of health and illness as a unified process. She viewed the concepts of person–environment energy field interaction and pattern manifestation as unique to the individual. Prigogine's Theory of Dissipative Structures was used to describe the dynamic, random fluctuations in a system as it experiences turbulence that propels the system toward change. Newman saw the experience of disruption as crucial for experiencing expanded consciousness. She also shared Bentov's view of the process of life as concerned with expanding the informational capacity or consciousness of the individual. From the synthesis of these perspectives and her personal caregiving experiences, she came to view time, space, and movement as interrelated phenomena that influence expanding consciousness or health. The nurse's role is to assist the individual to acknowledge and use power to move to higher or more inclusive levels of consciousness (i.e., health). Therefore, health is not the absence of disease; health is experienced even in the presence of a debilitating illness.

Newman's work suggests a new paradigm for nursing in which health is an evolving unitary pattern. Pattern identifies that the meaning of human–environment interaction and consciousness is the informational capacity of the individual (Newman, 2008). According to the THEC, health includes disease along with conditions that are not a disease. What is seen as a disease is merely the manifestation of the person's pattern, and that pattern is present before the disease manifests. Curing the disease does not change the underlying pattern. Health results from the person–environment interaction that leads to the expansion of consciousness. In this context, each client demonstrates unique patterns and relationships that evolve with all life processes moving toward expanded consciousness. Newman characterizes the THEC as in the unitary–transformative paradigm, which sees the whole of the client's context and views change as unpredictable and potentially transformative.

The THEC can be used to inform and guide clinical practice, health care administration, and nursing education. Newman's THEC has been used in multiple nursing roles, diverse cultures, and practice settings, from Japan to the United States and from birthing centers to health policy (Pharris, 2010). Clinically, pattern recognition has been explored in patients with mobility impairments and women with cancer (Endo, 1998). Moreover, the nature of nurse–family patterning has been explored by Litchfield (1993, 1999, 2005) and Tommet (2003).

Parse's Humanbecoming Paradigm

Rosemarie Rizzo Parse introduced her theory, then known as Man-Living-Health, in 1981. The original theory and its ensuing versions used several of Rogers's ideas and some from existential phenomenology. Health is viewed as the process of becoming, which is experienced via multiple dimensions, not just physical. Over time the theory evolved, and changes occurred, including the name change to *human becoming*, which later merged into *humanbecoming*. Another significant change was shifting from describing humanbecoming as a theory to describing it as a school of thought, or paradigm, for viewing health in general and nursing in particular. The current paradigm includes the assumption that personal meanings are chosen freely and placed in the person's values and priorities, and patterns of relationships are cocreated with the universe "co-transcending multidimensionally with emerging possibilities" (Parse, 1998, p. 29).

Parse's assumptions are based on the concepts of meaning, rhythmicity, and transcendence. Each concept is associated with a principle, and each principle has a practice dimension and a process. *Meaning* is concerned with the "what and how" the individual imagines, values, and communicates. The related principle explains that meaning is cocreated by languaging (or the way words are used), valuing, and imaging. *Rhythmicity* relates to processes and experiences characterized as dichotomies of revealing–concealing, enabling–limiting, and connecting–separating. *Transcendence* relates to the processes of powering, originating, and transforming. Powering refers to the person's ability to overcome difficulties. Originating involves the use of creative thinking to adapt to the world, and transforming occurs when the individual changes and creates a new path. The related principle states that patterns of rhythm are cocreated in patterns of revealing/concealing and enabling/limiting, which result in connecting/separating. Cotranscending involves new ways to begin the transformation process. These concepts of transcendence are synthesized to form the third principle described as "Cotranscending with the possibles is powering unique ways of originating in the process of transforming" (Fawcett, 2001, p. 126).

Humanbecoming is a frequent focus of nursing research, especially studies using qualitative methods. In both research and nursing practice, Parse suggests guidelines that include: eliciting and cocreating the client's perspectives; intent and priorities in becoming; and description of the experiences in the nurse/client relationships (Parse, 2010). Nursing services have been created using the guidelines and the principles of the Humanbecoming school of thought (Box 9.2).

Life Perspective Rhythm Model

In 1983, Joyce Fitzpatrick proposed the Life Perspective Rhythm Model based on Rogers's Science of Unitary Human Beings. The basic premise of the model is that meaningfulness is essential to health. Although this premise has remained unchanged, clarifications of the theory were published in 1989 and 2008 by Fitzpatrick and her graduate students.

Fitzpatrick proposes four indices of holistic human functioning: temporal, motion, consciousness, and perceptual patterns. Each of these is related to health patterns across the life span. According to this theory, health is basic to humans and is in a constant state of development. Therefore, health is a dynamic state or manifestation of person–environment interaction, identified by meaningfulness that is characterized by congruence, consistency, and integrity. Health is dependent on the meaningfulness of one's experiences as the person moves through life crises. Nursing in this context is focused on the person and the relationship with the meaning of health crisis experiences. As meaningfulness is a present-oriented concept, nursing interventions focused on present life experiences can be effective in facilitating optimal health (Pressler & Montgomery, 2012).

The model has been used extensively in research studies spanning the developmental spectrum, but with an emphasis in the geriatric population. Research using phenomenological or other qualitative methods are most suited to the theory. Little research has been conducted regarding direct educational or clinical care uses. However, the theory could be

---

BOX 9.2 Use of the Humanbecoming Theory in Research

Steven Bauman used the Humanbecoming Theory in an exploratory, descriptive study on the fathers of children with cleft lip and palate using three sets of questions: What does it mean to be a father? What are the relationship changes? And how has the view of the future changed? He then repeated the study with siblings. In both studies, Parse's Humanbecoming Theory was used to produce questions regarding the structuring of meaning, shifting patterns, and unfolding possibilities (Baumann & Braddick, 2016). The findings related to meaning included a need for information and facing limits and feelings. Shifting patterns included discomfort in being with some "others" and an increasing comfort with others. The unfolding possibilities reflected a mix of joy and sorrow.

used in settings where patterns of health could be observed over time or in creating systems or interventions where pattern support or change would enhance health and well-being.

 ## CONCLUSION

Although nurses have the skills to lead people to health, it is ultimately up to the individual to choose healthy behaviors and to engage with nurses and others who can assist them. In this chapter, frameworks that describe the process of attaining health and the nurse's role in those processes were explored. Nurse theorists have emphasized the concepts of adaptation, conservation of energy, goal setting, and person–environment interaction as essential to health. Although the decision to engage in behaviors and interactions that support health is ultimately the choice of the individual, the nurse plays a role in supporting, clarifying, and guiding the patient toward health. These frameworks can provide perspective and guidance as the nurse interacts with clients to achieve and maintain health. See Table 9.1 for a comparison of major health and illness frameworks.

TABLE 9.1 Comparison of Health and Illness Frameworks

Theory Name	Origin /Influences	Focus
King's Conceptual Frame of Reference	General Systems Theory	Interaction between personal, interpersonal, and social systems
King's Theory of Goal Attainment	King's Conceptual Framework	Transactions with professionals for goal attainment
Levine's Conservation Model	Problem-solving approach to nursing education	Four types of conservation: energy, structural integrity, personal integrity, and social integrity; choosing conservation enhances health
Neuman's Systems Model	Systems, Community Health	Interaction between systems with lines of defense maintaining homeostasis
Roy's Adaptation Model	Maslow's Human Needs, Humanism, Hans Selye, Helson's Adaptation level	Adaptation occurs via four modes: physiologic, self-concept, role function, and interdependence
Rogers's Science of Unitary Human Beings (SUHB)	Inseparability of people from their environment	Person–environment interaction and characteristics of interaction
Parse's Humanbecoming	SUHB Phenomenology	Cocreation of meaning resulting in health
Life Perspective Rhythm Model	SUHB	Health is a constant state of development identified by meaningfulness
Newman's Health as Expanding Consciousness	SUHB, Bentov, Prigogine	Person–environment interaction, pattern, expanding consciousness

◉ KEY POINTS

- King's Conceptual Framework is based on the concept of open, interacting personal, interpersonal, and social systems. Illness is an imbalance in/or between these systems.

- King's Theory of Goal Attainment is a middle range theory based on her conceptual framework. The main concepts are communication, growth and development, interaction, perception, role, space, stress, time, and transaction. A central assumption is that nurse-client transactions result in goal attainment.

- Levine's Conservation Model describes four areas of conservation (conservation of energy, structural integrity, personal integrity, and social integrity). Health is related to adaptation and conservation in all four areas.

- The Neuman Systems Model stems from her work in community mental health. The overarching concepts are human beings, environment, health, and nursing. The processes emphasized are stress and feedback. Lines of resistance are tools that the human system uses to manage stress and feedback.

- Roy's Adaption Model views health as an adaptation to the internal and external environment that is expressed through four modes: physiologic, self-concept, role function, and interdependence.

- Rogers's Science of Unitary Human Beings is based on the interaction between the person–environment energy fields. Energy fields, openness, pandimensionality, and patterning are the main postulates.

- Parse's Humanbecoming Paradigm is grounded in Rogers's Science of Unitary Human Beings and on the principles of patterns of rhythm, creating meaning, and cotranscending to begin the transformation.

- Newman's Theory of Health as Expanded Consciousness relies on Rogers's concepts of person–environment energy fields. The interaction between the person and environment energy fields manifests as pattern. Health is not the absence of disease, but a pattern of person–environment interaction that can be present even with the illness.

- Fitzpatrick's Life Perspective Rhythm Model is founded on four indices of holistic functioning that are temporal, motion, consciousness, and perceptual patterns.

REFERENCES

Alligood, M. R., & Tomey, A. M. (2002). *Nursing theory utilization and application* (2nd ed.). Philadelphia, PA: Mosby.

Baumann, S. L., & Braddick, M. (2016). On being a father or sibling in light of the human becoming family model. *Nursing Science Quarterly, 29*(1), 47–53. doi:10.1177/0894318415614902

Endo, E. (1998). Pattern recognition as a nursing intervention with Japanese women with ovarian cancer. *Advances in Nursing Science, 20*(4), 49–61.

Evans, C. L. S. (1991). *Imogene King: A conceptual framework for nursing.* Newbury Park, CA: Sage.

Fawcett, J. (2001). The nurse theorists: 21st-century updates: Rosemarie Rizzo Parse. *Nursing Science Quarterly, 14*(2), 126–131.

Fawcett, J. (2014). Thoughts about conceptual models, theories, and quality improvement projects. *Nursing Science Quarterly, 27*(4), 336–339.

George, J. B. (2002). *Nursing theories: The base for professional nursing practice.* Upper Saddle River, NJ: Prentice Hall.

King, I. M. (1981). *A theory for nursing: Systems, concepts, process.* Albany, NY: Delmar.

King, I. M. (1997). The King conceptual system and theory of goal attainment. *Nursing Science Quarterly, 10*, 180–185.

King, I. M., Sieloff, C., Killeen, M., & Frey, M. (2010). Imogene King's theory of goal attainment. In M. E. Parker & M. C. Smith (Eds.), *Nursing theories and nursing practice* (3rd ed., pp. 146–166). Philadelphia, PA: F. A. Davis.

Leach, M. J. (2006). Wound management: Using Levine's conservation model to guide practice. *Ostomy Wound Management, 52*(8), 74–80.

Leddy, S. K. (1995). Measuring mutual process: Development and psychometric testing of the person-environment participation scale. *Visions: The Journal of Rogerian Nursing Science, 3*, 20–31.

Leddy, S. K. (2003). A unitary energy-based nursing practice theory: Theory and application. *Visions: The Journal of Rogerian Nursing Science, 11*(1). Retrieved from http://www.biomedsearch.com/article/unitary-energy-based-nursing-practice/161397655.html

Levine, M. E. (1969). *Introduction to clinical nursing.* Philadelphia, PA: F. A. Davis.

Levine, M. E. (1973). *Introduction to clinical nursing* (2nd ed.). Philadelphia, PA: F. A. Davis.

Litchfield, M. C. (1993). *The process of health patterning in families with young children who have been repeatedly hospitalized.* Unpublished Master's Thesis, University of Minnesota, Minneapolis.

Litchfield, M. C. (1999). Practice wisdom. *Advances in Nursing Science, 22*(2), 62–73.

Litchfield, M. C. (2005). The nursing praxis of family health. In P. Picard & D. Jones (Eds.), *Giving voice to what we know: Margaret Newman's health as expanding consciousness in research, theory, and practice* (pp. 73–83). Boston, MA: Jones & Bartlett.

Mefford, L., & Alligood, M. (2011). Evaluating nurse staffing patterns and neonatal intensive care unit outcomes using Levine's conservation model of nursing. *Nursing Management, 19*(8), 998–1011. doi:10.1111/j.1365-2834.2011.01319.x

Meleis, A. I. (1997). *Theoretical nursing: Development and progress.* Philadelphia, PA: Lippincott.

Mock, V., Pickett, M., Ropka, M., Muscari, L., Stewart, K., Rhodes, V., … McCorkle, R. (2001). Fatigue and quality of life outcomes of exercise during cancer treatment. *Cancer Practice, 9*(3), 119–127. doi:10.1046/j.1523-5394.2001.009003119.x

Neuman, B. (1974). The Betty Neuman health care systems model: A total person approach to patient problems. In J. P. Riehl & C. Roy (Eds.), *Conceptual models for nursing practice* (pp. 94–104). New York, NY: Appleton-Century-Crofts.

Neuman, B. (1995). *The Neuman systems model.* Norwalk, CT: Appleton & Lange.

Neuman, B. (1996). The Neuman systems model in research and practice. *Nursing Science Quarterly, 9*, 67–70.

Neuman, B. (2002). Assessment and intervention based on the Neuman systems model. In B. Neuman & J. Fawcett (Eds.), *The Neuman systems model* (pp. 347–359). Upper Saddle River, NJ: Prentice Hall.

Neuman, B., & Young, R. J. (1972). A model for teaching total person approach to patient problems. *Nursing Research, 21*, 264–269.

Newman, M. (1994). *Health as expanding consciousness* (2nd ed.). New York, NY: National League for Nursing Press.

Newman, M., (2008) *Transforming presence: The difference that nursing makes.* Philadelphia, PA: F. A. Davis.

Parse, R. R. (1981). *Man-living-health: A theory of nursing.* New York, NY: Wiley.

Parse, R. R. (1998). *The human becoming school of thought: A perspective for nurses and other health professionals.* Thousand Oaks, CA: Sage.

Parse, R. R. (2010). Rosemarie Rizzo Parse's Humanbecoming school of thought. In M. E. Parker & M. C. Smith (Eds.), *Nursing theories and nursing practice* (3rd ed., pp. 277–289). Philadelphia, PA: F. A. Davis.

Pharris, M. D. (2010). Margaret Newman's theory of health as expanding consciousness. In M. E. Parker & M. C. Smith (Eds.), *Nursing theories and nursing practice* (3rd ed., pp. 290–313). Philadelphia, PA: F. A. Davis.

Pressler, J. L., & Montgomery, K. S. (2012). Fitzpatrick's rhythm model. In J. J. Fitzpatrick & M. W. Kazer (Eds.), *Encyclopedia of nursing research* (3rd ed., pp. 190–191). New York, NY: Springer Publishing.

Rogers, M. E. (1970). *An introduction to the theoretical basis of nursing.* Philadelphia, PA: F. A. Davis.

Rogers, M. E. (1986). Science of unitary human beings. In V. M. Malinski (Ed.), *Explorations on Martha Rogers' science of unitary human beings* (pp. 3–8). Norwalk, CT: Appleton-Century-Crofts.

Rogers, M. E. (1992). Nursing science and the space age. *Nursing Science Quarterly, 5*(1), 27–34.

Rogers, M. E. (1994a). Nursing science evolves. In M. Madrid & E. A. M. Barrett (Eds.), *Roger's scientific art of nursing practice* (pp. 3–9). New York, NY: National League for Nursing.

Rogers, M. E. (1994b). The science of unitary human beings: Current perspectives. *Nursing Science Quarterly, 7*, 33–35.

Roy, C. (1970). Adaptation: A conceptual framework for nursing. *Nursing Outlook, 18*, 42–45.

Roy, C. (2009). *The Roy adaptation model* (3rd ed.). Upper Saddle River, NJ: Prentice Hall.

Schaefer, K. M., & Potylycki, M. J. (1993). Fatigue associated with congestive heart failure: Use of Levine's conservation model. *Journal of Advanced Nursing, 18*(2), 260–268.

St. Ours, C., Bositis, A., Hall, S., & Mock, V. (2005). Using the Levine conservation model to guide an intervention trial of exercise to mitigate cancer treatment-related fatigue [Presentation Abstract]. *30th Annual Oncology Nursing Society Congress.* Retrieved from http://www.nursinglibrary.org/vhl/handle/10755/165361

Tommet, P. (2003). Nurse-parent dialogue: Illuminating the evolving pattern of families with children who are medically fragile. *Nursing Science Quarterly, 16*(3), 239–246.

Whitbourne, S. K., & Whitbourne, S. B. (2010). *Adult development and aging: Biopsychosocial perspectives* (4th ed.). Hoboken, NJ: Wiley.

10

Interpersonal and Family Frameworks

Kristina Henry and Lucretia Smith

Shared joy is a double joy; shared sorrow is half a sorrow.
—Swedish Proverb

Remember, we all stumble, every one of us. That's why it's a comfort to go hand in hand.
—Emily Kimbrough

KEY TERMS

Bioecological Family Theory
Family Conflict Framework
Family Systems Theory
feminist theories
Framework of Systemic
  Organization
group dynamics
Hackman's Multilevel
  Perspective
Humanistic Nursing
  Theory

Human-to-Human
  Relationship Model
  of Nursing
nurse–patient relationship
Nursing Process
  Discipline Theory
Olson's Circumplex Model
Realistic Group Conflict Theory
Resiliency Model of Family
  Stress, Adjustment, and
  Adaptation

Social Exchange Theory
Structural Family Theory
Theory of Goal Attainment
Theory of Interpersonal
  Relations
Tuckman's Five Stages of
  Group Development
Wheelan's Integrated Model
  of Group Development

LEARNING OBJECTIVES

1. Describe interpersonal relationship frameworks regarding attributes, assumptions, processes, tasks, and goals.

2. Explore the application of interpersonal relationship frameworks to nursing and other health care disciplines.

3. Discuss interpersonal relationship frameworks and how they relate to the nursing process and provision of patient care.

4. Compare and contrast the conceptual elements of group dynamics frameworks.

The foundational unit common to individuals, families, and groups is the interpersonal relationship. Human behavior resulting from interpersonal relationships is dynamic and often unpredictable. Therefore, interpersonal relationships must be flexible, adaptable, and resilient to prosper. The development and maintenance of interpersonal relationships are critical skills for living and thriving in society. Communicating with and empowering others, as well as developing caring and supportive family systems is the cornerstone of human development and life span goals. The value of interpersonal relationships and family is in the support and protection they afford, for without relationships, we live in isolation and are more vulnerable to a multitude of challenges and crises.

The art of nursing emphasizes the interpersonal relationship between the nurse and the patient. Establishing and maintaining a trusting and therapeutic relationship is a critical component of the *nurse–patient relationship*. Assisting patients and families to develop relationships is vital to health and wellness initiatives. The complexity of society and families has contributed to the development and usage of interpersonal frameworks to guide care in an increasingly multifaceted health care environment. In this chapter, frameworks related to interpersonal relationships, including those of families and groups, are explored.

◉ INTERPERSONAL RELATIONSHIP FRAMEWORKS

In this section, the focus is on frameworks that help us understand the nurse–patient relationship, its nature, the processes involved, and the expectations of nurse and patient during interactions.

Peplau's Theory of Interpersonal Relations

Hildegard Peplau has been revered as establishing the basis for psychiatric nursing through the development of the Theory of Interpersonal Relations (Peplau, 1952). The theory was inspired by several noted theorists including psychiatrist Henry Stack Sullivan and psychologist Abraham Maslow. The focus of this theory is the development of the nurse–patient relationship in a hospital setting. However, the phases of the nurse–patient relationship have been generalized to other health care settings.

The interpersonal relationship between the nurse and patient progress through four overlapping dynamic phases: orientation, identification, exploitation, and resolution (Peplau, 1952). The orientation phase consists of the patient seeking assistance, asking questions, and sharing his or her perception of the problem (Peplau, 1952). During the orientation phase, the nurse provides education and counseling to help the patient recognize the types of assistance and resources that may be needed. The nurse must also assess the patient's motivation and desire for participation in care. The orientation phase establishes the tone for the professional relationship and is focused on getting to know each other and establishing guidelines and goals. The identification phase occurs when the patient begins to respond to people involved in providing care and who the patient believes can meet his or her needs. The patient may engage with the nurse during the identification phase in one of three ways: by forming an interdependent relationship, a dependent relationship, or an independent relationship separate from the nurse. The exploitation phase is entered when the patient makes full use of the health care services needed. The resolution phase involves relinquishing dependencies and preparing for discharge. Providing discharge planning, identifying patient resources needed for discharge, and identifying strategies for future health care needs are common practices during the termination phase (Peplau, 1988).

The nurse–patient interpersonal relationship develops from a superficial to a deeper level of involvement as the patient goes through the admission process, intensive treatment, recovery and rehabilitation, and eventual discharge from care. The relationship initially begins with the nurse assuming the role of a stranger and expands to include the roles of teacher, resource person, counselor, surrogate, and leader (Peplau, 1988). The first role, as a stranger, is inherent in the orientation phase of the relationship. After the nurse and the patient complete the work of the orientation phase, they can enter the working phase. The remaining roles of teacher, resource person, counselor, surrogate, and leader are then used to assist the patient and family members to analyze and understand their behaviors and emotions and achieve health goals. The nurse does not solve problems for the patient but assists the patient in exploring solutions and making personal choices. Through these roles and therapeutic relationships, the nurse can promote the art of healing.

Nursing Process Discipline Theory

In 1961, Ida Jean Orlando developed the Nursing Process Discipline Theory, which is known today as the *nursing process*. The theory was developed through her research of nurse–patient interactions and relationships. Orlando studied thousands of nurse–patient encounters and was able to identify positive and negative interactions. Positive interactions were those in which the nurse thoroughly assessed the patient's perspective, behavior, and experience, and used the information to address the patient's specific needs. Through this analysis, Orlando established patient participation and the nurse–patient relationship as essential components to providing nursing care (Schmieding, 1984).

Orlando's theory describes nonlinear, reflective processes the nurse engages in during a patient–nurse encounter to meet the patient's needs. Interactions with the patient then produce cognitive and affective reactions in the nurse, described as the person's *process of action* (Orlando, 1972). During the process of action, a sequence occurs beginning with the nurse's perception of data through the senses. Perception then stimulates automatic thoughts by the nurse, which stimulates automatic feelings and concludes with personal actions.

The interaction among Orlando's action processes formed the foundation for what we know today as the five-phase nursing process: assess, diagnose, plan, implement, and evaluate. Assessment is the process of investigation and inquiry to determine the status and needs of the patient. It is accomplished through observation and examination. Diagnosis is defined as identification of primary needs to assist the patient. Planning is the process of collaborating with the patient to set goals to address the patient needs. Implementation is defined as the specific tasks, duties, and responsibilities that must be performed to meet the identified goals. Evaluation is the process of analyzing the outcome and answering the questions: Were the goals met? How could the process be improved? And do any alterations need to be made? Orlando's Nursing Process Theory helped to define the role of nursing and the integral role of the nurse–patient relationship in patient care.

Humanistic Nursing Theory

Paterson and Zderad (1976) developed the Humanistic Nursing Theory to describe the interactive and multifaceted characteristics of nursing. This theory is used to explore the phenomena of nursing, including its meaning and essence. It is based on the concept of the nurse sharing experiences and developing a relationship with the patient. Based on existentialism, the Humanistic Nursing Theory highlights nursing as a composition of lived experiences. Through lived experiences, nursing becomes a dynamic process experienced in the context of choices and relationships.

In clinical practice, when an individual or family is in need of health care, the nurse responds to meet the need in the pursuit of well-being. During this exchange, the nurse uses the skills, traits, education, and experiences acquired to assist the patient in an empathetic manner. He or she has made a commitment to assist others using professional roles, standards, and competencies as a guide. As the nurse is a blend of personal and professional experiences, each response and encounter are individualized. Thus, each nurse–patient relationship is individualized and distinct (Parker, 2001).

The exchange between nurse and patient is a lived experience by both parties. It is influenced by the unique experiences and perceptions of both the nurse and the patient. The Humanistic Nursing Theory focuses on the art of nursing, including human intimacy, and thus conflicts with the science-based approach in nursing, which focuses on tasks and quantitative evidence. This theory emphasizes the ever-changing and dynamic development of individuals throughout the life span. Therefore, each interaction is a product of the developmental process that uses the interactive, subjective, nurse–patient relationship (Meleis, 2012).

The Human-to-Human Relationship Model of Nursing

Joyce Travelbee, a nursing theorist, used existential concepts to describe and explain nursing and the human relationship experience. Her model called the Human-to-Human Relationship Model of Nursing values human accountability for personal choices and the process of continuous personal development. Through the nurse–patient relationship, the nurse assists the patient to cope with and understand personal experiences. In the human-to-human relationship, one person is seeking assistance, and the other is providing it. This exchange establishes the basis for meaningful interactions and relationships (Travelbee, 1966).

Travelbee explains the process of nursing through establishing nurse–patient rapport and relationship development. The relationship is based on the unique characteristics of both individuals. It establishes the basis for meaning and purposeful communication. Relationship development occurs in five phases: original encounter, visibility of personal identities, empathy, sympathy, and established rapport. In the original encounter, the nurse perceives the situation based on experience, media, and other influencing factors. The nurse uses these perceptions to form opinions that influence interactions. The visibility of identities, also called the *phase of emerging identities*, is when each person becomes familiar with the other and recognizes the person's uniqueness. The phase of empathy is characterized by a deeper knowledge of the other's inner experience. Empathy involves the mental and emotional understanding of the individual and precedes the demonstration of sympathy (Travelbee, 1964). Sympathy is the desire to help relieve another's discomfort and acknowledges the other person's stress. The final phase of the nurse–patient relationship is developing rapport, which is both a goal and an outcome of the relationship.

Through the nurse–patient relationship, seven basic concepts of the Human-to-Human Relationship Model of Nursing have evolved. Travelbee's Human to Human Relationship Model of Nursing has evolved to include the concepts of self-therapy, and targeted approach (Travelbee, 1966). *Suffering* is defined as a subjective mental or physical unease, discomfort, or pain. *Meaning* is the subjective reason that the individual attributes to the suffering experience. The *nursing role* is to assist the individual, family, or community to understand the experience. *Hope* is defined as an essential component in asking for assistance and indicates the desire that the future will be better. *Communication* between the nurse and the patient is critical for successful outcomes. *Self-therapy* is the ability of the patient to affect change through personal characteristics or attributes. Nurses also assist patients in self-therapy through education about available and appropriate resources to address their needs. This process is defined as a *targeted intellectual approach*.

Theory of Goal Attainment

Imogene King studied the development of nurse–patient interactions and transactions that she viewed as culminating in relationships. In this chapter, the discussion of King's Theory for Goal Attainment focuses on the key concept of the nurse–patient relationship (see Chapter 9). Through a process of sharing and communicating personal perceptions and attributes, the nurse and the patient develop a relationship to set and accomplish mutually agreed on goals.

The foundation of King's Theory of Goal Attainment is based on three coordinating systems: personal, interpersonal, and social systems (King, 1987). Personal systems comprise individuals; interpersonal systems consist of two or more people forming dyads, triads, or small groups; and social systems include families, organizations, and communities. Nurses play a valuable role in developing relationships and collaborating with the patient's personal, interpersonal, and social systems to establish and achieve the goals.

King proposed that communication and transactions between the nurse and patient result in more congruent perceptions for mutual understanding. This insight leads to relationship development and promotes congruency in patient-specific care and patient outcomes. The nurse–patient relationship is described as dynamic and flexible, and thus able to accommodate diverse life changes and experiences. Both the patient and the nurse bring critical knowledge, skills, and attributes to the relationship, which supports and strengthens the ability to achieve patient goals.

Social Exchange Theory

George Casper Homans, an American sociologist, developed the Social Exchange Theory in 1958. The foundation of this theory originated in economic systems frameworks and is rooted in cost and benefit analysis. As applied in a social context, Social Exchange Theory is based on the concept of rational choice and human behavior. The Social Exchange Theory is described as individuals analyzing the perceived costs and benefits or rewards and punishments resulting from social decisions. Individuals weigh the internal rewards and punishments for the relationships that they have established. The theory predicts individuals seek out and commit to a personal relationship with more perceived benefits and rewards and avoid people and relationships who have greater perceived costs or punishments.

Homans (1974) continued his sociological research and developed six propositions to explain social behaviors and exchanges:

- Success proposition refers to the person being more likely to repeat an action if it results in a reward.

- Stimulus proposition is when a past action resulted in a reward causing the person to be more likely to repeat the action given a similar situation.

- Value proposition is concerned with the perception of the reward as valuable, thereby making the person more likely to complete the action.

- Deprivation-satiation proposition occurs when a person who continually receives the same reward eventually perceives the reward as less valuable.

- The aggression-approval proposition is when an individual does not receive the expected reward or receives an unexpected punishment resulting in an emotional upset. However, if the reward is greater than anticipated or the expected punishment is not received, the person experiences positive emotions.

- Rationality proposition involves cognitive appraisal in which the individual analyzes the value and likelihood of receiving a reward before deciding to perform the action.

As relationships are dynamic experiences, the perceived cost and benefit fluctuates and is continually reevaluated. Rewards and costs are both subjective and objective. Rewards include affection, social support, satisfaction, and financial gains. Costs are defined as undesirability, illness, lack, and financial expenditures. As individuals weigh the benefits and costs, they determine whether to maintain or terminate the relationship.

The subjective nature of the cost and benefit analysis is dependent on personal expectations and perceived alternatives. If an individual has few social relationships or a history of abusive relationships, personal perceptions or cost and benefit analysis may be quite different from someone with an extensive history of positive relationships. The person with few social relationships may feel the alternative of loneliness is too great a cost for terminating a relationship, whereas the social person may see it as an opportunity to meet new people.

FRAMEWORKS RELATED TO FAMILY RELATIONSHIPS

Family relationships are usually the first and most basic relationships that humans experience. The nature of family relationships has been the object of study and theorizing in fields as diverse as advertising and nursing. The attributes of family membership including form, function, and interaction are frequently studied. The family frameworks presented later are from psychology and health-related disciplines.

Family Systems Theory

Ludwig Von Bertalanffy, an Austrian biologist, created the General Systems Theory that explored the science of organisms as complex, organized, and interactive (Von Bertalanffy, 1969). This holistic and dynamic view of organisms shifted the focus from a mechanistic, linear perspective. The Family Systems Theory applies the General Systems Theory in the social sciences and establishes a model to study the complex components and interactions of the family system as a whole, interdependent, and connected unit. A *family* is composed of individuals with personal histories, goals, and desires who share an emotional bond with the other family members. The Family Systems Theory focuses on the effect of changes in one family member on the other family members and the family unit as a whole (White, Klein, & Martin, 2015).

Each family member (subsystem) brings unique characteristics and attributes to the family. In a nuclear or traditional family unit, the mother, father, brother, and sister, all have specific roles that demonstrate a hierarchy of functioning and interaction patterns. Regardless of the family composition, each member of the family fulfills specific roles and tasks in the family system. When the family system operates optimally, equilibrium is established, which provides organization and role identity in the family. As family systems expand or members are added, the family relationships naturally become more complex.

Each family system has developed inclusive and exclusive boundaries. Open, inclusive boundaries experience external influences, while closed boundaries result in an isolated and contained atmosphere. All family systems are affected by external and internal influences to some degree. However, the operationalization of boundaries directly impacts the extent of influence. Life experiences may stress the organization of the family or roles of the family members. If a family member becomes ill or suffers an injury, that person's role in the family shifts and the entire family unit is affected. For this reason, family systems are dynamic and adaptable to meet changing needs and challenges.

On a broader level, the family is also a part of the community (supra system), so changes at the family level also impact the community supra system. It is important to acknowledge and anticipate the ripple effects of change when planning and implementing patient care. Effective interventions that use the Family Systems Theory approach and address the connectedness and interrelatedness of the subsystems, realize that change requires adjustments to these areas as well.

For a care provider, the Family Systems Theory is important for prioritization, planning, and implementing interventions. The provider must acknowledge and address the interconnectedness of the family units. Any changes to an individual or a unit in the family result in changes to the other units, as well as the family system as a whole. These relationships and interdependent interactions guide behaviors for the individual and the entire family unit. Family Systems Theory may be applied as the basis for research on family adaptation and recovery from substance abuse and dependence, traumatic events, and chronic illnesses.

Structural Family Theory

Salvador Minuchin, Montalvo, Guerney, Rosman, and Schumer developed the Structural Family Theory through their work with families in crisis (Minuchin et al., 1967). They describe the family as an interdependent unit comprising hierarchical subsystems (individuals). Any change or stressor in one subsystem affects the entire family unit. The family unit is dynamic and influenced by all interactions involving the subsystems. These subsystem interactions contribute to the adaptation and evolution of the unit, as the subsystems in the unit grow and develop simultaneously (Nichols & Schwartz, 2001).

The Structural Family Theory seeks to understand the intangible structure of the family including rules and hierarchy. The analysis of family structure enhances identification of dysfunctional family relationships. Once identified, the relationships can be addressed and adapted to more positive relationships. The identification and interpretation of dysfunctional family relationships result in a realignment or restructuring of the roles of each subsystem and the family unit as a whole.

The organization of the family unit is based on the interactions and specific roles of the subsystems. The organization defines the power and boundaries of the subsystems in the unit and provides the basis for a family function. Healthy families exhibit flexibility and adaptation when a stressor is introduced. However, dysfunctional families demonstrate behaviors ranging from enmeshment to disengagement, based on the family member's rigidity and ability to adapt to stressors. *Enmeshment* is described as undifferentiated roles or obsession with others, which leads to a loss of empowerment and autonomy. A mother may become enmeshed in the child's pursuits and goals, thus losing sight of her own goals. At the other extreme, *disengagement* is described as withdrawal from family interactions and relationships. An example would be a parent who is not concerned with a child's behavior even if those actions result in arrest or legal action. Thus, the nature of the family member's interactions, roles, power, and boundaries determine the flexibility and adaptation of the individual family members and the family unit as a whole.

Feminist Frameworks Related to Family

The traditional role of women in the family, along with their treatment by political, social, and organizational structures surrounding the family, has given birth to feminist scholarship. Known as *feminist theory*, this type of scholarship is defined by Gordon (1979) as "an analysis of women's subordination for the purpose of figuring out how to change it" (White & Klein, 2008, p. 107). Family, as defined by most empirical scientists, is not the focus of feminist frameworks. Rather, the family is often treated as a fabricated social structure that supports the ongoing privileged male role. This view of the family as a fabricated social structure gives rise to the notion of a "private sphere" where people, especially men, can escape public censure for wrongful behavior toward those who are vulnerable. These perspectives, among others, have been explored by feminist theorists and scholars.

One assumption underlying feminist frameworks is the idea that the experiences of women are of value. Historically, there have been some incidents where the ability of women to think rationally was in doubt (e.g., a woman's right to vote and limited career options for women). These cases should be treated as biased as they fail to recognize the many contributions of women to society (White & Klein, 2008). A second assumption is that all women's experiences, no matter what they are or how they are expressed, have value.

Third, understanding the differences between the genders is not sufficient. Research studies and theories must be judged by their ability to be emancipatory. Feminist theory delineates between sex (the biological element) and gender (the socially constructed element) of a person's identity. A derogatory generalization about a person, based on the sex of the individual, would be considered sexist, and actions that result from such generalization would be characterized as sexism.

The influence of feminist frameworks can be found in nursing practice and nursing research (Box 10.1). As a result of evidence-based practice, feminists' issues have found their way into clinical and administrative nursing as well. As nurses in a female-dominated profession, understanding and sensitivity to the ideas portrayed in feminist theories are an important consideration. Feminist perspectives influence the role of the nurse, the development of the nursing profession, and, in the case of sex/gender bias, impact the evaluation of research findings.

Olson's Circumplex Model

Building on Minuchin's research, Olson developed the Circumplex Model to establish an evidence-based, therapeutic approach to marriage and family therapy (Olson, 2000). The foundation of the theory includes the concepts of flexibility, cohesion, and communication. Healthy families demonstrate equilibrium with cohesion and flexibility, whereas unhealthy families demonstrate unequal or unstable levels of flexibility and cohesion, which result in dysfunctional family processes.

Healthy families must be flexible and adapt to change when necessary. In contrast, rigid families are unable to adapt or evolve with change. However, chaos can also result if the family is too flexible. Therefore, the goal is to achieve a balance or equilibrium with shared and agreed on rules and roles. Olson's Circumplex Model illustrates dynamic processes and fluctuations involved with family functioning, as well as the interrelationships among the concepts. Owing to these interrelated concepts, if one area shows improvement or decline, then it is likely to cause similar changes in the other areas.

Healthy families demonstrate an equilibrium in cohesion, which is described as an emotional connection and attachment. However, if families are too close, members may be enmeshed or too dependent on each other. In contrast, families lacking a bond or connection may be described as disengaged. The goal is to develop and maintain a balance of individual fulfillment along with a sense of familial emotional attachment to the family unit.

BOX 10.1 Using Feminist Theory to Research Cardiovascular Disease

McCormick and Bunting (2002) used feminist theory to look at research about women and cardiovascular disease. Using nine published peer-reviewed studies, they completed a critique using Bunting's Model of Feminist Critique. This model is concerned with moving from feminist principles to feminist praxis using the critique criteria given later as a method to evaluate literature. Overall the goal was to depict women in a way that acknowledges women's differences from men without making women appear inferior. The critique included: a purpose to benefit women, a valuing of women's experiences/needs, recognition of oppression of women, commitment to social change, and awareness of human diversity including women's strengths. The most problematic areas found were a commitment to social change and presenting women's strengths.

Olson describes communication as the foundation for establishing equilibrium, which involves the skills of listening, self-disclosure, and respect (2000). Families with balance in the areas of cohesion and flexibility demonstrate higher levels of communication skills. Therefore, interventions to improve family function using the Circumplex Model should specifically address communication skill development.

The Circumplex Model is based on the concepts of fluctuation and change and relies on therapeutic approaches that facilitate achieving balance. Children grow up, people change jobs, or relocate. As a result, the roles in the family shift. Thus, this model is designed to address family adaptation to environmental changes, as well as changing family demands. The Family Adaptation and Cohesion Scale (FACES) tool was developed to explore the dimensions of cohesion and flexibility regarding balanced and unbalanced attributes. FACES IV was found to have high construct and discriminant validity and was an accurate monitor of the family member's responses to therapy (Olson, 2011).

Family Conflict Framework

General social conflict frameworks date back to Thomas Hobbs, a social philosopher of the 1600s, who saw the basic state of nature as a war of all opposed to all (White & Klein, 2008). The family played an important part in social conflict as both the precursor and as a microcosm of class distinction and conflict. Family conflict frameworks are based on conflict in groups, and conflict among groups is considered to influence, and be influenced by, family interactions. Therefore, the basis of family conflict is disharmony in interpersonal relationships.

Conflict theory is based on the assumption that conflict between individuals and social groups is endemic and inevitable, making the management of conflict the primary concern. Underlying these assumptions are the ideas that self-interest usually motivates humans and the normal state of society is conflict, not harmony. Major concepts of the theory include conflict, the structure of the situation or the group, resources, negotiation, and consensus. The propositions that underlie conflict theory include resource inequity and structure as the basis for conflict. Negotiation, although more likely in egalitarian social structure, tends to favor the person in the family or the family unit with the greatest resources. The formation of coalitions between individuals and subgroups, or family units with a democratic group structure, may alter the outcome of resource-driven conflicts.

One criticism of the conflict theory is its attention to conflict and resolution, rather than its attention to the dialectical process of conflict and inequity. The theory has also been criticized for lack of scientific rigor and for inattention to inequalities that are not resource-based (White & Klein, 2008). However, this theory remains useful to nurses in the assessment of clinical and professional situations, especially those related to the family and the micro and macro environments of nursing roles.

Resiliency Model of Family Stress, Adjustment, and Adaptation

Families and family health have been historically viewed from an illness-based medical model. In the past, many therapists and health providers operated from the myth that there was a model of a healthy family and healthy families had no problems. Any deviation from the healthy family model was viewed as dysfunctional and risked damaging family members, especially children (Walsh, 2006). However, in the 1980s, the concept of resilience became the basis for a strengths-based view of health. Increasingly, family scientists are looking at family strengths, rather than *fixable deficiencies* and are studying methods of empowering the strength-based qualities in the families (Walsh, 2006).

The Resiliency Model of Family Stress, Adjustment, and Adaptation is used to explore the effects of challenges and rewards on the family (McCubbin, 1993). The assumptions of this model are that hardships and stressors are an inevitable part of life and families develop unique strengths to adapt and foster individual development and growth. Although stressors experienced by families have often been blamed for the deterioration and destruction of the family unit, the concept of resilience accounts for other families who experience the same stressors without damaging effects. The Resiliency Model is used to examine the differences between the adaptive and the maladaptive family and the family's adaptation to challenges experienced throughout the life span.

There are four components of the Resiliency Model of Family Stress, Adjustment, and Adaptation: the person, environment, health, and the role of nursing. The person is the individual unit in the family structure. The environment is described as an open system and is a component of the society and the community. Health is defined as the resiliency, flexibility, and adaptability of the family to specific crises throughout the life span. The role of the nurse is to advocate for the family by promoting understanding, recovery, and maximum functioning while supporting the family system.

McCubbin (1993) describes the Resiliency Model in two phases referred to as *adjustment* and *adaptation*. The adjustment phase involves changing in response to a stressor, assessing the family's vulnerability, and identifying patterns of family functioning. Once a critical appraisal of the stressors has been conducted, and the status of family functioning has been identified, the adaptation phase begins. The adaptation phase involves coping and problem solving, using family resources, and dealing with resistance. The result is either positive adjustment (i.e., *bonadjustment*), defined as maintaining positive patterns of family functioning, or maladjustment. In phase two, adaptation occurs. It begins with the family's experience of crisis, stressors, and transition, which leads to new patterns of family functioning. These new patterns include an appraisal of family capabilities, coping, and problem-solving abilities. Table 10.1 outlines the basic concepts of the phases of adjustment and adaptation.

The role of the nurse in the Resiliency Model is an advocate to promote health, recovery, and maximum functioning. The nurse can empower the family by enhancing the strengths of the family, fostering community relationships, and facilitating effective coping and problem

TABLE 10.1 Concepts of the Resiliency Model of Family Stress, Adjustment, and Adaptation Theory

Phase 1: Adjustment	Phase 2: Adaptation
Stressor	Family crisis
Family vulnerability	Family stressors and transitions
Established patterns of family functioning	New patterns of family functioning
Appraisal of stressor	Appraisal of family capabilities
Coping and problem solving	Coping and problem solving
Family resources or resistance	Social support and family resources
Bonadjustment: individual and family positive coping and resilience occur OR Maladjustment if resistance or if unable to cope	Bonadaptation: positive coping and adaptation occur OR Maladaptation with continued crisis and need for assistance

Source: McCubbin (1993).

solving. A primary goal for the nurse is to educate the individual and the family and provide support for a structured plan and process.

Bioecological Family Theory

An ecological theory of individual development was published in 1979 by Urie Bronfenbrenner. Since its introduction, the individual and family aspects of the theory have been developed and refined and have served as the basis for many studies. In its current form, the theory proposes five environmental systems in which the individual and the family develop. These are the microsystem, mesosystem, macrosystem, exosystem, and chronosystem. *Microsystem* consists of influences inside the person, while the *mesosystem* is the connections among the microsystems. The *macrosystem* refers to the culture surrounding the family. *Exosystems* are other social systems that influence the microsystem. The *chronosystem* connects all systems as it refers to the events occurring over the individual's life span and the socio-historical changes occurring in the community (Santrock, 2013).

Bronfenbrenner's theory is based on several assumptions. One assumption is that people live in both biological and social spheres and that they depend on their environment and one another. The other assumption is that temporal and spatial aspects are both constraints and resources for organizing and understanding human behavior and interactions (White & Klein, 2008). These assumptions have been used to understand the development of children and the effects of the person's life context and personal interactions on health. The theory can also be used to think about the health of all family members or the environmental influences on the health of any human. The use of Bronfenbrenner's Bioecological Family Theory to influence health policy is illustrated in Box 10.2.

The Framework of Systemic Organization

The Framework of Systemic Organization is a nursing theory focused on the family system about the community and other environmental influences (Friedemann, 1995). It is a holistic approach, highlighting well-being and balance in individual, family, and community interactions. Friedemann considers the definition of family as subjective to the individual. Families are not required to live together or be biologically linked. They are defined by the individual based on the function or roles in the family and the nature of the emotional bond. The framework defines family health as a dynamic process of response to external and internal changes, with the goal of reestablishing balance, stability, growth, control, and spirituality (Friedemann, 1995).

BOX 10.2 Using the Bioecological Theory for Policy Change

Greenfield (2011) used the Bioecological Systems Theory to "conceptualize a range of programs as aging-in-place initiatives and for describing their similarities and differences" (p. 1). The study is concerned with the quality and governing policy of national initiatives aimed to assist older adults to age in place. Eight initiatives were analyzed regarding the environment of initial change, the level of the environment to be changed, social systems and structures, the leadership of older adults, subgroups of older adults, and attention to transitions. The analysis highlighted the need for policies and programs that include older adults in the leadership of an initiative, and for specific attention to the needs specific to older adults when transitions occur. It also highlighted the common aims that could make a more influential statement about funding.

The underlying assumption of the model is that the world, environment, people, and families are open systems that strive for congruence. Congruence is an ideal rather than a reality, defined as an energy among systems that are compatible and attuned to each other. The systematic process is pictured as a circle with health at its center and the environment outside the circle. The external influences (spirituality, stability, control, and growth) and the internal influences (coherence, system maintenance, individualism, and system change) all act on health and each other.

Friedemann's model is used directly in family care, in the establishment of nursing care in acute care areas, and in research. It is frequently used in Europe as the basis of nursing education. As a practice level model, it has been used successfully in caring for families with a member receiving substance abuse treatment (Friedemann, 1994). Multiple family studies in the areas of chronic pediatric conditions, chronic pain, and geriatric care have used the framework (Köhlen, Beier, & Danzer, 2000; Pierce, 1997; Smith, & Friedemann, 1999).

◉ FRAMEWORKS RELATED TO GROUP DYNAMICS

Group dynamics frameworks are based on psychological, sociological, and anthropological premises. A group is defined as an entity that has identifying attributes and characteristics, independent of the individual members. Groups may be professional, personal, or social, or a combination. Whatever the type of group, it is common to contend with relational challenges such as competition and conflict. The phenomena of *group dynamics* have been used in a professional context in health care to explain group interactions, roles, behaviors, epidemiology of the disease, and health care disparities.

As health care continues to emphasize interprofessional collaboration, understanding group dynamics is becoming increasingly important for all members of the health care team. Shared goals and group cohesion become essential for optimal patient care. The study of group dynamics and leadership in the health care setting are intertwined. In Chapter 18, content useful in conjunction with teamwork and group dynamics is discussed.

Kurt Lewin was one of the first theorists to study group dynamics. He applied his change theories (see Chapter 4) to the process of group dynamics. He conceptualized groups as moving through the three stages of change: unfreezing, change, and refreezing (Lewin, 1947). Unfreezing is described as the process of challenging established thoughts and concepts while addressing defensive responses of the group members. The second stage, change, is marked by transition and confusion as established thoughts and concepts are challenged. The third and final stage, refreezing, is the integration of the change and the formalization of new thoughts, concepts, and patterns. In the refreezing stage, confusion is resolved as the group accepts the change as the norm (Lewin, 1947). Many of the following models stem from the original work of Kurt Lewin.

Tuckman's Five Stages of Group Development

Tuckman and Jensen (1977) developed the Four Stages of Group Development Theory to explain group dynamics and later expanded the theory to include five stages. In the five-stage theory, group development is described as moving through the stages of forming, storming, norming, performing, and adjourning. These stages are nonconsecutive, dynamic, and often chaotic as discussed subsequently.

The *forming* stage involves acquainting the group members with each other, including the group leader. During this stage, rules for interactions and behaviors are established, and members of the group are oriented to each other and the tasks or goals of the group. During this stage, members acknowledge potential conflicts. Stage two, *storming*, emphasizes the organization of tasks and the conflict resulting as individuals adapt their personal beliefs, ideas, and attitudes to meet the needs of the group. Structure, power, and leadership all contribute to conflict, whether it is apparent or not.

Stage three, referred to as *norming*, is characterized by individual members sharing contributions and the development of group cohesion (Tuckman & Jensen, 1977). Competition fears and questions must be addressed to progress at this stage. Active participation and shared leadership develop as group members begin to trust and acknowledge other members' contributions to the group. Conflict resolution and a sense of group belonging lead to maximum creativity and sharing of ideas. During the norming stage, the group members interact positively toward each other and accomplishing the group's tasks. However, members may also fear the foreseeable adjournment of the group and become resistant to change.

Stage four, *performing*, is not experienced by all groups (Tuckman & Jensen, 1977). It is characterized by the development of interdependence as the members adapt their roles to the needs of the group. At this stage, members are extremely loyal to the group, morale peaks, and optimal task performance and problem solving occur. The final stage, *adjourning*, involves the resolution of relationships and conclusion of tasks including planned dissolution of the group.

Wheelan's Integrated Model of Group Development

Susan Wheelan (1994) expanded on the research of Tuckman and Jensen and developed the Integrated Model of Group Development. She built on the stages described by Tuckman and Jensen, to include an examination of development as the group evolves. Through her work, she developed tools for application to group research including the Group Development Observation System (GDOS) and Group Development Questionnaire (GDQ). Both the GDOS and the GDQ are used to assess and analyze the developmental progress of the group. Wheelan's research indicates a significant correlation between the length of time the group has been in existence and the behavioral patterns of the group members, which supports group theories based on attainment of stages (Wheelan, 1994).

Wheelan (1994) identified the four stages of her theory as (a) dependency and inclusion, (b) counterdependency and fight, (c) trust and structure, (d) work and productivity. Stage one, *dependency and inclusion*, is explained as the members' reliance on the group leader for direction and organization. This stage focuses on concerns with member inclusion and member orientation to each other and the group's purpose. In stage two, *counterdependency and fight*, disagreement and conflict result as the group's purpose and procedures are clarified. The members establish a trusting culture for future conflict resolution and agree on group goals and functions. During stage three, *trust and structure*, group cooperation and commitment to open sharing, and communication are established. This stage emphasizes positive relationships and collaboration for group task accomplishment. Stage four, *work and productivity*, concentrates on group productivity and effective teamwork. The focus of energy is on task and goal accomplishment. Some groups have a distinct conclusion and experience a fifth and final stage of group termination. Thus, when the group achieves the goals, and there is no longer a need for the group, it is disbanded. This impending end may result in anxiety and fear, as well as an appreciation for fellow members and their experiences.

Hackman's Multilevel Perspective Theory

Psychology professor Richard Hackman combined multiple levels of analysis to study group dynamics at the micro-, meso-, and macro-levels (Hackman, 2003). He believed groups were based on individual, intergroup, and external influences. The micro-level is described as the individual, meso-level is the group, and macro-level is the organization, system, or community. He emphasized the complexity of groups and the need to look at the complete structure and function of the group in every context of the application.

Hackman (2003) applied his multilevel theory while studying airline crews. He found little variation at the micro- and meso-levels among the various airline crews. However, there was significant variation at the macro-level regarding the organizational function and structure. His research supports the assumption that external entities may affect the group as a whole. Therefore, for effective group analysis, it is essential to study the micro-, meso-, and macro-levels.

The application of this theory is based on analysis and evaluation of complex organizations. Studying the group dynamics and interactions at just one level ignores the potential opportunities and barriers at the other levels and results in an incomplete picture or perspective. Studying each level provides a more complete and broad analysis.

Using Hackman's Multilevel Perspective Theory, a study was performed on team leadership and its effect on individual performance at a large, complex organization (Chen, Kirkman, Kanfer, Allen, & Rosen, 2007). The results support the influence of leadership on each level, not just the macro-level. Leadership empowerment was found to be influential at each level and empowering at the macro level. These findings support the validity of Hackman's Multilevel Perspective Theory.

Realistic Group Conflict Theory

Realistic Group Conflict Theory (RGCT) is based on sociological and psychological principles developed from the research of Donald Campbell, an American social scientist (Campbell, 1965). RGCT explains how a conflict that arises from group competition for resources such as power, money, and social status, leads to controversy. The level of conflict directly correlates with the perception of the resource's value and availability, as well as discordant and unequal goals (Jackson, 1993).

An example of this theory is provided by the Robbers Cave Experiment described by Sherif, Harvey, White, Hood, and Sherif (1961). At a camp for adolescent boys in Oklahoma, researchers observed the campers' behaviors regarding group formation, competition, and intergroup cooperation. The researchers found that intergroup conflict occurred even in the absence of identifiable differences. Sherif and colleagues also noted that competition for resources among the groups resulted in hostility and conflict. Hostility and conflict were successfully reduced through collaboration toward a common goal.

RGCT has been used to explain conflict with racial integration (Jackson, 1993). The perception of one group as consuming limited resources (which negatively impacts the other group's lifestyle) leads to hostility and group conflict. The groups believe that the only solution is to eliminate the competition, either by improving the group's standing, diminishing the standing of the other group, or relocating to be further away from the competitor. In summary, according to the RGCT, conflict leads to discrimination and an imbalanced consumption of resources among the groups.

◉ CONCLUSION

This chapter has focused on the varied and complex interpersonal aspects of the nurse–patient relationship, family relationships, and group dynamics. As the concepts of patient, family, and groups are multifaceted and interconnected, defining these terms for use in research must be one of the first steps in research development and theory or model selection. To assist with this process and for purposes of organizational progression, we began the chapter with frameworks applicable to nurse–patient relationships and progressed to frameworks focusing on family and group relationships. As nursing is not limited to the care of the individual, a broader, holistic approach to the care of families and groups is warranted.

TABLE 10.2 Comparison of Group Dynamic Frameworks	
Group Dynamics Frameworks (Theorist)	**Principal Concepts**
Change Process Theory (Kurt Lewin)	Group dynamics Stages of change: unfreezing, change, and freezing
Five Stages of Group Development (Bruce Tuckman)	Five stage model for group behaviors: 1. Forming 2. Storming 3. Norming 4. Performing 5. Adjourning
Integrated Model of Group Development (Susan Wheelan)	Four stages of group behavior analysis: 1. Dependency and inclusion 2. Counterdependency and fight 3. Trust and structure 4. Work and productivity Final: dissolution of the group
Hackman's Multilevel Perspective (Richard Hackman)	Focus on creating and managing work groups based on micro-, meso-, and macro-level factors
Realistic Group Conflict Theory (Donald Campbell)	Based on sociological and psychological principles Explains conflict/competition among the groups for limited resources

A comparison of frameworks of group dynamics is provided in Table 10.2. These diverse frameworks describe and explain group change and group dynamics (Lewin's Change Theory), and stages of group behavior (Tuckman's stages of group development). The other frameworks have focused on stages of group behavior analysis (Wheelan's Integrated Model of Group Development), levels of influence (Hackman's Multilevel Perspective), and on understanding the motivations of competing groups (Campbell's Realistic Group Conflict Theory). Alone or in combination, these frameworks can be used in nursing research and to guide educators, clinicians, and nurse leaders when communicating and interacting with individuals, families, and groups.

KEY POINTS

- The Theory of Interpersonal Relations focuses on the nurse–patient relationship. The foundation of the theory explains interpersonal relationships in four dynamic phases: orientation, identification, exploitation, and resolution.

- Orlando developed the Nursing Process Theory through her research of nurse–patient interactions and relationships. She described the nurse–patient relationship as an essential component of the nursing process that includes assessment, diagnosis, planning, implementation, and evaluation.

- The Humanistic Nursing Theory is used to explore the phenomena of nursing. It highlights nursing as composed of lived experiences and relationships.

- Joyce Travelbee developed the Human-to-Human Relationship Model of Nursing to explain nursing through the human relationship experience. The nurse assists the patient to cope with and understand personal experiences through interactive relationships between the nurse and the patient.

- Imogene King described the Theory of Goal Attainment as a process of sharing and communicating personal perceptions and attributes through the nurse–patient relationship to develop and accomplish mutually agreed on goals.

- Social Exchange Theory is described as individuals analyzing the perceived costs and benefits or rewards and punishments of their social decisions.

- The Family Systems Theory (FST) involves the application of the General Systems Theory in the social sciences. FST is used to study the complex components and interactions of the family system as a whole, interdependent, and connected unit.

- Structural Family Theory describes the family as an interdependent unit comprising hierarchical subsystems (individuals). Any change or stressor in one subsystem affect the entire family unit.

- Feminist frameworks support the value and contribution of women in the family structure. They are used to analyze the role of women in the family.

- Circumplex Model established an evidence-based therapeutic approach to marriage and family therapy. Healthy families demonstrate equilibrium with cohesion and flexibility, whereas unhealthy families demonstrate unequal or unstable levels of flexibility and cohesion that result in dysfunctional family processes.

- Family Conflict Framework explains the influence of family and family interactions on conflict in groups and families.

- The Resiliency Model of Family Stress, Adjustment, and Adaptation explores the effect of stress on the family unit.

- The Bioecological Family Theory proposes five environmental systems in which the individual and the family develop: the micro-, meso-, exo-, macro-, and chronosystems. The theory is based on the assumption that people live in both biological and social environments.

- The Framework of Systemic Organization is a holistic approach focused on the family system about the community and other environmental influences.

- The phenomena of group dynamics have been used in health care to explain behaviors, epidemiology of diseases, and health care disparities. These concepts are explored through Change Process Theory, Five Stages of Group Development, Integrated Model of Group Development, Hackman's Multilevel Perspective, and Realistic Group Conflict Theory.

REFERENCES

Bronfenbrenner, U. (1979). *The ecology of human development: Experiments by nature and design.* Cambridge, MA: Harvard University Press.

Campbell, D. T. (1965). *Ethnocentric and other altruistic motives.* Lincoln: University of Nebraska Press.

Chen, G., Kirkman, B., Kanfer, R., Allen, D., & Rosen, B. (2007). A multilevel study of leadership, empowerment, and performance in teams. *Journal of Applied Psychology, 92*(2), 331–346. doi: 10.1037/0021-9010.92.2.331

Friedemann, M. L. (1994). Evaluation of a family intervention with rehabilitating substance abusers. *International Journal of Nursing Studies, 31*(1), 97–108.

Friedemann, M. L. (1995). *The framework of systemic organization: A conceptual approach to families and nursing*. Thousand Oaks, CA: Sage.

Gordon, L. (1979). The struggle for reproductive freedom: Three stages of feminism. In Z. Eisenstein (Ed.), *Capitalist patriarchy and the case for socialist feminism* (pp. 107–136). New York, NY: Monthly Review Press.

Greenfield, E. A. (2011). Using ecological frameworks to advance a field of research, practice, and policy on aging-in-place initiatives. *Gerontologist, 52*(1), 1–12.

Hackman, J. (2003). Learning more by crossing levels: Evidence from airplanes, hospitals, and orchestras. *Journal of Organizational Behavior, 24*, 905–922.

Homans, G. C. (1958). Social behavior as exchange. *American Journal of Sociology, 63*(6), 597–606.

Homans, G. C. (1974). *Elementary forms of social behavior* (2nd ed.). New York, NY: Harcourt Brace Jovanovich.

Jackson, J. (1993). Realistic group conflict theory: A review and evaluation of the theoretical and empirical literature. *Psychological Record, 43*(3), 395–415.

King, I. M. (1987). King's theory of goal attainment. In R. R. Parse (Ed.), *Nursing science: Major paradigms, theories, and critiques* (pp. 107–113). Philadelphia, PA: W. B. Saunders.

Köhlen, C., Beier, J., & Danzer, G. (2000). They don't leave you on your own: A qualitative study of the home care of chronically ill children. *Pediatric Nursing, 26*(4), 364–371.

Lewin, K. (1947). Frontiers in group dynamics: Concept, method, and reality in social science: Social equilibria and social change. *Human Relations, 1*(1), 5–41.

McCormick, K. M., & Bunting, S. M. (2002). Application of feminist theory in nursing research: The case of women and cardiovascular disease. *Health Care for Women International, 23*(8), 820–834. doi:10.1080/07399330290112344

McCubbin, M. A. (1993). Family stress theory and the development of nursing knowledge about family adaptation. In S. L. Feethan, S. B. Meister, J. M. Bell, & C. L. Gillis (Eds.), *The nursing of families* (pp. 46–58). New Bury Park, CA: Sage.

Meleis, A. (2012). *Theoretical nursing: Development & progress*. Philadelphia, PA: Lippincott Williams & Wilkins.

Minuchin, S., Montalvo, B., Guerney, B. G., Rosman, B. L., & Schumer, F. (1967). *Families of the slums*. New York, NY: Basic Books.

Nichols, M. P., & Schwartz, R. C. (2001). *Family therapy: Concepts and methods*. New York, NY: Allyn & Bacon.

Orlando, I. J. (1961). *The dynamic nurse-patient relationship: Function, process, and principles*. New York, NY: Putnam.

Orlando, I. J. (1972). *The discipline and teaching of nursing process: An evaluative study*. New York, NY: Putnam.

Olson, D. H. (2000). Circumplex model of marital and family systems. *Journal of Family Therapy, 22*, 144–167.

Olson, D. H. (2011). FACES IV and the circumplex model: A validation study. *Journal of Marital and Family Therapy, 3*(1), 64–80.

Parker, M. (2001). *Nursing theories and nursing practice*. Philadelphia, PA: F. A. Davis.

Paterson, J., & Zderad, L. (1976). *Humanistic nursing*. New York, NY: Wiley.

Peplau, H. E. (1952). *Interpersonal relations in nursing*. New York, NY: G. P. Putnam.

Peplau, H. E. (1988). *Interpersonal relations in nursing*. London, UK: Macmillan.

Pierce, L. (1997). The framework of systemic organization applied to older adults as family caregivers of persons with chronic illness and disability. *Gastroenterology Nursing, 20*(5), 168–175.

Santrock, J. W. (2013). *Life-span development* (14th ed.). New York, NY: McGraw-Hill.

Schmieding, N. J. (1984). Putting Orlando's theory into practice. *American Journal of Nursing, 84*(6), 759–761.

Sherif, M., Harvey, O. J., White , B. J., Hood, W., & Sherif, C. W. (1961). *Intergroup conflict and cooperation: The robber's cave experiment*. Norman, OK: The University Book Exchange.

Smith, A. A., & Friedemann, M. L. (1999). Perceived family dynamics of persons with chronic pain. *Journal of Advanced Nursing, 30*, 543–551.

Travelbee, J. (1964). What's wrong with sympathy? *American Journal of Nursing, 64*(1), 68–71.

Travelbee, J. (1966). *Interpersonal aspects of nursing*. Philadelphia, PA: F. A. Davis.

Tuckman, B., & Jensen, M. (1977). Stages of small group development revisited. *Group and Organizational Studies, 2*(4), 419–427.

Von Bertalanffy, L. (1969). *General system theory*. New York, NY: George Braziller.

Walsh, F. (2006). *Strengthening family resilience*. New York, NY: Guilford Press.

Wheelan, S. (1994). *Group processes: A developmental perspective*. Boston, MA: Allyn & Bacon.

White, J. M., & Klein, D. M. (2008). *Family theories*. Los Angeles, CA: Sage.

White, J. M., & Klein, D. M., & Martin, T. F. (2015). *Family theories: An introduction* (4th ed.). Los Angeles, CA: Sage.

CHAPTER 11

Needs-Based Frameworks

Rhea Faye Felicilda-Reynaldo and Lucretia Smith

Everyone needs help. That's the human condition.
—Max Allan Collins

KEY TERMS

agency
automatic actions
care agent
deliberate actions
Gordon's Functional Health
   Patterns & Nursing
   Diagnoses

Henderson's Nursing
   Needs Theory
Maslow's Hierarchy
   of Needs
Nightingale's
   Environmental Theory

Orem's Self-Care
   Deficit Theory
Orlando-Pelletier's Nursing
   Process Discipline Theory
Roper–Logan–Tierney Model
   for Nursing

LEARNING OBJECTIVES

1. Summarize the attributes of each needs-based framework of care.

2. Compare concepts and unique attributes in the needs-based frameworks.

3. Discuss the uses of each needs-based framework in the roles of educator, clinician, leader, and researcher.

Nursing is concerned with meeting the patient's needs. Although some frameworks reviewed in this chapter offer solutions and plans for meeting needs, many are concerned with answering the "why" question. That is, why nursing exists and what is the purpose of nursing. The concepts in these needs-based frameworks address a range of issues regarding not only meeting the patient's health needs but also meeting the human needs from a holistic perspective.

Nurses practicing in advanced roles will notice the needs-based frameworks discussed in this chapter addresses a range of internal and external factors. Internal physiological changes and internal cognitive, emotional, and spiritual issues, as well as external environmental and sociocultural influences, are addressed. With this breadth of coverage, using these frameworks in clinical practice can provide a foundation for nursing care and a framework for meeting the patient's holistic needs. Addressing patient needs in this manner enhances clinical practice and the delivery of quality care in today's patient satisfaction–driven health care system.

◉ NEEDS-BASED FRAMEWORKS

The origins of nursing and health care can be found in meeting human needs. This is evident from Nightingale's articulation of the canons of nursing to more modern developments such as nursing diagnosis classification. Understanding, categorizing, and prioritizing needs as well as identifying interventions to meet those needs is important and valued in nursing and other health care disciplines. The perspectives of nursing, psychology, and sociology have been influential in the development of our understanding of human needs.

Although the frameworks discussed later may differ in how needs are viewed, or in the origins and motivations of the needs, and the categorization of needs, they share a commonality. These human-needs frameworks represent a spectrum of needs. In this spectrum, we find human needs ranging from essential, required, or prerequisite to those that are desired but not essential. At the required end of the spectrum, needs are given priority as they are foundational to health. At the nonessential end of the spectrum, those needs are not necessary for life but make life more fulfilling and enjoyable. Unfulfilled nonessential needs can also impact health and the individual's psychological, social, emotional and spiritual well-being. Human needs are integral to the human condition and impact professional nursing practice in all specialty areas. Therefore, understanding human needs through various theoretical perspectives can be invaluable to the profession.

Nightingale's Environmental Theory

Nightingale is considered as the mother of modern nursing. She is also considered the first nurse researcher, epidemiologist, and theorist. However, when she presented her observations and recommendations during the Crimean War in the book, *Notes on Nursing: What it Is and What it Is Not*, she did not intend to present this information as a "theory." Her work, now known as the Environmental Theory, facilitated the evolution of nursing into a respected vocation, then into a profession. Although the interventions outlined in her book were focused on manipulating the patient's environment, they also reflect the patient's needs for nutrition, water, rest, hygiene, and fresh air.

Nightingale (1860/1969) believed a person had the capacity to self-heal. In that context, the nurse was responsible for changing the environment to make it conducive to a patient's self-healing. Nightingale mentions two kinds of environment, the external and the internal. The external environment refers to things or circumstances outside of the person's body that could affect healing. Examples include the temperature of the room, the noise level on a nursing unit, and cleanliness of the environment. Internal environment refers to things or circumstances inside the body that could influence the quality of a person's self-healing process. Examples of the internal environment include amount and quality of food, water, fresh air, and hope.

Nightingale's Environmental Theory of nursing is based on 13 canons, which are guidelines for the provision of patient care. Each of these canons demonstrates the application of physical, mental, and external environmental care practices that meet the patient's needs and promote health and healing. One of Nightingale's central guidelines for nursing care revolves around maintaining cleanliness of the environment. This was exemplified in the canon of "cleanliness of rooms and walls." The canon of "health of houses" emphasized clean air, clean water, effective and efficient drainage of waste, and adequate lighting. The maintenance of ventilation and warmth required nurses to keep the temperature of the room moderate and comfortable for the patient and ensure the patient breathed air that was clean and free of odor. The canon "bed and bedding" focused on providing comfort measures such as a comfortable bed and clean, dry, and wrinkle-free bedding. In the canon "personal cleanliness," nurses were to assist patients with maintaining hygiene and grooming.

Adjusting light and noise for patients were also two of the 13 canons (Nightingale, 1860/ 1969). They include the adjustment of lighting for patient comfort, avoiding noise that was startling to the patient, and keeping the noise level to a minimum to facilitate the patient's rest. Providing variety in the patient's environment would help distract the patient from boredom. Nightingale was concerned with the patient's food intake and recommended that the patient's preferred foods be included in the nutritional care plan. When conversing with the patients, she instructed nurses to avoid "chattering hopes and advices" (1860/1969, p. 95), meaning nurses should abstain from the meaningless conversation and should not give advice without basis. Although not specifically stated as a canon, Nightingale believed patient teaching and promoting health was essential even for people who were not sick (Bolton, 2006).

In the final canon, Nightingale encouraged nurses to observe the sick and note the patient's progress toward healing through regular documentation of observations. Observation helps the nurse manage patient care that Nightingale referred to as "petty management." Documentation of observations and nursing care helps nurses to provide continuity and management of patient care.

Nightingale's theory is deeply embedded in current nursing practice standards. Her canons provided the starting point for the evolution of nursing practice. Since the initial inception of Nightingale's work, there have been many language updates to the 13 canons as science, medicine, and nursing advanced. However, the concepts in the canons are still relevant for meeting the patient's spoken and unspoken needs.

Maslow's Hierarchy of Needs

Abraham H. Maslow (1943) first presented the Hierarchy of Needs Theory as a way to describe what motivates people to act. Maslow proposed people strive to meet their lowest level needs before they pursue higher level needs (Harrigan & Commons, 2015). A pyramid provides the symbol of the needs hierarchy. The base of the pyramid represents a person's lower-level or deficit needs, and the top of the pyramid represents the higher level needs (Harrigan & Commons, 2015). The human needs progress as follows: physiological, safety, love and belongingness, self-esteem, and self-actualization (Maslow, 1943).

The lowest level of need, physiological, is directly observable in the environment (Harrigan & Commons, 2015). Physiological needs refer to actions and resources needed for the body to function and maintain homeostasis. Some examples of these needs include air, food, water, sleep, and excretion (Thielke et al., 2012). As physiological needs are of primary importance for existence, a person's motivation to satisfy this level is quite high (Thielke et al., 2012).

The next level, safety, is acted on when the person's physiological needs have been met (Maslow, 1970). When achieving this level, people want to protect themselves from physical or emotional harm (Thielke et al., 2012). Safety needs include security, protection, stability, dependency, structure, and freedom from anxiety and fear (Finsterwalder, 2010). Maslow (1943) proposed the idea that people living in the modern world usually have their safety needs satisfied if they live in peaceful and stable societies. Thus, the need for security is usually felt only when it is threatened or destroyed, such as war, natural catastrophes, crime waves, epidemics, or societal disintegration (Finsterwalder, 2010; Maslow, 1943; Thielke et al., 2012).

When persons long to be members of social structures, they are pursuing their need for love and belongingness (Harrigan & Commons, 2015). At this level, people want to love and be loved and find acceptance from other people (Maslow, 1970; Thielke et al., 2012). To meet this need, people communicate, show affection, and build relationships with other people, such as spouses, children, friends, or neighbors (Finsterwalder, 2010; Thielke et al., 2012). In addition to building relationships, people want to fit into the social group to which they believe they belong (Datta, 2013). Moreover, because of this need, people make choices regarding their neighborhoods, daily transportation use, and their appearance.

On meeting the first three need levels, persons then seek self-confidence and the respect of others (Harrigan & Commons, 2015). This represents the need for self-esteem. Maslow (1943) believed self-esteem had two sides: self-esteem garnered intrinsically and self-esteem to which outside sources contributed. Datta (2013) identified three aspects of extrinsic self-esteem, which are attention (i.e., appearances), status (i.e., fame and glory, dignity, and dominance), and recognition (i.e., reputation or prestige, and importance). There are also three dimensions of intrinsic self-esteem: professional achievement (i.e., mastery and competence), personal enrichment (i.e., self-indulgence and aesthetics), and rearing children to be globally competitive (i.e., independence and freedom; Datta, 2013; Maslow, 1970).

The highest level in the human needs hierarchy is self-actualization. Maslow (1943) described this need as "what a man *can* be *must* be" (p. 382). Self-actualized people pursue self-fulfillment by unlocking creativity, seeking morality, and pursuing truth (Harrigan & Commons, 2015; Thielke et al., 2012). Those who achieve this level are true to their nature (Datta, 2013). As all the lower level needs have been satisfied, the person can engage in activities to find meaning in them or to find meaning in life.

Since its conception, Maslow's Hierarchy of Needs has been used in multiple fields of study. The primary use of the theory was in psychology as a way to explain people's motivation and behaviors (Maslow, 1943). In the field of health care, the theory has been used to determine patient-need priorities (Silvestri, 2014). In gerontology, Maslow's Hierarchy of Needs has been used to determine how health-related technology can help older adults achieve their needs (Thielke et al., 2012). In the field of business, it has been used to determine how to align customer service with customer needs (Finsterwalder, 2010).

Scholars have found that with the change of times, updates of the theory may be needed. Maslow expanded on his work to seek answers related to the motivation of self-actualized people (Guest, 2014). He believed that intrinsic values such as "truth, goodness, perfection, excellence, simplicity, elegance, and so on" (Maslow, 1969, p. 4) would motivate self-actualized people. Guest (2014) proposes the hierarchy should be updated to include intrinsic values as the highest level.

Although Guest proposed an expansion of the hierarchy, Harrigan and Commons (2015) sought to make Maslow's theory more practical and measurable. They believed Maslow's Hierarchy of Needs could be measured by giving numerical values to actions, which were aimed at meeting the needs of the hierarchy. They reinterpreted needs as stages and categorized actions by whether they were primary or secondary reinforcers of motivation, as a person moved from one stage to another. According to the tool, the higher the score, the better the social perspective (Harrigan & Commons, 2015).

Henderson's Nursing Needs Theory

Virginia Henderson developed the Nursing Needs Theory to describe the focus of nursing and to assist with setting goals in patient care (Henderson, 1966). The basis of the Nursing Needs Theory is reflected in her definition of nursing "to assist the individual, sick or well, in the performance of those activities contributing to health or its recovery (or to a peaceful death) that he would perform unaided if he [sic] had the necessary strength, will or knowledge. And to do this in such a way as to help him [sic] gain independence as rapidly as possible" (Henderson, 2006, p. 26). She identified 14 needs, which when met, facilitated the patient's independence and functioning. Each need is discussed subsequently.

Similar to Maslow's Hierarchy of Needs, Henderson incorporated physiological, safety, and higher order needs. However, unlike Maslow, the emphasis was not on the prioritization of needs. Instead, Henderson described these needs regarding patient actions or behaviors, and she delineated more specific and holistic needs than in Maslow's Hierarchy of Needs. For example, Henderson (2006) identified physical-based needs as: (a) breathe normally, (b) eat and drink adequately, (c) eliminate body wastes, (d) move and maintain desired postures, (e) sleep and rest, (f) select and wear suitable clothing, (g) maintain normal body temperature, (h) keep the skin clean and protected. These physical needs not only incorporate the patient's actions but imply that control, choice, and/or adaptation processes are involved in meeting the need.

Henderson addressed safety in the ninth need, which involves avoiding danger in the environment. In addition, safety is incorporated in several physical needs such as maintaining body temperature by adjusting exposure to the environment and protecting the skin. The remaining needs represent what Maslow referred to as higher order needs. However, Henderson identified several needs Maslow did not specify, such as: (a) communicate with others, (b) worship as one chooses, (c) engage in work that provides a sense of accomplishment, (d) engage in recreation, and (e) learn and discover to achieve proper development.

Application of Henderson's Needs Theory is seen in clinical practice, education, administration, and research. Her definition of nursing is operationalized by assisting the patient in performing activities to meet a holistic set of needs. Emphasis is placed on individualized patient care. In nursing education, her theory can be used to design and develop curricula and teach nursing skills in clinical practice. Similarly, nurse administrators can use Henderson's needs theory to evaluate the extent to which their health care setting is meeting patient needs. In nursing research, Henderson (1991) cautioned that it is important for nurses to study nursing functions and approaches to basic nursing care to prevent stagnation and to provide validation for nursing's actions. Henderson's Needs Theory can provide a framework for studying and classifying nursing care.

Orem's Self-Care Deficit Theory

During the 1950s, Dorothea Orem began searching for the characteristics of nursing that were unique to nursing. During that decade she collected and categorized those characteristics based on her experience, and succinctly defined nursing as, "The inabilities of people to care for themselves at times when they need assistance because of their state of personal health" (Orem, 1995, p. 5). With the help of other nurse theorists, the idea grew. Propositions and relationships were formed, and her theory was published in 1971. Over the years the theory underwent modifications including reformulation of the concept of self-care requisites, the development of a practice guide (Denyes, Orem, & Bekel, 2001), and the inclusion of spiritual self-care (White, Peters, & Schim, 2011).

Orem proposed three separate but interrelated theories that constitute the Self-Care Deficit Theory (Orem, 2001). These "constituent theories" include Nursing Systems Theory, Self-Care, and Self-Care Deficit. The Nursing Systems Theory begins with the central idea that when nurses perform actions (single or systemic) for legitimate patients by prescribing, designing and providing care, a nursing system is formed. These systems regulate the self-care of an individual and evaluate the relationship between the individual's demand for care and his or her ability to perform that care. The central idea of the Self-Care Theory is that care of self and care of dependents are learned behaviors for the purpose of regulating human structural integrity, function, and development. In cases where self-care is done by another, as in children or other dependents, the caregiver is called the *care agent*. However, the ability to care for either self or dependents is called *agency*. The central idea of the constituent Theory of Self-Care Deficit is that people benefit from nursing as a result of health-related limitations that make them incapable of caring for themselves. Each constituent theory is based on propositions and presuppositions as depicted in Table 11.1.

Simply stated, Orem's philosophy of nursing declares that there are behaviors necessary for self or dependent care. These behaviors may include everything from remaining hydrated to the performance of complex therapies in crisis situations. When the ability, or agency, of the self (or caregiving other) does not have the ability to perform the behaviors, nursing fills that self-care agency deficit.

Orem's theory continues to be useful in research, education, and practice. Nursing researchers have fertile soil in this complex model and have studied multiple aspects of the three constituent theories, their relationships, propositions, and presuppositions (Box 11.1). An example of an advanced practice model for psychiatric nursing based wholly on Orem's principles was reported by Grando (2005). A survey of baccalaureate nursing programs found the majority of those using a nursing theory to structure the curriculum used Orem (Taylor & Hartweg, 2002). Overall, nurse educators from a variety of types and levels of nursing programs have found Orem's theories useful in structuring curriculum for educational programs (Berbiglia, 2011).

Orlando-Pelletier's Nursing Process Discipline Theory

Ida Jean Orlando-Pelletier used empirical data as the starting point of her theory development. She observed nursing situations with the goal of determining what constitutes effective nursing practice (Orlando, 1990). Her theory is one of the first to present essential components of how nursing worked and is one of the early nursing theories addressing relationships with other people in the nursing system (Schmieding, 1988).

Orlando-Pelletier's nursing process is triggered by patient behavior. A patient's need for nursing care is reflected in the patient's behavior. She noted that there is a positive relationship between the length of time a patient experiences a need and the level of distress the patient feels because of the unmet need. The longer the time the patient is experiencing the need, the higher the level of distress the patient experiences. A patient's need for help usually stems from the inability to complete activities usually done independently (Orlando, 1990). The need for help could be because of physical limitations, negative effects on the environment, or situations where the patient is unable to communicate needs. Nurses should continually assess for changes in the patient's behavior to determine whether it indicates a need for help.

Sensory perception of a change in patient's behavior stimulates the nurse to react to the change. Orlando-Pelletier stated that the nurse's reaction follows the sequential pattern of perception of behavior through senses, conversion of perception into an automatic thought, and conversion of the thought into feelings about the patient's distress (Orlando, 1990). For confirmation of accuracy, the nurse shares her reaction with the patient. The process of sharing creates a climate where the patient can comfortably share his or her need for help with the nurse (George, 2011).

When the nurse receives a positive confirmation that his or her perceptions, thoughts, and feelings reflect the patient's distress, the next step is to act on the distress (nursing action). The goal of nursing care in Orlando-Pelletier's theory is to provide immediate help to meet the patient's need. The concept of immediacy is central to her theory. Orlando-Pelletier described two types of nursing actions: automatic and deliberative (Orlando, 1990). She describes the latter as based on the professional function of the nurse. *Automatic actions* are initiated without thought to the patient's immediate need, while *deliberative actions* directly benefit the patient through the resolution of the distress. Part of the action step is for the nurse to evaluate whether the care provided is effective in relieving the patient's need (Orlando, 1990).

Orlando-Pelletier is often critiqued by nursing scholars as the theory does not apply to nursing care situations that require long-term planning and education for the resolution of patient needs. The theory is most applicable in acute illness situations where nurses can

TABLE 11.1 Propositions and Presuppositions in Orem's Self-Care Deficit Theory

Constituent Theory	Summary of Propositions	Summary of Presuppositions
Theory of Nursing System	1. Legitimate recipients of nursing are people with inadequate care because of condition or nature of requirements. 2. The design of nursing seeks and confirms information, makes judgments about demands, agency, or dependence. 3. Nursing is compensatory and localized. 4. Nursing confines itself when learning can overcome certain limitations. 5. Nursing system structure varies depending on the demands and deficits of the legitimate recipients.	1. Nursing is a practical health service. 2. Nursing is an art involving designing and providing nursing care. 3. Nursing is result-achieving in interpersonal and social arenas. 4. The results of nursing are movement to positive health/well-being.
Theory of Self-Care Deficit	1. People who take action have specialized capabilities. 2. Caregivers are conditioned by age, development, experience, sociocultural orientation, health, and resources. 3. The relationship between the ability to care and the care demand can be determined. 4. The relationship between care ability and care demand are defined as equal to, less than, or more than. 5. Nursing is legitimized when demand exceeds patient's abilities, or a future deficit can be foreseen. 6. Deficit or projected deficit equals social dependency which legitimates a nursing relationship. 7. A deficit may be permanent or transitory. 8. Deficits may be eliminated. 9. Type of deficit guides the selection of the intervention.	1. Self-care requires management in stable or changing environment. 2. Self-care is affected by valuation of care measures. 3. Quality of care rests on culture and educability of community groups. 4. Deficit of care is affected by lack of knowledge about specific conditions. 5. Societies provide aid for socially dependent people. 6. Dependent people in institutions need the direct help of others. 7. Direct care is either age-related or not. 8. Direct care is meant to provide assistance irrespective of age. 9. Nursing is one of the social groups that provide care.

(continued)

TABLE 11.1 Propositions and Presuppositions in Orem's Self-Care Deficit Theory (*continued*)

Constituent Theory	Summary of Propositions	Summary of Presuppositions
Theory of Self-Care	1. Materials for care are materials essential for life (e.g., air, food). 2. Conditions provided or maintained by self-care are the safe engagement of human functions. 3. Materials and conditions needed for self-care must be required for human life, development, structural integrity, and functioning. 4. Self-care is performed with good intent but may fall short because of limitations. 5. Self-care includes an estimation of what can and should be done, a decision about what will be done, and the production of care through deliberate action. 6. It is work or labor that requires time, energy, finances, and willingness. 7. It is an action system with reliable information and reliable connections among actions. 8. Performance of care is developed over time and becomes habit.	1. People have adequate skill and motivation for effective daily care of self and dependents. 2. Self-care requires the availability, procurement, preparation, and use of resources. 3. Means and procurement of care are cultural and vary between families. 4. Action takes place in the context of stable or changing life situations. 5. Experience enables knowledge of care. 6. Available and communicated knowledge enables care.

Source: Orem (2001).

BOX 11.1 Using Orem's Self-Care Deficit Theory in Baccalaureate Nursing Education

Orem's model has often been used as a structure for educating students in diverse educational programs. To clarify the use of the theory in nursing education, Berbiglia (2011) identified content and criteria for the model's use in training baccalaureate level nurses. Berbiglia offers curriculum threads of caring, self-care agency, self-care requisites, health, nurse agency, nursing system, and nursing process that are based on the model. The threads are content specific for each of four levels: beginning, intermediate, and advanced undergraduate, and a graduate level. A discussion of Orem's original curriculum map is presented as an underpinning for the proposed use. Further exploration of both the importance of theory-based education and the Self-Care Deficit Theory in baccalaureate education is suggested (Berbiglia, 2011).

monitor patients for changes in behavior. Several studies have indicated that the theory can be applied to leadership and management situations in nursing (Laurent, 2000; Schmieding, 1988). See Box 11.2, which summarizes the use of the Nursing Process Theory in nursing leadership.

Roper–Logan–Tierney Model for Nursing

In 1980, a trio of British nurses, Roper, Logan, and Tierney, developed a model for nursing that linked nursing care with people's lifestyle (Tierney, 1998). Roper and colleagues recognized that an individual's need for nursing was usually short term. Therefore, it was important for nurses to value the person's current lifestyle preferences and activities. Building on Henderson's definition of nursing, Roper et al. (1980) defined nursing as "helping people to prevent, alleviate, solve, or cope with problems (actual or potential) related to the activities of living" (p. 37). By emphasizing prevention, their definition added to the scope of nursing practice. Unlike other frameworks that focused on nursing activities to meet patient needs, Roper's model focused on the activities performed by the patient (Roper et al., 2000).

The central concepts of the model are activities of living, factors influencing the activities of living, the person's level of dependence or independence in engaging in activities of living, life span factors, and individualizing nursing (Box 11.3). The theory categorizes factors that influence the patient's ability to perform activities of living into (a) biological, (b) psychological, (c) sociocultural, (d) environmental, and (e) politico-economic factors (Tierney, 1998).

Similar to Henderson's theory, there is no attempt to prioritize needs. However, the Roper–Logan–Tierney Model adds to our understanding of the nature of nursing by adding factors that influence activities of living while providing a continuum of dependence and independence. The concept of life span is overarching. It impacts the person's abilities and needs regarding activities of living, factors that influence the activities of living, and factors influencing the person's dependence and independence. The model culminates with the concept of individualized nursing, which uses the nursing process to assess, plan, implement, and evaluate nursing care.

Gordon's Functional Health Patterns and Nursing Diagnoses

Marjory Gordon was among the first to recognize and propose a resolution to the need for a common language by which nurses could categorize, justify, and share their work. Gordon believed the standardized language was a necessity and the result of nurses' autonomy and accountability (Herdman & Gordon, 2000). The initial work of the North American Nurses

---

BOX 11.2 Orlando's Model and Nursing Leadership

Laurent (2000) distinguishes nursing management from nursing leadership, then discusses the lack of an organized model specific to nursing leadership. According to the author, the nurse manager focuses on what is to be done and the processes by which they are done. A leader is one whose focus is the leader–follower relationship and the involvement of those followers in the processes of doing. Orlando's model stresses the importance of the relationship, the sharing of the assessment, and the verification of the truth of the assessment, which occurs as part of the relationship. The plan of action is then made based on the assessment of the patients' needs, making the role of the leader that of a guide rather than that of a controller (Laurent, 2000).

BOX 11.3 Activities of Living in the Roper–Logan–Tierney Model for Nursing

- Maintaining a safe environment
- Communicating
- Eating and drinking
- Eliminating wastes
- Cleaning and dressing the body
- Controlling body temperature
- Mobilizing the body
- Working and playing
- Sleeping
- Expressing sexuality
- Dying

Source: Tierney (1998).

Diagnosis Association (NANDA) committee, of which Gordon was a part, resulted in an alphabetized approved list of nursing diagnoses. This list was the initial attempt to answer the need for a common nursing language. Subsequently, Gordon arranged the diagnoses by health patterns she had developed over the course of many years as a teaching tool for health assessment. This model, known as Gordon's Functional Health Patterns, acted as a way to categorize nursing diagnoses and even as a structure to guide the nurse's assessment of the patient's environment and needs.

This model emphasizes the connection between diagnostic judgment and therapeutic judgment. According to Gordon (1994), there are 11 functional health patterns. They are: health perception/health management, nutritional/metabolic, elimination, activity/exercise, sleep/rest, cognitive/perceptual, self-perception/self-concept, role/relationship, sexuality/ reproductive, coping/stress-tolerance, and value/belief patterns, and each of the health patterns includes an individual, family, and community category. In each of these categories, a health history and an examination is completed to gather assessment data. When identifying health patterns, the nurse also notes any interaction among the functional health categories.

Dysfunctional health patterns are those patterns noted when a constructed pattern differs from the norms of development, social–cultural, and personal baseline values. Those patterns can be a change from a functional to a dysfunctional pattern, a stabilized dysfunctional pattern, or a stabilized developmental dysfunctional pattern. The relationships among dysfunctional patterns are of particular interest when causal relationships can be established. The construction of a pattern could also include the presence of a risk state.

Using the patterns (especially dysfunctional patterns) found in the functional health assessment tool, the nurse notes the specific nursing diagnoses found in the health function categories. The nurse is then led quickly and efficiently to potentially useful nursing plans and interventions. The most common criticism of this approach is that nurses do the work and do it well, whether they use the same language or not (Griffiths, 1998). Researchers have found evidence both for and against a common language and the use of uniform assessment measures. In particular, much research has been conducted on the efficacy of using the Functional Health Patterns Model as a tool for assessment in different settings and populations (Decker & Knight, 1990; Dunne, Coates, & Moran, 1997; Nettle et al., 1993; Recker & O'Brien, 1992).

◉ CONCLUSION

Meeting patient needs is the foundation of the frameworks discussed in this chapter. Nightingale provided the foundation and the impetus for organizing and planning nursing care designed to meet patient needs. Although the frameworks developed post-Nightingale vary according to prioritization (e.g., Maslow compared to Henderson or Roper, Logan, & Tierney) and components of specific population needs (as in Orlando-Pelletier), nurses find that meeting the patient's needs consumes the larger part of the working day.

As the quality of health care is in part evaluated by patient satisfaction (Al-Abri & Al-Balushi, 2014), it is important to note that care for the needs of a patient is the most basic element of patient satisfaction. The frameworks reviewed in this section use the processes of planning, delivering, and evaluating care as a foundation for addressing the patient's needs, which contribute to patient satisfaction and quality of care. Individually, these frameworks provide organized ways of thinking about patient needs and anticipating, meeting, and evaluating the success of patient care efforts. See Table 11.2 for a comparison of needs-based frameworks.

TABLE 11.2 Comparison of Needs-Based Frameworks

Theory	Author/Discipline	Unique Attributes
Hierarchy of Needs	Maslow/ Psychology	Presents pyramid of five needs categories. Before progressing to higher needs, lower needs must be met.
Environmental Theory	Nightingale/ Nursing	Identifies what patients need from a nurse (13 canons). Healing is enhanced by manipulating the internal and the external environment.
Nursing Needs Theory	Henderson/ Nursing	Identifies 14 needs, not prioritized. Focuses on patient actions that promote holistic health.
Model for Nursing	Roper, Logan, Tierney/ Nursing	Identifies 12 activities of living in five categories. Focuses on individualized influences of patient behaviors and prevention.
Nursing Process Theory	Orlando-Pelletier/ Nursing	Describes processes used to provide nursing care. Identifies two types of nursing actions: automatic and deliberative.
Self-Care Deficit Theory	Orem/ Nursing	Actions necessary for health are supplemented by nursing when people are not able to carry them out for themselves.
Functional Health Patterns	Gordon/ Nursing	Categorizes 11 functional health patterns. Guides patient assessment, categorizes nursing diagnoses. Provides a framework for the nursing process.

⊙ KEY POINTS

- Nightingale's Environmental Theory dates from 1860 and consists of 13 canons, which have formed the basis of most nursing care and theorizing since that time.

- Maslow's Hierarchy of Needs originated from the field of psychology and is used to determine the prioritization of needs deficit and higher-order needs.

- Henderson's Nursing Needs Theory describes 14 needs of the patient that, when met, facilitates the patient's independence and functioning.

- Orem's Self-Care Deficit Theory is composed of three theories that delineate self-care actions, self-care deficit, and nursing systems used to correct the deficit.

- Orlando-Pelletier's Nursing Process Theory stresses the essential components of effective nursing and the goal of nursing care to provide immediate help for the patient's needs.

- The Roper–Logan–Tierney Model for Nursing is focused on prevention and emphasizes the actions/behaviors of the patient rather than those of the nurse.

- Gordon's Functional Health Patterns is an assessment tool. It is often associated with the process of making nursing diagnoses.

REFERENCES

Al-Abri, R., & Al-Balushi, A. (2014). Patient satisfaction survey as a tool towards quality improvement. *Oman Medical Journal, 29*(1), 3–7. doi:10.5001/omj.2014.02

Berbiglia, V. A. (2011). The self-care deficit nursing theory as a curriculum conceptual framework in baccalaureate education. *Nursing Science Quarterly, 24*(2), 137–145. doi:10.1177/0894318411399452

Bolton, K. (2006). Nightingale's philosophy in nursing practice. In M. R. Alligood & A. Marriner-Tomey (Eds.), *Nursing theory: Utilization and application* (3rd ed., pp. 84–95). St. Louis, MO: Mosby.

Datta, Y. (2013). Maslow's hierarchy of basic needs: An ecological view. *Oxford Journal: An International Journal of Business & Economics, 8*(1), 53–67.

Decker, S., & Knight, L. (1990). Functional health pattern assessment: A seasonal migrant farmworker community. *Journal of Community Health Nursing, 7*(3), 141–151.

Denyes, M. J., Orem, D. E., & Bekel, G. (2001). Self-care: A foundational science. *Nursing Science Quarterly, 14*(1), 48–54.

Dunne, K., Coates, V., & Moran, A. (1997). Functional health patterns applied to palliative care: A case study. *International Journal of Palliative Nursing, 3*(6), 324–329.

Finsterwalder, J. (2010). On shaky grounds? Customer needs and service provision after a major disaster in the light of Maslow's hierarchies. *New Zealand Journal of Applied Business Research, 8*(2), 1–28.

George, J. B. (2011). *Nursing theories: The base for professional nursing practice.* Upper Saddle River, NJ: Pearson.

Gordon, M. (1994). *Nursing diagnosis: Process and application.* St. Louis, MO: Mosby.

Grando, V. (2005). A self-care deficit nursing theory-practice model for advanced practice psychiatric/mental health nursing. *Self-Care, Dependent-Care & Nursing, 13*(1), 4–8.

Griffiths, P. (1998). An investigation into the description of patients' problems by nurses using two different needs-based nursing models. *Journal of Advanced Nursing, 28*(5), 969–977.

Guest, H. S. (2014). Maslow's Hierarchy of Needs: The sixth level. *The Psychologist, 27*(12), 982–983.

Harrigan, W. J., & Commons, M. L. (2015). Replacing Maslow's needs hierarchy with an account based on stage and value. *Behavioral Development Bulletin, 20*(1), 24–31.

Henderson, V. (1966). *The nature of nursing: A definition and its implications for practice, research, and education.* New York, NY: Macmillan.

Henderson, V. (1991). *The nature of nursing: A definition and its implications for practice, research, and education: Reflections after 25 years.* New York, NY: National League for Nursing.

Henderson, V. (2006). The concept of nursing. *Journal of Advanced Nursing, 53*(1), 21–31. doi:10.1111/j.1365-2648.2006.03660.x

Herdman, T., & Gordon, M. (2000). Notes on NDEC. The evolving role of DRC: Impact on collaboration with NDEC and other research groups. Nursing Diagnosis Extension and Classification ... Diagnosis Review Committee. *Nursing Diagnosis, 11*(4), 176–178.

Laurent, C. (2000). A nursing theory for nursing leadership. *Journal of Nursing Management, 8*(2), 83–87. doi:10.1046/j.1365-2834.2000.00161.x

Maslow, A. H. (1943). A theory of human motivation. *Psychological Review, 50,* 370–396.

Maslow, A. H. (1969). The farther reaches of human nature. *Journal of Transpersonal Psychology, 1*(1), 1–9.

Maslow, A. H. (1970). *Motivation and personality.* New York, NY: Harper & Row.

Nettle, C., Pavelich, J., Jones, N., Beltz, C., Laboon, P., & Pier, P. (1993). Family as client: Using Gordon's health pattern typology. *Journal of Community Health Nursing, 10*(1), 53–61.

Nightingale, F. (1860/1969). *Notes on nursing: What it is and what it is not.* New York, NY: Dover.

Orem, D. E. (1995). *Nursing: Concepts of practice* (5th ed.). St. Louis, MO: Mosby.

Orem, D. E. (2001). *Nursing: Concepts of practice* (6th ed.). St. Louis, MO: Mosby.

Orlando-Pelletier, I. J. (1990). *The dynamic nurse-patient relationship: Function, process, and principles.* New York, NY: National League for Nursing.

Recker, D., & O'Brien, C. (1992). Using Gordon's functional health patterns to organize a critical care orientation program. *Focus on Critical Care, 19*(1), 21–25, 28.

Roper, N., Logan, W., & Tierney, A. (1980). *The elements of nursing: A model for nursing based on a model of living.* Edinburgh, UK: Churchill Livingstone.

Roper, N., Logan, W., & Tierney, A. (2000). *The Roper-Logan-Tierney model of nursing.* Philadelphia, PA: Elsevier.

Schmieding, N. J. (1988). Action process of nurse administrators to problematic situations based on Orlando's theory. *Journal of Advanced Nursing, 13*(1), 99–107. doi:10.1111/1365-2648.ep13102266

Silvestri, L. A. (2014). *Saunders' comprehensive review for the NCLEX-RN examination* (6th ed.). St. Louis, MO: Elsevier Saunders.

Taylor, S. G., & Hartweg, D. (2002, November). Nursing theory use in baccalaureate programs in the United States (#27). Proceedings of the Seventh International Self-Care Deficit Nursing Theory Conference: The practice of nursing: Using and extending the self-care deficit nursing theory, Atlanta GA.

Thielke, S., Harniss, M., Thompson, H., Patel, S., Demiris, G., & Johnson, K. (2012). Maslow's hierarchy of human needs and the adoption of health-related technologies for older adults. *Ageing International, 37,* 470–488.

Tierney, A. (1998). Nursing models: Extant or extinct? *Journal of Advanced Nursing, 28*(1), 77–85.

White, M. L., Peters, R., & Schim, S. M. (2011). Spirituality and spiritual self-care: Expanding self-care deficit nursing theory. *Nursing Science Quarterly, 24*(1), 48–56. doi:10.1177/0894318410389059

Physiological Frameworks

Lucretia Smith

The bottom line is that the human body is complex and subtle, and oversimplifying ... can be hazardous to your health.
—Andrew Weil

KEY TERMS

Adaptation to Chronic
  Pain Theory
allele
automatic processing
Biobehavioral Model of
  Altered Dysregulation in
  Circadian Systems
Cellular Immunity
  Theory
chromosome
Chromosome Theory of
  Inheritance
Classical Immunology
Clonal Selection
  Theory
cognitive-evaluative
  dimension
controlled processing
Danger Model
Developmental Origins
  Theory
Distraction and Coping
  with Pain Model
dominant trait

Dynamical Systems
  Approach Endogenous
  Pain Control Theory
epigenetics
gametes
Gate Control Theory of Pain
gene
Generalized Motor
  Program Theory
genetic drift
genetic mutation
genome
genotype
Germ Theory
Internal Dynamics Model
Koch's postulates
law of dominant traits
law of independent
  assortment
law of segregation
mitosis
Model for the Development
  of Dependence-Related
  Lesions

natural selection
network hypothesis
Neuroendocrine-Based
  Regulatory Fatigue
  Model
Optimal Control Theory
Pattern Theory
phenotype
Physical Stress Theory
Piper Integrated
  Fatigue Model
sensory-discriminative
  dimension
Specificity Theory
Spielman's Three-Factor
  Insomnia Model
Symmetrical Immune
  Network Theory
symmetrical inhibition
symmetrical killing
symmetrical stimulation
Theory of Balance
  Between Analgesia and
  Side Effects

1. Summarize attributes of selected frameworks related to human physiological phenomena.
2. Compare and contrast the theoretical explanations of physiological phenomena.
3. Discuss the use, by nurses and others, of theories of disease causation, physiological processes, response to stressors, and disease defense.

Nurses, especially as they grow into an advanced practice role, use physiological theory in many varied ways, from predicting short- and long-term disease processes to predicting outcomes of prescription medication and other therapies. Although these frameworks are well supported, they are not unalterable facts and may represent only a limited perspective. The nurse is cautioned to use a mindset that is open to diverse frameworks and evaluate research that tests physiological phenomena and its application to clinical practice, thereby assisting the patient in attaining optimum wellness.

This chapter reviews a selection of physiological theories that may be used by nurses, especially those in advanced practice roles. Because the role functions of clinicians are many and varied (e.g., caregiver, teacher, advocate, guide, leader, and change agent), each nurse also has additional models that guide clinical practice. The aim of this writing is to introduce the nurse to a broad scope of physiological frameworks that can be used to guide nursing care and enhance the wellness possibilities for patients.

The structure of this chapter begins with the genetic frameworks, followed by causation of disease, and ends with frameworks related to physical stress responses. It is hoped that this organization aids the reader in exploring the multiplicity of physiological frameworks and choose those most appropriate for practice. Due to the technical and rapidly evolving nature of these frameworks, the reader is referred to the References section at the end of the chapter for further exploration.

◉ GENETIC AND GENOMIC FRAMEWORKS

Genetics is the study of how characteristics are transmitted to offspring, the role of genes in the inheritance of traits. *Genes* are a set of instructions composed of DNA that function together for building a specific protein. *Genomics* involves the study of the *genome* or the entire structure of DNA/RNA within an organism (Genetic Science Learning Center, 2016). In this section, the progression of the study of genetic science is briefly reviewed, beginning with Mendelian inheritance and concluding with the subject of genomics.

Mendelian Inheritance

The basis of genetic theory stems from the work of Gregor Mendel in the 1860s. Mendel originally conducted research on the propagation of plant life (i.e., peas) to establish how various traits of peas could be reproduced. He discovered three laws of inheritance (Reid & Ross, 2011). First is the *law of segregation* that describes what happens to *alleles* that constitute a gene when they separate from each other during the formation of *gametes*. Second is the *law of independent assortment* that explains that an organism has many different genes, but each includes a code for a different *phenotype* or physical expression. Third is the *law of dominant traits* that purports that in every pair of alleles, one is more likely to be expressed (i.e., dominant) than the other. At the time, Mendel's ideas were not widely accepted but later were found to be translatable to other life forms.

Mendelian inheritance was explained further through the work of scientists Sutton, Boveri, and Flemming in the early 1900s (Paweletz, 2001; Satzinger, 2008). Sutton and

Boveri, working independently, discovered that *chromosomes* carry the genetic information that is passed on to offspring and that chromosomes are present in all dividing cells. They found that chromosomes occur in matched pairs with one pair from the mother and the other pair from the father. They also discovered that proper development of the embryo requires the presence of all chromosomes. Flemming, a physician and biologist, studied the process of cell division and how the chromosomes are distributed to subsequent cell nuclei. He referred to this process division as *mitosis*. These scientific findings paved the way for the development of the *Chromosome Theory of Inheritance* discussed in the following.

Chromosome Theory of Inheritance and Gene Theory

The geneticist, Thomas Morgan, build his work upon previous research by Mendel, Sutton, Boveri, and Flemming, and integrated that knowledge to form the Chromosome Theory of Inheritance (O'Connor & Miko, 2008; Reid & Ross, 2011). Through the study of inheritance traits in fruit flies, Morgan discovered that the transmission of certain genes was determined by the transmission of the X chromosome. His research confirmed that sex-linked characters were inherited.

Sturtevant, an assistant on Morgan's research team, began looking closely at the chromosomal material and was able to map the placement of the genes on the chromosomes of fruit flies (Farrell, 2012). As a result of Morgan's research, the inheritance of genetic traits was linked to the behavior of chromosomes. In 1933, Morgan received the Nobel Prize in Medicine for his work in establishing the Chromosomal Theory of Inheritance (O'Connor & Miko, 2008). In 1946, Muller, another student of Morgan's, received the Nobel Prize for demonstrating that x-rays can damage DNA and cause mutations. Beadle, another student of Morgan's, won the Nobel Prize in 1958 for furthering the theory to include a direct link between enzyme reactions and the behavior of genes (Farrell, 2012).

Gene theory, a component of chromosome theory, continued to develop in scientists' work with bacteria. The theory's original form proposed a linear process for producing genetic material from DNA, to RNA transcription, to protein synthesis without feedback. This linear model gave rise to the notion that the genes had the final say about human development. However, when the complete genome was mapped, there were about 25,000 genes and at least three times that number of proteins, making the concept of one gene per protein obsolete (Capra & Luisi, 2014). The genomic map also revealed evidence of rogue genes breaking away, replicating themselves, and reinserting themselves into the chromosome. In addition to this finding, support was found for the idea that RNA, which contains a copy of the genetic data from a strand of DNA, was being reprogrammed while in route to the cytoplasm where protein synthesis would occur.

Models of Population Genetics

The study of *population genetics* evolved from the culmination of several diverse frameworks including Darwin's Theory of Evolution, Mendelian Inheritance, Morgan's Chromosome Theory of Inheritance, and the Mathematical Theory of Probability. Combining this history with advances in medicine and artificial intelligence in the late 1900s enabled the first proposed sequence of the human genome to be published in 2001 (Christiansen, 2008). Genomic science continues to move beyond basic gene theory (in which the placement of the genes represents the whole of inheritance) to a network of relationships within and outside the DNA sequence, which defines trait inheritance (Horne et al., 2013).

Population geneticists view evolution as variation in the genetic material of a population that occurs over time (Stanford, 2012). Factors involved in population genetics include natural selection, genetic mutation, random genetic drift, and migration of people into or out of the population (Genetic Science Learning Center, 2016). *Natural selection* occurs when individuals in a population enjoy greater longevity or reproduction advantages over others with different genotype attributes. In other words, the changes in the *genotype* or the genetic material of the cell produce changes in the phenotype that may or may not be advantageous. Either way, the changes will have an effect on individuals within the population who share the same genetic information. *Genetic mutation* is a spontaneous and random source of genetic variation in populations. *Genetic drift* is a phenomenon that complicates the study of genetic variation in populations. It refers to chance fluctuations in gene frequency and expression that can lead subpopulations of a species to diverge genetically. *Migration* opposes this trend and tends to make groups more alike. Therefore, when immigrants are genetically different from the population they are entering, this will cause the population's genetic composition to be altered.

Epigenetics

A related theory, epigenetics, was developing simultaneously with genomic mapping. *Epigenetics* (i.e., the study of inherited traits that cannot be explained by changes in DNA sequence) has found that environmental influences have the ability to silence or activate specific genes. The linearity of the original gene theory is changing due to the discovery of genetic feedback loops both inside and outside the human body (Capra & Luisi, 2014). Challenges for researchers studying epigenetics include the transient nature of the epigenetic changes. Specifically, the environmental factor that triggered the silencing or activation of a gene may be reversed or changed when the individual is no longer exposed to the trigger or when exposed to a different environmental stimulus.

Another avenue for research is in the area of epigenetic inheritance. The complexity of the human genome provides the potential for many mutations that could cause a genetic change. As a result, a challenge to establishing epigenetic inheritance is the possibility of a true genetic change accounting for what was thought to be an epigenetic change (Genetic Science Learning Center, 2016). Another condition that must be satisfied is the passage of an epigenetic change through to the fourth generation. This is required to rule out the effects of direct exposure to the environmental condition. For example, a pregnant mother who is exposed to an environmental condition has already potentially exposed three generations. In this case, the mother is the first generation, the fetus second, and the fetus' reproductive cells are the third generation. Therefore, transmission to the fourth generation is necessary to support epigenetic inheritance.

Nurses in practice will find information on genetic frameworks useful in multiple areas of client disease and intervention, from targeted prescribing to environmental assessment. The applications to research and policy development have nearly endless possibilities. Nursing has the potential for significant contributions to the generation of evidence useful for nursing practice and local to global health policy.

● DISEASE CAUSATION FRAMEWORKS

Developmental Origins Theory

In the early 1980s, studies regarding mortality from coronary disease explored multiple data sets for possible causes or contributing factors for heart disease. Interestingly, strong correlations were found in the geographic epidemiologic data (Barker, 2007). These data made a strong case that the conditions surrounding prenatal and birth conditions of a given population were significantly correlated with the incidence of fatal coronary incidents (Barker, 2007). The resulting Developmental Origins Theory included any and all events of the perinatal experience.

The Developmental Origins Theory proposes that outcome concepts such as specific diseases or disease propensity, in general, are related to the perinatal stage of life. More recently, the inclusion of familial inheritance patterns, as a result of perinatal situations, has become a concept of interest. Further investigation of the theory suggests the in utero environment affects not only the adult life of the fetus but may also program the genes in such a way that the effects become intergenerational (Sinclair, Lea, Rees, & Young, 2007).

According to Sullivan, Hawes, Winchester, and Miller (2008), nursing has not sufficiently applied this theory to its utmost potential. Nursing research by Winchester, Sullivan, Roberts, & Granger (2016) focused on the epidemiologic evidence that obstetric conditions are correlated with adult disease (Box 12.1). In both practice and research, the investigation of perinatal conditions either current or past can improve nursing's professional approach and the level of patient care. Given the purposes of the theory are to predict disease, its course, and the human responses to disease, this theory continues to be relevant to nursing.

Germ Theory

Germ theory, or disease transmission theory, has been believed in some form or another for centuries (Karamanou, Panayiotopoulos, Tsoucalas, Kousoulis, & Androutsos, 2012). Before Socrates, disease causation was deeply embedded in religion, followed by the combination of religion and "miasmas," or poisonous vapors from the environment that invaded the body. An architect during the Roman Empire pointed out the dangers of swampy areas and miasmas, and a Roman physician suspected miasmas as the contagious agent in plagues. Perhaps the most brilliant application of contagion and epidemiological principles was found in early biblical history surrounding the spread and control of skin diseases such as leprosy. During the Byzantine period (the 5th to the 15th century CE), breathing and direct contact by an afflicted person were believed to cause disease.

The concept of germs was first mentioned during the 16th century by Fracastoro, who pictured germs as chemical substances rather than an organism (Karamanou et al., 2012). Despite the work of Fracastoro, scientists during the 17th century continued to adhere to the theory of spontaneous generation that purported that living organisms, such as maggots and fleas, arose from inanimate objects. During that period, Redi, an Italian physician, sought to disprove the theory of spontaneous generation. However, it was not until the 1800s, when Pasteur demonstrated that we are surrounded by living organisms, that germ theory was taken seriously. Then, in the late 1800s, Robert Koch, a microbiologist, demonstrated that a specific microbe was responsible for a specific disease and established a set of rules used to determine if an organism causes a disease. *Koch's postulates* or rules should apply to all cases of the causative organism. According to the postulates, the organism must be prepared and maintained in a pure culture to avoid inadvertent cross contamination. Even after several

---

BOX 12.1 Research Using Developmental Origins Theory

The Developmental Origins Theory proposes the idea that perinatal conditions affect the health of the infant into adulthood. This proposition was supported by the research of Winchester, Sullivan, Roberts, and Granger (2016). The researchers collected the cortisol levels in the saliva of 23-year-old people ($n = 180$) and correlated those levels with the perinatal circumstances of the subjects. Striking differences between the cortisol levels were found between those who were of normal gestational age and weight and of those who were premature with low birth weight and morbidities. Interestingly, the socioeconomic status of the people both during the study and during their perinatal period was a statistically significant factor in the research, with the lowest socioeconomic statuses at the highest risk for disease.

generations in culture, the organism should be capable of producing the original infection, and the organism should be retrievable from an inoculated animal and able to be cultured again.

Germ theory is becoming more inclusive and accepting a wider array of causation than a single microbe for a single disease. Dove (2013) notes, "There are more microbial genomes within us than we have human cells. We're a walking ecosystem" (p. 763). Attenborough (2012) believes that multifactorial causes, in addition to modes of transmission, are becoming more realistic than single cause explanations or transmission modes. However, since Koch's rules of causality were disseminated, efforts to develop similar rules of causality and test the multicausality nature of disease have been limited, despite the rise in the availability of knowledge and technology (Inglis, 2007).

The Theory of Etiological Certainty

An example of current thinking is the theory of etiological certainty that uses molecular methods along with more current, inclusive argument styles to build a case for causation. This theory is based on the assertions described in the following.

> Assertion 1: [There is] congruence or reproducible correlation of a taxonomically defined life form with the clinicopathological and epidemiological features of infection.
> Assertion 2: [There is] consistency of the demonstrable biological response in the subject to an encounter with the prospective infective agent.
> Assertion 3: [There is] progressive or cumulative dissonance as an explanation for pathophysiological processes at every known level of biological organization in the subject.
> Assertion 4: [There is] curtailment of that pathophysiological process on the deliberate introduction of a specified biomedical intervention...an initiator of or primer for cumulative dissonance...[is] known as "priobes." Priobes are the sufficient and necessary antecedent causes of a pathophysiological process manifesting as an infectious disease. (Inglis, 2007, p. 56)

The germ theory is used by nurses to provide primary, secondary, and tertiary prevention of disease, communicable or otherwise. The historical progression of this theory is a reminder that theory and knowledge are not static. All nurses whether clinicians, educators, or administrators need to function within a frame of evidence that supports their practice.

⊙ IMMUNOLOGICAL FRAMEWORKS

This section of the chapter deals with how the human body responds immunologically to stress and reaches for wellness. Under this heading, a host of theories from physics, chemistry, biology, could be included. However, only a small sample of the many theories that have been proposed regarding immunological stress and physical health and illness is presented.

The body, in response to the disease causation mentioned previously and the stressors noted in the following, compensates for, or fights off, those influences and attempts to move toward wellness. Research and theorizing about how the body is able to do this have resulted in theories of immunology. The progression of this theoretical knowledge is highlighted beginning with Classical Immunology, Symmetrical Immune Network Theory, and culminating in the Danger Model.

Classical Immunology

During the late 1800s, two opposing theories of immunology were proposed (Silverman, 1989). The first, by Elie Metchnikoff, is referred to as *Cellular Immunity Theory*. This theory holds that the phagocytes are responsible for the body's immune response by attacking and destroying intruding particles. The second, referred to as Humoral Theory, was introduced by Robert Koch and Emil von Behring. The *Humoral Theory* proposed that the immune system is active outside the cell, which is in the "humor." The theory concerns the creation of "side chains" by a cell that defends the cell before damage can reach it. In 1908, both the parties of the opposition co-won the Nobel Prize in medicine. Today's scientists recognize that both models, acting simultaneously, fight disease.

Building on the work of Niels Jerne, Frank Burnet developed the *Clonal Selection Theory*. Jerne had proposed that all antigen patterns were available to the body except antiself. However, Burnet suggested that there was a self/nonself component that triggered the immune response (Burnet, 1976). Accordingly, those things that were identified by the body as "self" would not trigger an immune response, and those things that were "nonself" would trigger a response. In 1970, Bretscher and Cohn proposed a complex process of two-signal activation of the T cells. In the language of the theory, the concepts of "self" and "nonself" continue to have a strong influence on immunology.

Symmetrical Immune Network Theory

In the mid-1970s, using updated discoveries regarding autoimmunity and the help of computer-assisted mathematical modeling, Jerne (1974) proposed a *network hypothesis*. This was in contrast to previous theories that portrayed the immune characteristics as residing in a single cell. In the network hypothesis, the cells of the immune system are interconnected and recognize and respond to each other in addition to identifying and responding to foreign substances. Also, according to the network hypothesis, cells of the immune system are regulated by each other. Thus, a complex array of sets and subsets of cells are proposed. Instead of residing in a single cell, an entire system of cells containing the characteristics was proposed. This hypothesis was supported by a surge of research through the early 1980s resulting in several mathematical models. However, those models did not fit with the emerging genetic mapping and fell out of favor.

However, in 2008, Hoffmann revisited the network hypothesis and proposed a Symmetrical Immune Network Theory. This theory suggests there are symmetrical interactions between cells. Three interactions were proposed: symmetrical stimulation, inhibition, and killing. *Symmetrical stimulation* is where the cells have cross-linked receptors creating responses in one another. The second interaction, *symmetrical inhibition*, uses those cross-links to inhibit the responses. Lastly, *symmetrical killing* involves the direct killing of antigen-specific cells. This symmetry answered many of the questions raised in the genetic mapping of the immune system.

The Danger Model

Matzinger (2002) proposed a theory wherein the immune system does not identify self and nonself-intrusion. Instead, it distinguishes between dangerous and safe by either recognizing "alarm" signals from injury or stress in the body or by the memory of known pathogens. At the root of the theory are molecular patterns secreted by stressed cells. These patterns are both on the surface of the cell and secreted into the extracellular space. These molecule patterns and the patterns of known pathogens are recognized by specific receptors. The receptors are not only on the surface of cells involved in immunity but also in the cytoplasm. The stimulation of the receptors activates the immune system cell that will process antigens, increase the regulation of molecules, and give the antigen to the T cells.

Nurses use the mechanisms described in these frameworks on a daily basis to research the human response to immunity and treat insults to the system. Artificial immunity conferred by immunization of employees and patients is formulated as a result of these theories. Although the immune theories have been greatly simplified in this chapter, their impact on patient care and health and illness is evident. Keeping abreast of new developments enables the nurse to use emerging research in practice, policy making, and leadership activities in which nurses engage (Aickelin & Cayzer, 2002).

◉ MOTOR AND SKELETAL STRESS FRAMEWORKS

While immunologists theorized about how the body fought off intrusion, there were cases in which the immune system did not respond at all and other situations where more than immunity appeared to be involved. This provided the impetus for other disciplines to explore how insults to the body were being addressed and how they impacted the person's ability to achieve wellness. The following theories address some of the body's efforts to protect and rebuild itself. Some of these efforts occur outside of the immune system; others occur in conjunction with immune responses previously discussed.

The Physical Stress Theory

The Physical Stress Theory (PST) was first proposed by Mueller and Maluf (2002). It is an integration of current practice and research in the discipline of physical therapy. This theory is based on the idea that the interventions used in physical therapy are an attempt to modify the physical stress placed on the body tissues; in some cases, to increase the stress (as in the case of exercise), and in other cases to decrease the stress (as in the case of some orthotic devices).

The basic premise of PST is: Changes in the relative level of physical stress cause a predictable adaptive response in all biological tissue. Physical stress is described as a composite value of magnitude, time, and direction. There are 12 fundamental principles underlying the theory, such as,

> Changes in the relative level of physical stress cause a predictable response in all biological tissues. . . . Physical stress levels that exceed the maintenance range result in increased tolerance of tissues to subsequent stresses . . . [and] excessively high levels of physical stress result in tissue injury. (Mueller & Maluf, 2002, p. 39)

In addition to these principles, the theory has four factors that affect the level of stress on the tissue and the response of the tissue to the stress. These are movement and alignment factors (e.g., posture), extrinsic factors (e.g., gravity), psychosocial factors (e.g., social support), and physiological factors (e.g., age; Mueller & Maluf, 2002).

The following theories represent the subsets of PST reviewed by Li (2013) and summarized here. They are offered as an overview of multidisciplinary possibilities, especially relevant for nurses working in advanced roles.

Optimal Control Theory

Movements, especially of the joints of the body, are ultimately controlled by the central nervous system (CNS), which is rich and complex. The CNS is able to accomplish tasks involving motion in multiple ways. When building models to describe the movement and assist in reaching optimal motor ability, this variety of possibilities (also called *degrees of freedom*) interferes with both the mathematical and the practice focus of *the best way* to reach optimal motor ability (Li, 2013).

The Optimal Control Theory seeks to "solve" the degrees of freedom problem by finding, in a single joint making a single motion, which variables can be varied and which cannot. The theory specifies the variables of time, force, impulse, energy, and jerk influence physical control (Li, 2013). Using these parameters, the cost of energy for each movement is balanced with the control needed for smooth movement. The theory postulates that the best condition for optimal control (smooth and efficient movement) is the state of constant stiffness. While this is a useful theory for the control of a single joint, it is based on linear geometry, and the musculoskeletal system generally has multiple joint motions occurring simultaneously in multiple geometric planes.

Dynamical Systems Approach

The Dynamical Systems Approach was proposed in 1990 by three physical therapists involved in researching motor movement (particularly the stepping reflex) in infants (Kamm, Thelen, & Jensen, 1990). They sought to characterize how movement is coordinated and developed in infants. The underlying assumption is that biological organisms are complex, multidimensional, cooperative systems and that no single subsystem has priority in effecting the behavior of the system. For infant leg movements, such as the stepping reflex, the multiple subsystems and their component parts work cooperatively. The Dynamical Systems Approach also considers the context of the behavior and the task as influencing factors. Both the general context (e.g., postural, gravitational, social aspects) and the nature of the task are important organizing influences.

This approach deals with how movement is coordinated and contends that most human movement has a predictable pattern. Using mathematical modeling, research around this theory has been trying to apply the mathematical model to the range of complexity in human movement. The criticism of this theory is that there is no effort to include the integrative process around coordination and the interaction of the activated brain areas during coordinated movement (Li, 2013).

Generalized Motor Program Theory

The Generalized Motor Program Theory was developed by Schmidt and Lee (1999). It is based on the assumption that there are programs of movement "stored" in the CNS. Those programs are, with practiced movement, integrated into generalized patterns. These patterns are then used in both familiar and unfamiliar movement. Although the unfamiliar movements are not executed in exactly the same manner, they have components recognizably similar to the familiar movements.

In the Generalized Motor Program Theory, certain parameters have to be supplied to stimulate the execution of movements (Schneider & Schmidt, 1995). The motor controller gets the information of certain parameters and identifies the motor program to perform the unique activity. In contrast to the Dynamical Systems Approach, the CNS is seen as an integral part of the organization of motor control (Li, 2013).

Internal Dynamics Model

Like the Generalized Motor Program, the Internal Dynamics Model relies on the assumption that the CNS is an integral component of the human's underlying strategy of motor control. However, instead of a "library" of general movement patterns, the CNS learns inverse dynamic models, that is CNS, using past experience, learns to calculate the energy and muscle dynamics needed to accomplish tasks using internal and external conditions. In this case, full limb dynamics, rather than movement, form the shape of the model. These theories also suggest that inverse dynamic models can be incomplete or may fade over time if the conditions around the movement change (Li, 2013).

Nursing, like physical therapy and occupational therapy, is concerned with the response of the human body to stress and how human bodies are able to create and sustain motion. The specific effects of stress to the body (both positive and negative) are of concern, and these principles can be applied to many nursing situations especially those encountered with limitations of client movement or in which a client's neurological or musculoskeletal system must relearn movement as a result of a stressor. Each of the motor and skeletal stress theories provides parameters within which to intervene and conduct research regarding the expectations and limitations of human movement.

Model for the Development of Dependence-Related Lesions

Over the course of modern nursing and medicine, there have been multiple attempts to quantify the risk that a patient will develop a pressure ulcer or other breach in integumentary defense. The Model for the Development of Dependence-Related Lesions (MDDRL) was proposed in 2013 by García-Fernández, Agreda, Verdú, and Pancorbo-Hidalgo. They reviewed 56 scales commonly used to quantify that risk and discovered 83 risk factors that could be classified into 23 risk dimensions. These dimensions formed the basis of a middle range theory, which identifies the mechanism and predicts the occurrence of seven types of dependence-related lesions.

The MDDRL names and defines seven types of lesions and mixed lesions. These are pressure lesions, moisture lesions, friction lesions, combined pressure–moisture, pressure–friction, moisture–friction lesions, and multifactorial lesions. The main etiologic factors are specified as moisture, friction, pressure, shear, and adjuvant factors. Each of these etiologic factors has a dimension; for example, in the etiology of pressure, the decreased capacity of repositioning is the dimension. Each dimension is associated with risk factors. To follow the previous example, a risk factor for the dimension of decreased repositioning capacity could be obesity. Interestingly, this model does not place reduced tissue tolerance in the category of etiology. Instead, it acts as a coadjuvant factor that predisposes the body to the development of the lesions.

The integrity of the skin may be adversely affected by multiple stressors to the body. A breach in skin integrity will call on multiple resources within the body such as nutrition, hydration, circulation, and oxygenation, to compensate. The nurse's ability to correctly assess the condition and manage risk dimensions is essential for the prevention of dependence-related lesions. The approach to lesion treatment and therapy is also determined by the causative mechanisms, and treatment should be adapted according to the etiological factors involved (García-Fernández et al., 2013, p. 37). Providing assessment and direct intervention for the health of the integumentary system is a major concern for nurses in clinical settings. The nurse clinician can use this model to assess for etiological factors, provide interventions to manage those factors, and provide adequate physical resources to support skin integrity.

◉ FRAMEWORKS FOR UNDERSTANDING PAIN MECHANISMS

Pain is a physiological response to various physical insults that usually acts as a protective mechanism against further damage and as a warning that something has gone wrong. However, some pain appears to happen for unknown reasons. The following theories concern the origins and reasons for pain, mechanisms of pain production, and the relief of pain.

Gate Control Theory of Pain

The first modern theories of pain (i.e., those that were proposed after the discovery of neurons and the mapping of the nervous system) were Specificity Theory and Pattern Theory. *Specificity Theory* posits neuroreceptors specific to each pain sensation, while *Pattern Theory* proposes that any sensation is transmitted by all receptors, and the pattern of receptor transmission is the cause of pain sensation (Moayedi & Davis, 2013). Melzack and Wall (1965) then proposed the Gate Control Theory, which uses data supporting both the Specificity and Pattern Theories.

The Gate Control Theory proposes that specific sensory (afferent) fibers exist and the signals from those afferent fibers are transmitted to the substantia gelantinosa, the dorsal column, and to transmission cells. The "gate," which is the substantia gelatinosa located in the dorsal horn, modulates the signals from the afferent fibers to the transmission cells. The gate is controlled by the pain fibers; the large fibers close the gate, and small fibers open the gate. The gate is also controlled by some activities in the brain. For example, when the transmissions reach a particular threshold, the gate is opened and pain is experienced.

After conducting additional research, Melzack and Casey (1968) updated the theory to include multiple dimensions of the human experience that modify the sensation of pain and the elicited behaviors. The specific dimensions were categorized as sensory-discriminative, affective-motivational, and cognitive-evaluative. The *sensory-discriminative dimension* is concerned with processing information about the intensity, time, and space aspects of pain. In the brain, the reticular formation, limbic system, and brain stem mediate the *affective-motivational dimension*. The *cognitive-evaluative dimension* is concerned with learned responses to the experience of pain that may block, modulate, or enhance the perception of pain. While these dimensions can operate somewhat independently, the majority of their actions are interactive.

Adaptation to Chronic Pain

The Adaptation to Chronic Pain Theory is a middle range theory based on the Roy Adaptation Model discussed in Chapter 9 (Dunn, 2005). This theory identifies contextual variables such as age, gender, and race which, along with pain intensity, directly affect the ability to cope. The effects of pain intensity on the outcomes such as functional ability, depression, and spiritual well-being are mediated by coping mechanisms. In addition, both pain intensity and the contextual variables have direct effects on the outcome measures. For example, when an injury around a joint first occurs, it is usually the intensity of pain that restricts its function. Other contextual factors related to age, for example, may also affect the intensity of pain and joint mobility. Then, coping mechanisms used by the individual may either improve or impede the recovery of joint mobility and function. This theory and its underlying research base give direction to nurses in all clinical specialties for managing pain. It increases the nurse's understanding of pain and offers a variety of contributing factors that can be addressed to influence pain outcomes. See Box 12.2 for a test of this model in older adults.

This model depicts chronic pain as a multidimensional stressor that negatively affects individuals not just physically but psychologically, and spiritually as well (Dunn, 2005). It is important for the nurse to consider both focal and contextual stimuli when assessing pain, as they can influence the individual's behavioral response to pain. Dunn recommends that the nature of the focal and contextual variables be considered when planning care for older adults who report chronic pain. Furthermore, those with high pain intensity levels may benefit from multiple interventions in both religious and nonreligious coping categories.

Endogenous Pain Control Theory

Endogenous control of pain was proposed by Basbaum and Fields in 1978. Using opiate agonists, they traced the activation of cells to the dorsal horn of the spinal cord where pain-transmission neurons are inhibited by opiate-like compounds, endorphins. This system is activated by cognitive factors, electrical or chemical stimuli, and by the pain itself.

BOX 12.2 Testing the Adaptation to Chronic Pain Theory

Dunn (2005) used multiple validated assessment tools to create the conceptual variables for the Adaptation to Chronic Pain Theory. The focal stimuli were identified as chronic pain; contextual variables were age, gender, and race. The contextual variables were hypothesized to impact total pain intensity, the use of religious coping and nonreligious coping strategies, and the individual's functional ability and spiritual well-being. Structural equation modeling was used to test the network of relationships depicted in the model. Figure 12.1 shows the best model fit of this research. Interestingly, there were no significant pathways between the demographics and the perception of pain intensity, neither of the coping strategies (religious and nonreligious) mediated any of the three health outcomes, and the relationship between pain intensity and depression was mediated by functional ability. Subjects who reported higher pain intensity had lower spiritual well-being scores, were more functionally disabled and depressed, and used religious and nonreligious coping strategies more often than those with lower pain intensity. In this study, the age, gender, and race of the elders did not affect pain intensity levels but did have a direct impact on the health outcomes.

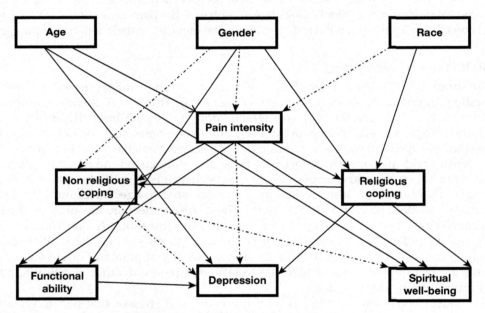

FIGURE 12.1 Model of best fit for Adaptation to Chronic Pain Theory.

Source: Adapted from Dunn (2005).

The theory describes a pain-suppression system that operates at three levels: midbrain, medulla, and spinal cord (Basbaum & Fields, 1978). The midbrain may be activated by opiates, electrical stimulation, or by psychological factors. Activation of the midbrain excites neurons of the medulla, some of which contain serotonin. In the medulla, the neurons specifically inhibit the firing of trigeminal and spinal pain-transmission neurons. A negative feedback loop exists in which the output (i.e., the perception of pain) of the pain-transmission neurons contributes to activating the pain-suppression system.

Distraction and Coping With Pain Model

The model by McCaul and Malott (1984) is based on two assumptions. First, that cognition mediates the pain experience and, second, humans have a limited capacity for focusing attention on different stimuli. The principles of the model propose that distraction reduces distress and distraction techniques that require more attention are more effective. Several principles relate to the intensity of pain including distraction, which is most effective with low-intensity pain. Distraction is more effective than alternative sensation (e.g., ice or heat) for mild pain, but the reverse is true for more intense pain.

The concepts of controlled and automatic processing of painful stimuli are important considerations for using this model. *Controlled processing* occurs when the individual is focused on performing a task that requires the use of short-term memory. This process is also characterized as having limited capacity. In contrast, *automatic processing* is not limited by capacity. It refers to certain tasks that demand minimal attention or awareness, and do not require concentrated effort. For distraction to reduce distress, the pain perception must use a controlled, rather than an automatic, process. McCaul and Malott (1984) hypothesize that the distracting task must be a type that requires controlled processing and reduces the capacity of the system to process pain.

Theory of Balance Between Analgesia and Side Effects

Good (1998) proposed a theory that established the goal of pain control as obtaining a balance between analgesia and the side effects of analgesia. The theory was based on the 1992 pain management guidelines published by the Agency for Healthcare Policy and Research. Although guidelines were based on research, the authors recommended additional research to validate the use in clinical practice. This required that the guidelines be in a testable format of a middle range theory, which led to the development of the Theory of Balance Between Analgesia and Side effects.

The theory is based on several assumptions. First is that physicians and nurses have current knowledge of acute pain management and are able to collaborate. Second, pain medication should be warranted, and third, treatment for side effects should be provided when indicated. Another assumption involves the context in which the theory is used. Good (1998) notes, "The theory is designed to direct treatment of moderate to severe acute pain after operative procedures or trauma, in adults who are able to learn, set goals, and communicate their symptoms" (p. 121). The pain theory does not address pain in children, older adults, and those with opioid tolerance.

Three concepts that produce the outcome of balance between analgesia and side effects are identified. First is multimodal intervention such as the interaction between medication, pharmaceutical adjuvants, and nonpharmaceutical adjuvants. Next is providing attentive care that involves assessment, intervention, and reassessment. Third is patient involvement in care that incorporates teaching and goal setting. The combination of these three concepts form the central concept of the theory, the balance between analgesia and side effects (Good, 1998).

◉ SLEEP DISTURBANCE AND FATIGUE FRAMEWORKS

Sleep is a physiological phenomenon that also benefits the psychological and behavioral dimensions of humans. The most cohesive theories about sleep and fatigue have been developed from studies of cancer patients. Otte and Carpenter (2009) reviewed those theories, and a summary of those they considered well supported is presented here.

Biobehavioral Model of Altered Dysregulation in Circadian Systems

The Biobehavioral Model of Altered Dysregulation in Circadian Systems was proposed as a basis for quantification of psychological functioning as related to the physical system changes (Carlson, Campbell, Garland & Grossman, 2007). The model focuses on identifying and explaining mechanisms that contribute to disturbances in the sleep–wake cycles. The basic concepts of the theory begin with psychological functioning such as in the individual's stress, depression, and mood. These psychological functions interact with the endocrine system (i.e., to regulate cortisol and melatonin), the autonomic nervous system (resulting in sympathetic nervous system catecholamine production), and the sleep system (measured by sleep duration and quality). The outcomes of the model embrace the quality of life, well-being, treatment adherence, fatigue, disease progression, and survival, all of which are affected by the interaction of the physiological systems and psychological functioning.

This model was proposed using an extensive literature review of both psychological and physiological contributors to sleep problems in women. The authors of the model then compared the psychological status and biological systems (including endocrine, autonomic systems, and sleep) of healthy women and women with breast cancer. They assessed the subjects such as psychological and biological functioning, levels of stress, and the presence of mood disturbances. The findings indicated that, although the sleep disturbances and global sleep quality differences between the groups were significant, lower dopamine levels in the women with cancer was the only significant biological difference. The total symptoms of distress were significantly higher in women with cancer as were total mood disturbances (Carlson et al., 2007). The model was supported by the findings that psychological factors and sleep disturbances are higher in women with cancer (although not all of the biological markers were supported). Also, the measures of wellness, depression, and anxiety were significantly more problematic in the women with breast cancer.

Spielman's Three-Factor Insomnia Model

Spielman's Three-Factor Insomnia Model, also called the *3P Model of Insomnia*, is built on a time continuum (Spielman, & Glovinsky, 1991). Predisposing factors, the first P, are the things that make a person more likely to experience insomnia. These factors extend across the biopsychosocial spectrum and include biological factors (i.e., hyperarousal, hyperreactivity), psychological factors such as anxiety, worry, or preoccupation, and social factors such as the sleeping behaviors of one's mate. The second P stands for precipitating events. These events often induce limited periods of difficulty sleeping. Like predisposing factors, they cross the biopsychosocial spectrum and generally represent acute changes affecting sleep such as illness or injury, or waking up to care for a sick infant. Perpetuating activities are the third P, and these are responsible for developing chronic insomnia. Activities such as prolonged time in bed or watching television in bed have been found to encourage insomnia. Also, maladaptive cognitions about sleep may cause the perpetuating activity or produce fear of the upcoming night resulting in a self-perpetuating cycle (Ebben & Spielman, 2009).

The strengths of Spielman's model are the clear treatment recommendations it provides. By identifying the predisposing, precipitating, and perpetuating factors, the nurse will be able to target interventions that address those factors. Other strengths of the model include its conceptualization of how both acute insomnia and chronic insomnia develop.

Neuroendocrine-Based Regulatory Fatigue Model

Payne (2004) described this neuroendocrine model as a multidimensional model useful in the intervention for fatigue in chronic illness. The model proposes that any stress on the endocrine system produces biological consequences that can be traced backward from fatigue.

Antecedents to fatigue are considered either physiological or psychological. The physiological antecedents include demographics, patient profile, disease process, the treatment, pain, age, menstrual status, endocrine system, hematologic system, circadian rhythm, and altered nutrition. Psychosocial antecedents include depression, inadequate social support, lack of spirituality, sense of cultural deficit, impaired coping, and an environment that is either chaotic or inadequate (Payne, 2004).

The antecedents of the stress, either psychological or physiological, are the targets of interventions for fatigue (Otte & Carpenter, 2009). The interventions may include acupressure, acupuncture, massage, pharmaceuticals, therapeutic touch, diet, exercise, distraction, restorative attention, virtual reality, spirituality, light therapy, ethnic or cultural adaptation, adequate coping skills, improved environment, and individualized social support. The interventions then either influence physical biomarkers that influence fatigue or directly influence fatigue. The physical biomarkers include endocrine-based chemicals, specifically: tryptophan, serotonin, melatonin, thyroid-stimulating hormone (TSH), T4, hormones, cytokines, cortisol, endorphins, and catecholamines (i.e., norepinephrine, epinephrine, and adrenocorticotropic hormone [ACTH]; Payne, 2004).

The model proposes that, although fatigue is multidimensional, the interventions for fatigue may be supported by common metabolic pathways or mechanisms. Further, the model supports the idea that multiple symptoms may be connected to the endocrine system and interventions targeting the neuroendocrine system may relieve clusters of symptoms.

Piper Integrated Fatigue Model

This model was proposed to assist cancer patients. The Integrated Fatigue Model suggests that both subjective and objective symptoms of fatigue are influenced by physical, environmental, and psychological factors. The symptoms are categorized into physiological, biochemical, and behavioral components. As fatigue becomes chronic, the symptoms occur more often in combination (Otte & Carpenter, 2009).

The Piper Fatigue Scale was revised after testing on a sample of women who have survived breast cancer (Piper et al., 1998; Piper, Lindsey, & Dodd, 1987). In the revised tool, the total number of items were reduced from 31 to 22, and the number of subscales reduced from five to four. The resulting subscales are: behavioral/severity, affective meaning, sensory, and cognitive/ mood components. Piper and colleagues acknowledge that fatigue is extremely common in persons with cancer. Therefore, accurate assessment tools are needed.

While these theories address fatigue and insomnia in cancer patients, many of the principles should be studied for generalizability to other populations. The concepts of insomnia and fatigue are problematic in multiple client groups that experience chronic disease, pain, anxiety, or other mental health issues. These physiological frameworks and principles may be helpful to nurse clinicians and educators practicing in diverse patient care settings as they provide guidance for assessment and identification of modifiable contributing factors.

● CONCLUSION

Nurses' view of client care should be holistic. The purpose of this chapter is to provide building blocks for the physiological care of the whole person. Only a sample of the frameworks that contribute to our base of knowledge in the physiological realm is presented in this chapter. It is imperative that the nurse appreciates the continual growth of physiological research that supports and expands our understanding of physiological functioning and its interrelationships to psychological, emotional, and social dimensions of the person. See Table 12.1 for a comparison of the physiological frameworks.

TABLE 12.1 Characteristics of Physiological Frameworks

Physiologic Category	Framework	Characteristics
Genetics/genomics	Mendelian Inheritance	Inheritance of traits based on laws of segregation, independent assortment, and dominant traits.
	Chromosome Theory of Inheritance Gene Theory	Transmission of certain genes is linked to the X chromosome; explains the process of producing genetic material from DNA.
	Model of Population Genetics	Variation in genetic material occurs over time and is based on natural selection, genetic mutation, random genetic drift, and migration of individuals in and out of the population.
	Epigenetics	Concerned with environmental influences that can activate or inhibit gene expression.
Disease causation	Developmental Origins	Disease causation begins in the perinatal environment and includes multiple feedback and risk loops.
	Germ Theory	Concerned with understanding the microbial world as both cause and cure of human disease processes; based on Koch's postulates of disease causation.
	Etiological Certainty	Uses molecular methods and logical argument to explain disease causation; based on four assertions including the concept of priobes as an antecedent to disease.
Immunological frameworks	Classical Immunology	Identifies the phagocytic response to intruding substances, development of side chains outside the cell for cellular defense, and triggering of the immune response by recognizing substances such as "nonself" and activating T cells.
	Symmetrical Immune Network	Network hypothesis notes the interconnectedness of the immune system and three types of simulation, symmetrical, inhibition, and killing.
	Danger Model	Recognizes alarm signals from injured or stressed cells; the molecular pattern secreted by these cells is recognized by receptors that activate antigen production.

(continued)

Physiologic Category	Framework	Characteristics
TABLE 12.1 Characteristics of Physiological Frameworks (*continued*)		
Motor skeletal stress	Physical Stress Theory	Change in physical stress results in predictable adaptive responses; stress and tissue response is affected by movement/alignment, extrinsic factors, psychosocial and physiological factors.
	Optimal Control	Focuses on the variables of time, force, impulse, energy, and jerk as influencing physical control.
	Dynamical Systems	Multiple subsystems work cooperatively to produce movement; no single system has a dominant influence.
	Generalized Motor Program	Programs of movement are stored in the CNS and used in executing both familiar and unfamiliar movements.
	Internal Dynamics	The CNS learns movements using inverse dynamic models such as past experiences to calculate the energy and muscle dynamics needed to perform a task.
	Dependence-Related Lesions	Identifies seven mechanisms of dependent lesions and predicts their occurrence.
Pain mechanisms	Gate Control	Describes transmission of pain stimuli to the dorsal horn that modulates pain fibers; influenced by sensory/discriminative, affective/motivational, and cognitive/evaluative dimensions.
	Adaptation to Chronic Pain	Identifies contextual variables (age, gender, race) that affect coping.
	Endogenous Pain Control	Pain-suppression system operates on three levels, the midbrain, medulla, and the spinal cord.
	Distraction and Coping	Based on two assumptions, cognition mediates pain, and people have a limited capacity to focus on different stimuli.
	Balance Between Analgesia and Side Effects	Based on pain management guidelines; used to guide treatment of adults with moderate to severe pain who are able to learn, set goals, and communicate symptoms; incorporates multimodal interventions, attentive care, and patient involvement.

(*continued*)

TABLE 12.1 Characteristics of Physiological Frameworks (*continued*)		
Physiologic Category	**Framework**	**Characteristics**
Sleep and fatigue	Biobehavioral Dysregulation in Circadian Rhythms	Psychological functions have a reciprocal relationship with the endocrine, autonomic, and sleep systems.
	Spielman's Three-Factor Insomnia Model	Based on a time continuum, identifies three predisposing factors, precipitating events, and perpetuating activities.
	Neuroendocrine Regulatory Fatigue Model	The antecedent of stress, both physiological and psychological, are the focus of interventions; the focus is on interventions for fatigue in chronic illness.
	Piper Integrated Fatigue Model	Fatigue is influenced by physical, environmental, and psychological factors; symptoms are categorized as physiological, biochemical, and behavioral; as fatigue becomes chronic, symptoms occur more often in combination.

CNS, central nervous system.

◉ KEY POINTS

- The theory of genetics has been enlarged by the mapping of the genome and the growth of epigenetic discoveries.

- Gregor Mendel's laws of inheritance and Charles Darwin's idea of natural selection were the underpinnings of Chromosome Theory, which grew into population genetics.

- Population genetics, now using the mapping of the human genome, proposes multiple inheritance/chromosomal pathways, in addition to environmental influences.

- The theories of Developmental Origins and Germ Theory comprise the most common grand theories about disease causation. They also theorize about the health-protecting aspects of development and microbes.

- Developmental Origins Theory proposes the perinatal experience, the family inheritance patterns, and the interaction between them can predict the occurrence of disease. These factors may also alter genetic material to increase the likelihood of disease in future generations.

- Germ Theory in some form has existed for centuries in the form of direct transmission disease. In current thinking, multifactor causation of disease includes not only germs, but also includes modes of transmission, susceptibility, environment, and a host of other possible contributors.

- The body's response to stress is generally an effort to regain health. The theories of stress responses like motion, immunology, pain, and sleep offer explanations for this phenomenon and interventions to assist the body to wellness.

- The network hypothesis recognizes "teamwork" among cells.

- The Symmetrical Theory defines the roles/responsibilities of "team members," and the Danger Theory includes cells that are targets of disease as part of the "team."

- Skeletal stress theories explain how the body responds to positive and negative stress to carry out the physiological functions of the body.

- The Model for the Development of Dependence-Related Lesions focuses on the importance of the integumentary system of the body and the assessment of its function.

- The Gate Control Theory of Pain explains the cellular level operations of the neurological system in the production and maintenance of the pain sensation.

- The Adaptation to Chronic Pain and Distraction and Coping Theories propose physical mechanisms, environmental contributors, and effective interventions that assist in coping with pain.

- Sleep and fatigue theories are generally proposed in light of disease processes such as cancer. They focus on the physical and environmental causes of sleeplessness and fatigue and suggest interventions to increase overall health.

REFERENCES

Aickelin, U., & Cayzer, S. (2002). The danger theory and its application to artificial immune systems. In *Proceedings of the 1st Internet Conference on Artificial Immune Systems* (pp. 141–148), Canterbury, UK. Retrieved from http://www.hpl.hp.com/techreports/2002/HPL-2002-244.pdf

Attenborough, F. T. (2012). To rid oneself of the uninvited guest: Robert Koch, Sergei Winogradsky and competing styles of practice in medical microbiology. *Journal of Historical Sociology, 25*(1), 50–82.

Barker, D. P. (2007). The origins of the developmental origins theory. *Journal of Internal Medicine, 21*(5), 412–417. doi:10.1111/j.1365-2796.2007.01809.x

Basbaum, A. L., & Fields, H. L. (1978). Endogenous pain control mechanisms: Review and hypothesis. *Annals of Neurology, 4*(5), 451–462. doi:10.1002/ana.410040511

Bretscher, P., & Cohn, M. (1970). A theory of self-nonself discrimination. *Science, 169*(3950), 1042–1049. doi:10.1126/science.169.3950.1042

Burnet, F. M. (1976). A modification of Jerne's theory of antibody production using the concept of clonal selection. *CA: A Cancer Journal for Clinicians, 26*(2), 119–121. doi:10.3322/canjclin.26.2.119

Capra, F., & Luisi, P. L. (2014). *The systems view of life: A unifying vision.* New York, NY: Cambridge University Press. doi:10.1017/CBO9780511895555

Carlson, L. E., Campbell, T. S., Garland, S. N., & Grossman, P. (2007). Associations among salivary cortisol, melatonin, catecholamines, sleep quality and stress in women with breast cancer and healthy controls. *Journal of Behavioral Medicine, 30*, 45–58.

Christiansen, F. B. (2008). *Theories of population variation in genes and genomes.* Princeton, NJ: Princeton University Press.

Dove, A. (2013). Microbiomics: The germ theory of everything. *Science, 340*(6133), 763–765. doi:10.1126/science.opms.p1300075

Dunn, K. (2005). Testing a middle-range theoretical model of adaptation to chronic pain. *Nursing Science Quarterly, 18*(2), 146–156.

Ebben, M. R., & Spielman, A. J. (2009). Non-pharmacological treatments for insomnia. *Journal of Behavioral Medicine, 32*(3), 244–254.

Farrell, C. (2012). Thomas Hunt Morgan. In Salem Press (Ed.), *Great Lives from History: Scientists & Science* (pp. 657–660). Amenia, NY: Salem Press.

García-Fernández, F. P., Agreda, J. S., Verdú, J., & Pancorbo-Hidalgo, P. L. (2013). A new theoretical model for the development of pressure ulcers and other dependence-related lesions. *Journal of Nursing Scholarship, 46*(1), 28–38. doi:10.1111/jnu.12051

Genetic Science Learning Center. (2016, March 1). Basic genetics. Retrieved from http://learn.genetics.utah.edu

Good, M. (1998). A middle-range theory of acute pain management: Use in research. *Nursing Outlook, 46*(3), 120–124.

Hoffmann, G. W. (2008). Immune network theory. Retrieved from http://www.phas.ubc .ca/~hoffmann/book/Immune%20Network%20Theory.pdf

Horne, S. D., Abdallah, B. Y., Stevens, J. B., Liu, G., Ye, K. J., Bremer, S. W., & Heng, H. Q. (2013). Genome constraint through sexual reproduction: Application of 4D-genomics in reproductive biology. *Systems Biology in Reproductive Medicine, 59*(3), 124–130. doi:10.3109/19396368.2012.754969

Inglis, T. J. (2007). Principia ætiologica: Taking causality beyond Koch's postulates. *Journal of Medical Microbiology, 56*, 1419–1422. doi:10.1099/jmm.0.47179-0

Jerne, N. K. (1974). Towards a network theory of the immune system. *Annales d' immunologie, 125C*(1–2), 373–389.

Kamm, K., Thelen, E., & Jensen, J. (1990). A dynamical systems approach to motor development. *Physical Therapy, 70*(12), 763–775.

Karamanou, M., Panayiotakopoulos, G., Tsoucalas, G., Kousoulis, A. A., & Androutsos, G. (2012). From miasmas to germs: A historical approach to theories of infectious disease transmission. *Le Infezioni in Medicina: Rivista Periodica di Eziologia, Epidemiologia, Diagnostica, Clinica e Terapia Delle Patologie Infettive, 20*(1), 58–62.

Li, K. (2013). Examining contemporary motor control theories from the perspective of degrees of freedom. *Australian Occupational Therapy Journal, 60*(2), 138–143. doi:10.1111/1440-1630.12009

Matzinger, P. (2002). The danger model: A renewed sense of self. *Science, 296*(5566), 301–305. doi:10.1126/science.1071059

McCaul, K. D., & Malott, J. M. (1984). Distraction and coping with pain. *Psychological Bulletin, 95*(3), 516–533. doi:10.1037/0033-2909.95.3.516

Melzack, R., & Casey, K. L. (1968). Sensory, motivational, and central control determinants of pain: A new conceptual model. In D. Kenshalo (Ed.), *The skin senses* (pp. 423–439). Springfield, IL: C. C. Thomas.

Melzack, R., & Wall, P. D. (1965). Pain mechanisms: A new theory. *Science, 150*, 971–979.

Moayedi, M., & Davis, K. D. (2013). Theories of pain: From specificity to gate control. *Journal of Neurophysiology, 109*(1), 5–12. doi:10.1152/jn.00457.2012

Mueller, M., & Maluf, K. (2002). Perspective: Tissue adaptation to physical stress: A proposed "physical stress theory" to guide physical therapist practice, education, and research. *Physical Therapy, 82*(4), 383–403.

O'Connor, C., & Miko, I. (2008) Developing chromosome theory. *Nature Education, 1*(1), 44. Retrieved from http://www.nature.com/scitable/topicpage/Developing-the-Chromosome-Theory-164

Otte, J. L., & Carpenter, J. S. (2009). Theories, models, and frameworks related to sleep-wake disturbances in the context of cancer. *Cancer Nursing, 32*(2), 90–104. doi:10.1097/01.NCC.0000339261.06442.7d

Paweletz, N. (2001). TIMELINE: Walther Flemming: Pioneer of mitosis research. *Nature Reviews Molecular Cell Biology, 2*(1), 72–75. doi:10.1038/35048077

Payne, J. K. (2004). A neuroendocrine-based regulatory fatigue model. *Biological Research for Nursing, 6*, 141–150.

Piper, B. F., Dibble, S.L., Dodd, M. J., Weiss, M. C., Slaughter, R. E., & Paul, S. M. (1998). The revised Piper Fatigue Scale: Psychometric evaluation in women with breast cancer. *Oncology Nursing Forum, 25*(4), 677–684.

Piper, B. F., Lindsey, A. M., & Dodd, M. J. (1987). Fatigue mechanisms in cancer patients: Developing nursing theory. *Oncology Nursing Forum, 14*, 17–23.

Reid, J. B., & Ross, J. J. (2011). Mendel's genes: Toward a full molecular characterization. *Genetics, 189*(1), 3–10. doi:10.1534/genetics.111.132118

Satzinger, H. (2008). Theodor and Marcella Boveri: Chromosomes and cytoplasm in heredity and development. *Nature Reviews. Genetics, 9*(3), 231–238. doi:10.1038/nrg2311

Schmidt, R. A., & Lee, T. D. (1999). *Motor control and learning: A behavioral emphasis*. Urbana-Champaign, IL: Human Kinetics.

Schneider, D. M., & Schmidt, R.A. (1995). Units of action in motor control: Role of response complexity and target speed. *Human Performance, 8*(1), 27–49.

Silverman, A. A. (1989). *History of immunology*. New York, NY: Academic Press.

Sinclair, K. D., Lea, R. G., Rees, W. D., & Young, L. E. (2007). The developmental origins of health and disease: Current theories and epigenetic mechanisms. *Society of Reproduction and Fertility Supplement, 64*, 425–443. doi:10.5661/RDR-VI-425

Spielman, A. J., & Glovinsky, P. (1991). The varied nature of insomnia. In P. J. Hauri (Ed.), *Case studies in insomnia* (pp. 1–16). New York, NY: Plenum Press.

Stanford Encyclopedia of Philosophy. (2012). Population genetics. Retrieved from https://plato .stanford.edu/entries/population-genetics/#PopGenModEvo

Sullivan, M., Hawes, K., Winchester, S., & Miller, R. (2008). Developmental origins theory from prematurity to adult disease. *Journal of Obstetric, Gynecologic & Neonatal Nursing, 37*(2), 158–164. doi:10.1111/ j.1552-6909.2008.00216.x

Winchester, S. B., Sullivan, M. C., Roberts, M. B., & Granger, D. A. (2016). Prematurity, birth weight, and socioeconomic status are linked to atypical diurnal hypothalamic-pituitary-adrenal axis activity in young adults. *Research in Nursing & Health, 39*(1), 15–29. doi:10.1002/nur.21707

Psychological Frameworks

Kristina Henry

There is no medicine like hope, no incentive so great, and no tonic so powerful as expectation of something better tomorrow.
—Orison Swett Marden

Adaptation Model of Nursing
Bandura's Social Learning Theory
Behavioral Theory
Biological Theory
Bowlby and Parkes's Four Phases of Mourning
Bowlby's Attachment Theory
Continuing Bonds Theory of Grief
coping

Evolved Psychological Mechanism
General Adaptation Syndrome
grief
Humanistic Theory
Kübler-Ross Grief Cycle
Lindemann's Crisis Theory
Psychodynamic Theory
psychological adaptation
Psychological Resilience Theory
Rando's Six R Process of Mourning

Self-Determination Theory
Self-Esteem Theory
Social Learning Theory
stress
Theory of Analytical Psychology
Theory of Natural Selection
Tidal Model
Trait Theory
Transactional Model of Stress and Coping
Worden's Four Tasks of Mourning

LEARNING OBJECTIVES

1. Explore historical development and modern application of psychological theories in patient planning and care.
2. Describe psychological theories in terms of attributes, assumptions, and applicability to patient planning and care.
3. Compare and contrast psychological theories as applied to patient planning, care, and research.

The profession of nursing is based on the concept of providing holistic care to humans; this includes a comprehensive approach to addressing physical and psychological needs. Nurses must have an understanding of psychological concepts and theories to develop patient-specific plans of care, as well as plans of care designed to emphasize human motivation, behavior, and psychological development. This chapter focuses on psychological concepts and frameworks applicable to nursing care, such as personality development, stress, coping, and grief. These psychological concepts and frameworks reflect the holistic scope of nursing practice and are applicable in diverse health care settings. Theory development is reviewed, as well as examples of relevance in nursing practice and research.

○ PERSONALITY FRAMEWORKS

Many psychologists have studied *personalities* to understand the human psyche. Several theories have been developed to explain personality, including biological, behavioral, psychodynamic, humanistic, and trait-learning theories. In health care, these theories have become the basis for designing and developing patient-specific care. To optimize patient outcomes, nurses must understand human behavior. Personality theory development gained momentum in the early part of the 20th century and continues to develop. The development of personality theory experienced significant overlap; however, the order of presentation in this chapter reflects the developmental chronology.

Psychodynamic Theories

Psychodynamic theorists, such as Sigmund Freud, Erik Erikson, and Alfred Adler explain personality formation based on childhood experiences and unconscious psyche. Psychodynamic theorists focus on the early childhood influence of perceptions, relationships, and personal experiences, as well as the conscious and unconscious mind on personality development. A major component of the child's perceptions, relationships, and personal experiences is related to the parent's influence. Thus, in psychodynamic theories, parental influence is seen as critical to personality development (Cervone & Pervin, 2008).

Freud described three components of personality: id, ego, and superego. The id represents urges and instincts such as hunger, sex, and aggression. The superego represents moral and ethical principles, the conscience. Both the id and the superego represent the unconscious mind. The ego represents the conscious mind and regulates the id and superego with reality and decision making. The ego essentially moderates between the id and superego (Cervone & Pervin, 2008; Freud, 1990).

Erikson described personality development as progressive. He believed an individual must successfully navigate the challenges of one stage of development to graduate to the next stage. For instance, the first stage is trust versus mistrust. The infant who successfully develops trust will also develop a sense of hope to progress through the rest of the stages (Cervone & Pervin, 2008). Erikson's theory of Psychosocial Development is discussed in greater detail in Chapter 6.

Adler studied the effect of birth order on personality development (Adler, 1928). He proposed that the first-born children tend to be more serious, high achieving, and goal oriented, whereas the middle-born children have a range of personality possibilities but tend to be less serious and less goal driven, and may seek direction from the first-born child. The youngest child is more outgoing, not afraid to test the limits. Alder notes that other birth order factors that should be considered are the spacing in years among siblings, the total number of children, and the changing circumstances of the family over time. Adler identified birth order (oldest, middle, youngest) as influential on personality development but not absolute. A combination of factors as described here interacts to affect personality development.

Theory of Analytical Psychology

Carl G. Jung, a student of Freud, did not agree with the concept of sex as a central motivator of human behavior and instead focused on the concept of general life energy (Jung, 2006). Jung also disagreed with the theory of personality development based on childhood experiences and believed personality evolved throughout the life span toward self-realization.

He believed in the unique characteristics of each individual and the equilibrium of the conscious and unconscious psyche.

Jung described the mind as having conscious and unconscious components. The conscious component is the ego and consists of personal thoughts, feelings, memories, and perceptions. In contrast, the unconscious is more complex and consists of both personal and collective attributes. This unconscious component includes forgotten experiences and emotions, such as events that occurred in childhood and may or may not ever be brought to the conscious mind. The collective unconscious is the basis of the personality. The collective unconscious is described as an archetype or symbol shared by people or a society. Jung saw the collective unconscious as a universal symbology belonging to the species, such as a language (2006).

Through the conscious and unconscious mind, individuals react and respond to the environment. Therefore, the individual personality continues to develop through the life span. Understanding personality development is an essential component in providing health care for the individual client. In health care, Jung's Theory of Analytical Psychology is easily generalizable and may be applied to behavioral change and the planning of care.

Trait Theory

The Trait Theory explains personality development through general and wide-ranging personal attributes. Traits are described as stable characteristics, thoughts, or behaviors with some being more dominant than others. For instance, some individuals are quiet and shy, while others are outgoing and sociable. The focus of this theory is identifying and describing personality traits in the development of the individual.

One of the first psychologists to study trait theory related to personality development was Gordon Allport (1937). He described three levels of personality traits: cardinal, central, and secondary. Cardinal traits determine the primary behaviors of an individual. They frame the desires and drives of the person. An example of a cardinal trait is a desire for money and wealth. Central traits are general attributes or characteristics found in varying levels in all people. They determine our behavior but are not as significant as cardinal traits. An example of a central trait would be generosity. Secondary traits are personal likes and dislikes that make each person unique, such as if one likes to exercise or not, or prefers to be around others over solitude.

Many scales and tools have been developed to measure and study personality trait development. The Myers–Briggs Type Indicator and Eysenck Personality Questionnaire are two common personality tools.

Biological Theory

The Biological Theory of Personality Development explains that innate personality traits and aspects of personality are present at birth. These inherited traits are often described as an individual's disposition or temperament. For example, does the person tend to be happy and pleasant or tend to display sullen and irritable qualities? Studies of identical and fraternal twins raised together and raised apart have served as a major methodology for teasing out the effect of environment on personality development and thereby demonstrate this genetic influence on personality.

Psychologist Hans Eysenck was one of the most well-known researchers to study the biological influence of personality development. He believed aspects of personality were linked to genetics and were inheritable. In 1947, he wrote the classic text titled *Dimensions of Personality* in which he described the personality dimensions of neuroticism and extroversion. Eysenck asserted that the degree of cortical arousal was the root of introvert and extrovert attributes. He hypothesized that introverts have high cortical arousal and therefore avoid people and stimulation, whereas extroverts have low cortical arousal and seek interaction and stimulation (Depue & Collins, 1999). He then added a third dimension, psychoticism, defined as the degree of aggression and hostility, to form a three-factor biological model of personality.

Behavioral Theories

Behavioral, social learning theorists believe that personality development is the result of an individual interacting with the environment. B. F. Skinner and John B. Watson are two of the more notable behavioral theorists (Mischel, 1993). They believe that individual characteristics are the result of variations in personal encounters in the course of the life span. Characteristics are learned through personal experience or by observing others. Rewards or punishments may facilitate or hinder the process of personality development.

Behavioral concepts and theories were developed from initial studies of animals and conditioning to stimuli. Animals were repeatedly exposed to a neutral stimulus, such as a bell ringing, and to a natural stimulus, such as food. Eventually, the natural stimulus was removed, and the animal continued to respond to the neutral stimulus. This pairing of stimuli with a conditioned response established a mechanism for shaping behavior that became known as *operant conditioning*. These behavioral concepts provide an explanation for how people acquire new behaviors or learn (see Chapter 7). Behavioral and social learning theories are instrumental in the treatment of psychological conditions such as neuroses and phobias. Repetitive exposure to the stimulus eventually results in a conditioned response. Thus, when an individual with a fear of dogs is repetitively exposed to a dog, the person may become desensitized and reconditioned. Eventually, the individual could create a new conditioned response (i.e., no fear) when exposed to a dog.

Humanistic Theories

The humanistic approach, also called *humanism*, developed in the 1950s due to dissatisfaction with behaviorism and psychoanalytic perspectives that were the prevailing schools of thought. Humanism values the individual's subjective experiences and emphasizes motivation to achieve self-actualization. In 1962, Abraham Maslow published *The Psychology of Being* in which he describes the humanistic approach as the third force in psychology denoting it as an alternative to psychoanalysis and behaviorism. *Humanistic theorists*, such as Carl Rogers and Abraham Maslow, focused on individualism, personal choice, and subjective experiences in personality development. They believed individuals have an instinctive motivation for growth and development toward self-actualization, a position in stark contrast to behaviorism's emphasis on external stimuli and positive and negative reinforcement (Rogers, 1957).

Another difference between humanism and its theoretical predecessors is its grounding in personal perceptions and the present, rather than past events or childhood experiences. The personal perceptions of the present are subjective and include relationships and experiences, which are based on the individual's free will. People respond to their environment and subjective experiences. The environment is constantly changing and the individual's personality develops according to his or her perception of this changing reality. Humanistic Theory has also provided a framework for understanding the motivation for learning. See Chapter 7 for more detail on humanistic theory.

Bandura's Social Learning Theory

Body image is an essential component of self-esteem and psychological development. Albert Bandura (1986) used the Social Learning Theory to explain the individual's development of body image. He noted that children would witness adult's self-degrading behavior related to body image. Those observations coupled with societal influences would lead to the children eventually learning similar behaviors. Bandura's Social Learning Theory focuses on observational learning and emulation of experiences for maturational development.

In applying this theory, familial and media influences are believed to affect children in either a positive or negative manner. The culture in which the child develops influences his or her self-concept and perception. Children are raised observing parental self-criticism regarding body image. The praise, fame, and monetary rewards associated with successful models and celebrities set unrealistic and unreasonable expectations for children. These experiences create aspirations for an unrealistic ideal persona that negatively affects the child's development of self-esteem and body image.

In one study, Social Learning Theory served as a framework for examining ethical and professional behaviors for business students (Hanna, Crittenden, & Crittenden, 2013). Bandura's theory was used to analyze factors that influenced the development of ethical standards for business students from diverse backgrounds and cultures. See Chapter 7 for an overview of Social Learning Theory in education.

Self-Esteem Theory

In 1969, psychotherapist Nathaniel Branden identified the Self-Esteem Theory and published the first edition of *The Psychology of Self-Esteem*. Although not an official collaborative project, Branden's writing does reflect the theories and style of his mentor, Ayn Rand. Branden saw self-confidence, self-respect, and an awareness of personal values as the essence of self-esteem that he identified as critical factors in the psychology of the individual. According to Branden (2001), psychological conditions such as depression and anxiety result from lack of self-esteem and self-confidence.

Branden elaborated on the Self-Esteem Theory to address approaches to psychotherapy. He stressed the value of psychotherapists using their personal morals and principles to influence and guide client's self-esteem development. He describes using sentence-completion exercises as an effective application method (Branden, 2001). For example, the therapist would provide the patient with a sentence stem such as "When I look in the mirror ...." The patient finishes the sentence, thus providing a focus for a therapeutic conversation. This process enables the therapist to analyze patient's beliefs and mental states.

A variety of therapeutic modalities reflects Branden's influence. For example, providers utilize Branden's Self-Esteem Theory to promote self-help and autonomy in psychotherapy analysis and treatments. Branden's theory has had a significant influence on the development of the popular culture of self-help strategies and the prevalence of self-help classes. The use of self-help strategies and understanding the role of self has become essential in a society challenged with limited access to mental health.

Bowlby's Attachment Theory

John Bowlby, a British psychologist, studied the psychological connection and attachment between humans. As a psychoanalyst, he was influenced by Lorenz's study of imprinting in baby geese. Lorenz (1935) discovered a critical period after birth in which the goslings would bond with the first object seen after birth, referred to as *imprinting*. Bowlby described the attachment of the infant to the caregiver as an innate and instinctual response or psychological adaptation, triggered by the need for safety and security. Bowlby further described the presence of attachment behaviors in infants and the effect of attachment on the child's social and emotional development. Children who experience severe caregiver mistreatment or neglect are more susceptible to social development irregularities. For example, a child who has been neglected may experience reactive attachment disorder in which the child fails to establish healthy patterns of relationships with the caretaker or the parent. Although

Bowlby's theory was initially ascribed to infants and children, it was later extended to apply to adults as well (Bowlby, 1980).

Attachment Theory is explained using four basic concepts: safe haven, secure base, proximity maintenance, and separation distress (Bowlby, 1980). Safe haven refers to the child's reliance on a caregiver for comfort when frightened or threatened. A secure base is when the caregiver provides a reliable and stable foundation for the child's development. Proximity maintenance is when the child is supported and empowered to explore but is still able to maintain a close relationship with the caregiver. Separation distress is described as a state in which the child is discontent as a result of separation from the caregiver (Bowlby, 1980).

Other researchers further developed the Attachment Theory through the study of infant and mother attachment patterns and analyzing their responses to threats and separations. Mary Ainsworth and colleagues developed and tested an assessment procedure for infants between the ages of 1 and 2 years called the "strange situation protocol" (Ainsworth & Bell, 1970; Ainsworth, Blehars, Water & Wall, 1978). In this protocol, the child is observed playing while caregivers and strangers enter and leave the room. Four patterns of attachment behavior were noted: secure attachment, anxious–ambivalent, anxious–avoidant, and disorganized–disoriented. The secure attachment relationship pattern is based on the child's ability to securely explore the environment knowing the caregiver will meet the child's needs. This is believed to be a result of responsive and attentive caregiving. The anxious–ambivalent attachment relationship pattern is expressed by a cautious and guarded child. The child demonstrates extreme distress and anxiety with caregiver separation. This relationship is often the result of unpredictable caregiving patterns. The anxious–avoidant relationship pattern is conveyed as the child ignores the caregiver and expresses minimal emotion toward the caregiver regardless of presence. This pattern is more likely to manifest when the child receives no response from the caregiver regardless of communication of needs of the child. In the final pattern, referred to as the disorganized–disoriented relationship pattern, the child presents irregular patterns typically associated with stress. Often, this relationship pattern is the result of unresolved trauma or grief of the caregiver.

Self-Determination Theory

Psychologists Edward Deci and Richard Ryan studied intrinsic motivation related to personal development (Deci & Ryan, 2002). They described the Self-Determination Theory as a process of individual internal motivation to achieve self-realization. The focus is on continual psychological growth and development through relationships.

Deci and Ryan believe three primary components are essential for self-growth: competence, relatedness, and autonomy. Competence is an individual's ability to learn and master skills and meet needs. Relatedness is the feeling of being connected to others and possessing a sense of belonging. Autonomy involves feeling empowered or in control of one's personal behaviors and goals. These components can be negatively impacted by providing extrinsic rewards for intrinsically motivated behaviors. As people become conditioned to expect an extrinsic motivation, they feel less autonomous and competent. This diminishes individual growth and stalls the process of self-determination. Deci and Ryan (2002) explain that the best way to promote competence, relatedness, and autonomy for self-determination is to supply unexpected constructive feedback. The positive encouragement supports and enhances these three essential components.

According to the Self-Determination Theory, relationships can impede or facilitate inherent characteristics of humanity that intrinsically motivate growth and development. For example, inherent characteristics that influence motivation may be natural curiosity, perseverance, or desire. Relationships and experiences alter the development of these characteristics throughout the life span. As with other theories presented, the Self-Determination Theory can be applied in health care to planning individualized treatments and care.

TABLE 13.1 Comparison of Foundational Concepts of Personality Frameworks	
Framework (Theorist)	**Foundational Concepts**
Biological Theory (Eysenck)	• Concerned with innate personality traits (disposition or temperament) linkage to genetics or heredity
Behavioral Theory (Skinner, Watson)	• Individual characteristics due to variations in personal encounters during the life span • Rewards or punishments may facilitate or hinder the process
Psychodynamic Theory (Freud, Erikson, and Adler)	• Development based on childhood experiences and unconscious psyche • Freud: id, superego, ego • Erikson: progressive development in stages • Adler: effect of birth order on personality development
Humanistic Theory (Rogers, Maslow)	• Focused on individualism, personal choice, and subjective experiences • Emphasizes personal development
Trait Theory (Allport, Eysenck)	• Explains personality development through stable personal attributes
Theory of Analytical Psychology (Jung)	• Personality evolves through the life span • Determined by the individual's unique characteristics and the equilibrium of the conscious and unconscious psyche
Self-Determination Theory (Deci, Ryan)	• Intrinsic motivation related to personal development • Focus on continual psychological development through relationships • Competence, relatedness, and autonomy are essential for self-growth
Self-Esteem Theory (Branden)	• Concepts of self-confidence, self-respect, and an awareness of personal value contribute to self-esteem

However, the use of external motivators (e.g., monetary rewards or gifts) needs to be used with caution when implementing care. To maximize results and focus on long-term growth, providing encouragement and positive support is the better option. The key aspects of the Self-Determination Theory and other personality frameworks discussed in this section are outlined in Table 13.1.

OVERVIEW OF STRESS AND COPING

Stress is a generic term used to explain mental, physical, or emotional burden on the body. Everyone experiences stress. Stress can be acute or chronic, resulting in negative physical and psychological effects such as aging or illness (Folkman, 2013). Interestingly, stress can result from both positive experiences such as a wedding or birth of a child, as well as negative experiences such as a divorce or job loss. Regardless of the type and source of stress, each person adapts or copes with stress in his or her own manner.

Stressful life events such as acute crises or hardships also affect family functioning. Families cope with these events or prolonged challenges by restructuring. For instance, if a child is sick, the family must adapt to meet the needs of the child perhaps by the parent staying home to care for the child. This restructures the family and affects family roles and dynamics. Further discussion of family stress is found in Chapter 10.

Stress is a subjective experience and may result in behavioral and psychological changes. Lazarus explained stress as being personally significant and demanding, thus requiring excessive coping skills (1977). Behavioral changes could involve changes in eating habits, smoking, or nail biting. Psychological changes could result in concerns with anxiety and depression, or lead to physical changes such as heart disease and hypertension.

Individuals must develop appropriate coping skills and strategies to deal with and adapt to stress. *Coping* is a subjective response to address or alleviate stress. As people are diverse, their coping strategies reflect this diversity. Individuals develop coping skills on both a conscious and unconscious level. On a conscious level, coping strategies may include engaging in physical activity, seeking support from friends or family, or using drugs or alcohol. On the unconscious level, common coping strategies may be related to diet, such as eating more or less to alleviate stress or developing a habit such as nail biting.

Coping strategies may have both negative and positive effects on the individual. If the person routinely chooses substance abuse as his or her coping strategy, this may lead to negative or detrimental consequences and even exacerbate the stress. However, if the individual routinely chooses a physical activity, such as running or swimming, this may lead to positive outcomes such as physical fitness and enriching experiences and relationships.

Although coping is largely a subjective process specific to the individual, research has attributed variations in coping strategies to gender differences, learned behaviors, and age. For instance, gender differences are seen in how women and men manage stress. Women tend to internalize stress, which may lead to increased incidence of depression (Rosenfield & Mouzon, 2013). However, men tend to externalize stress, which may lead to aggressive behaviors or substance abuse. An individual's environment may affect the coping strategies and learned behaviors as well. People in a supportive and caring environment may choose more effective and positive coping strategies, while someone in a negative or abusive environment may make detrimental choices such as substance abuse (Cohen, Evans, Stokols, & Krantz, 2013). Age differences are also found in coping strategies of children and adults. In response to stress, children may need more assistance with problem solving than adults and may develop attachment issues (Jensen, Ellestad, & Dyb, 2013). The diversity represented in coping strategies necessitates nurses to choose an appropriate theory to guide nursing care that is relevant to patient-specific needs.

General Adaptation Syndrome

The General Adaptation Syndrome (GAS) Theory is considered the foundation for stress research. Many physiological and psychological theories are based on concepts developed from the GAS. Hans Selye was an endocrinologist, who, through the study of rats, described the GAS and the physiological effects of stress on the body. When exposed to a stressor, the person is stimulated and experiences the fight or flight response of hyperarousal. If continuously exposed at a low level, the person becomes conditioned to the stressful stimuli and eventually may no longer be stimulated. The GAS Theory describes the process of learning to adapt to chronic stressful stimuli and thrive in a stressful environment. However, sustained and chronic exposure to stress can eventually lead to physiological changes, disease, and even death (Selye, 1955 & 1956). An individual with a stressful career diagnosed with chronic hypertension may have experienced a physiological response consistent with those described by the GAS.

Selye (1956) described the GAS in three main stages: alarm, resistance, and exhaustion. The alarm stage is an initial reaction and response to the stressor. The resistance stage is experienced with continued exposure to the stressor as the body adapts to the stress. The exhaustion stage is the body's response to continued high-stress exposure and resource depletion. With continued exposure to the stressor, this stage is manifested by disease or possibly death (Szabo, Tache, & Somogyi, 2012).

Psychological Adaption

Psychological adaptation is based on the evolution of human behavior and is also referred to as *evolved psychological mechanism* (EPM). The evolutionary changes result from current needs, historical needs, or consequences from another EPM. These changes assist the individual in accommodating to the environment. Traditionally, evolutionary psychologists have studied the relationship between human behaviors and the environment searching for population trends (Buss, 2004). This research has assisted public health nurses in identifying methods to approach public health threats.

Charles Darwin established one of the most common psychological adaptation theories with the Theory of Natural Selection. His research focused on understanding adaptation in relation to survival in a specific environment. For instance, an animal must adapt to the environment or it will perish as a result of natural selection. David Buss (2004) expanded these concepts and outlined six characteristics of EPMs.

Through the study of psychological adaptation, specific behaviors are analyzed for meaning. Psychological concepts, such as mental and emotional responses, are examined related to the social and cultural environment. For instance, if an individual is repeatedly exposed to a sound, the individual will adapt to the environment and no longer hear the sound. This adaptation is true for nurses working on units with call lights. Nurses become immune to the sounds of alarms beeping and noise of the unit, while the patients are made alert and anxious by the noises.

Adaptation Model of Nursing

Sister Callista Roy developed the Adaptation Model of Nursing (1980) to explain an individual's unique balance of coping with life stressors. She described people as bio-psychosocial beings, constantly interacting with the environment. Each person adapts to stress through the use of one or more of the four modes of adaptation (i.e., physiological, self-concept, roles, and interdependence). The goal is for the individual to find a unique balance between these modes when adapting to stress. Originally, Roy developed the model solely with the individual patient in mind; however, as this model evolved, it was expanded to address families and communities (1980).

Roy described the nurse's role in promoting adaptation to stimuli or stressors to improve or maximize the quality of life. Promoting adaptation is accomplished through a six-step nursing process including behavior assessment, stimuli assessment, nursing diagnosis, goal setting, intervention, and finally evaluation. Each of these steps leads to the ultimate goal of adaptation. This nursing theory is based on a holistic view of the individual, family, and community to achieve a balance through adaptation for health and quality of life.

The assessment of the behavioral response to a stimulus determines whether the response is an adaptive or ineffective coping strategy. When conducting a stimuli assessment, each stimulus is examined based on whether it is immediate or acute. The nurse determines whether it applies to a specific situation and identifies any contributing beliefs or attitudes. Based on behavioral and stimuli assessments, the nurse assigns a nursing diagnosis and begins setting goals. Goals are set in collaboration with the individual and must be realistic and attainable. After the goals are determined, the intervention is implemented to address the stimuli or stressor. The final step is the evaluation of the process and revision if necessary.

Roy's Adaptation Model has been applied in many areas of research. One example involves the study of veteran's adjustment to lower extremity amputation (Azarmi & Farsi, 2015). The model, as summarized in Box 13.1, was used to validate characteristics of the model.

BOX 13.1 Research Application of Roy's Adaptation Model

In a study of veterans with lower extremity amputation, Roy's Adaptation Model was used as a basis for education and adjustment support. Findings of the study validated the use of the model to facilitate physiological and role adaptation; however, it was not effective in self-concept and interdependence categories (Azarmi & Farsi, 2015). Another researcher studied death and dying using Roy's Adaptation Model. This study expanded the theory to include aspects of spirituality and meaning in relation to the death and dying experience (Dobratz, 2014).

Psychological Resilience Theory

Psychological resilience was first popularized by clinical psychologist Norman Garmezy (1973) and was later expanded by developmental psychologist Emmy Werner (1989), in a study of children raised in adverse environments. A cohort of children in Hawaii, who were raised in poverty by parents suffering from mental illness, were sampled. Two thirds of the children grew up exhibiting destructive behaviors such as drug abuse and chronic unemployment, whereas one-third did not exhibit destructive behaviors and were described by Werner as resilient.

The Psychological Resilience Theory is based on an individual's coping with personal challenges or stress. Individuals demonstrate resilience in everyday life by dealing with a variety of challenges in relationships, health, and work. Since everyone experiences challenges and adversity at some point in time, the Psychological Resilience Theory focuses on the ability of the individual to deal successfully with the challenges through the use of effective coping processes.

Resiliency qualities are believed to be developed and are not necessarily an inherent trait. Many factors contribute to an individual's resiliency such as the ability to set and complete goals, self-confidence, awareness of personal strengths, communication and problem solving, as well as the ability to manage impulses and emotions. Research supports resilience as promoting or protecting an individual in an adverse environment and may be assisted by positive social factors, such as supportive family and friends (Herrick, Stall, Goldhammer, Egan, & Mayer, 2014). See Box 13.2 for a synopsis of Herrick et al.'s study using the Psychological Resiliency Theory.

In research, the theory has been applied to studying the phenomenon of personal success and adaptation following extreme personal traumas such as terrorism and natural disasters (Winter, Brown, Goins, & Mason, 2016). The results have been incorporated into the assessment, planning, and implementation of optimal nursing care for clients experiencing trauma. Assisting clients to develop resiliency will reduce long-term effects of stress and assist them to cope with other adversities as well (Winter et al., 2016).

The Tidal Model

The Tidal Model was developed as an interprofessional approach to mental health care and recovery through personal empowerment (Barker, 2000). As mental illness and challenges are known to hinder and suppress individual development and growth, the Tidal Model emphasizes personal strengths and power in delivering mental health care. The adaptation of care to meet the fluctuating needs of the individual characterizes the core concepts of the Tidal Model.

In the Tidal Model, the person is represented by three domains: self, world, and others. A domain is "a sphere of control or influence: a place where the person experiences or acts out

> **BOX 13.2 Research Application of Resilience Theory**
>
> A consortium, including the Fenway Institute of Boston and the University of Pittsburgh Center for Lesbian, Gay, Bisexual, and Transgender Health Research, established a guide to HIV prevention interventions in gay male communities based on resilience concepts. The consortium created a model to address the strengths of the specific community and ultimately impact health promotion efforts by using established community resilience models as frameworks for success (Herrick et al., 2014).

aspects of private or public life … a place where someone lives" (Tidal Model, *A Model of the Person*, 2015, para. 1). The "self" domain is where the person experiences private, subjective thoughts and feelings. It is where emotional pain is first experienced and where the clinician focuses when helping the individual deal with distressing thoughts and feelings. Through personal interaction with the clinician, the individual can share aspects of his or her "self" domain and move into the "world" domain. When the individual's thoughts and feelings are shared with another, thus making private aspects public, the person is acting within the "world" domain. The "others" domain is engaged when the person participates in interpersonal relationships. This is where the person may be influenced by others, and may, in turn, influence others. Throughout these domains, the clinician and client move through the processes of discovery, information sharing, and solution finding (Tidal Model, 2015).

The use of an interprofessional team facilitates meeting the unique needs of individuals by empowering the individuals to explore meaning in their experiences. The physician, pastor, social worker, and family members, all play an integral role as the individual develops, adapts, and progresses. The ability of the team to meet the diverse needs of the individual promotes patient-specific quality care. The basis of the Tidal Model is to help individuals to be resourceful and see the crisis or stressor as an opportunity to explore their individual story and develop goals. Key considerations for implementation of the Tidal Model include: being transparent, showing genuine interest, learning from the individual, allowing the individual to be the expert in his or her own care, accept that change is constant, and valuing the perspective of the individual. The primary goal is to assist the individual to develop resources and to discourage dependence (Buchanan & Barker, 2008).

Transactional Model of Stress and Coping

The Transactional Model of Stress and Coping is a guide to analyze coping processes in response to stress. Stressful experiences are determined by subjective perceptions of the person, the nature of the environment, and available resources (Cohen, 1984; Lazarus & Cohen, 1977). The model consists of a primary and secondary appraisal process in which the individual engages during the coping process.

Primary appraisal occurs when the individual evaluates an event or situation and decides whether the event is stressful or not. The individual's initial assessment of the stressor or event is influenced by subjective experiences related to the event, such as whether it is viewed as a negative, positive, traumatic, or irrelevant event. The secondary appraisal involves assessing the actions or actual coping efforts aimed at problem management and emotional regulation. The optimal outcome is to return to functional status and emotional health. Nurses may use the Transactional Model of Stress and Coping to assess and evaluate an individual's response to stress and the individual's help-seeking and help-acceptance behaviors. As nurses provide education and develop treatment plans, this model is helpful in designing patient-specific care.

Lindemann's Crisis Theory

Crisis Theory is a general theory based on psychological and behavioral responses to any subjective catastrophic event or disaster. The idea of crisis originated in 1944 through the work of psychiatrist Erich Lindemann. Later it was further explored by Gerald Caplan at Harvard University (1964). A crisis is an acute subjective event causing an imbalance and disorganization in normal coping and function. In a crisis, the individual's usual modes of coping or problem solving are no longer available or effective. A crisis is temporary and may last 4 to 6 weeks. During this time, the individual is often more willing to seek professional assistance and engage in new problem-solving techniques (Caplan, 1964; Lindemann, 1944).

Lindemann further described crisis as a change or changes to an individual's equilibrium that causes acute disorder and disruption (1944). There are two primary results of a crisis: (a) the development of adaptive solutions or coping strategies and return to a state of equilibrium, or (b) the use of maladaptive solutions or coping strategies in which the individual does not return to the same level of equilibrium.

Rapoport (1962), a social worker who studied with Lindemann, expanded the crisis theory and categorized crises into three main types: developmental, role transition, or accidental. Essentially, a developmental crisis is based on growth and development of the individual such as occurs in puberty. Role transition crisis involves a major life transition such as empty nesting or retirement. Accidental crises are unexpected or perilous events such as natural disasters. Awareness of these categories enhances our understanding of crisis. Moreover, in the case of developmental and role crises, they may be used to anticipate future crises.

According to Caplan, there are four phases of a crisis. In phase one, an individual experiences anxiety as the result of a stressful event. If coping mechanisms are not effective, a crisis will occur. In phase two, the anxiety and stress escalate. During phase three, the anxiety continues to escalate, and the individual may ask for assistance. The absence of support or lack of adequate coping mechanisms will increase the risk of crisis. Phase four is the process of active crisis where the person experiences unproductive behaviors. The individual is often frightened, disorganized, and unproductive. During active crisis, the goal is to assist the individual to resolve the immediate problem and achieve stability and balance (Caplan, 1964). See Figure 13.1 for a graphic depicting Caplan's Four Phases of Crisis.

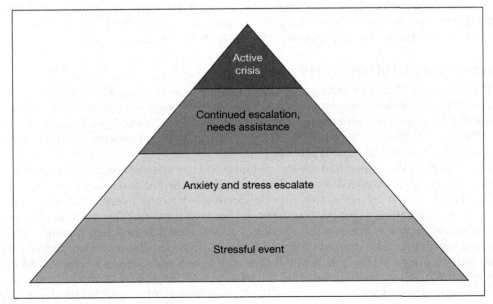

FIGURE 13.1 Caplan's Four Phases of a Crisis.

> **BOX 13.3 Research Application of Crisis Intervention Theory**
>
> Langsley, Kaplan, and Pittman (1968) studied treatments for patients in crisis versus inpatient treatment at a mental health hospital. Through their research, family crisis therapy proved to be an effective alternative. Patients experienced shorter hospitalizations and were less likely to experience readmission. Their social functioning and development of coping skills were improved as well. This study established a viable alternative for inpatient crisis therapy, as well as an initial model for other forms of crisis intervention therapies. It provides a foundation for crisis intervention therapies.

Crisis intervention programs have developed based on the original crisis concepts described by Lindemann (1944) and Caplan (1964). The purpose of crisis intervention is to alleviate symptoms of crisis such as stress and anxiety while limiting the time frame and gravity of the crisis. Through this process, the individual develops problem-solving and coping strategies (Caplan, 1964). Intervention programs and strategies are based on specific needs, circumstances, and populations. For instance, Langsley and Kaplan studied interventional programs related to families in crisis. Patients with early outpatient family interventions and therapy were treated more effectively than patients with acute hospitalization (Langsley, Kaplan, & Pittman, 1968). See Box 13.3 for a study comparing patients in crisis to patients in an inpatient mental health setting.

As a nurse, the goal in crisis response is to assist the individual in making decisions and in expressing feelings in a productive manner. The nurse must remain non-judgmental and supportive. The focus is to reinforce the strengths of the individual and encourage active participation and empowerment in crisis resolution. The individual must learn new coping strategies and regain a level of function.

FRAMEWORKS FOR UNDERSTANDING GRIEF

Grief is an emotional response to a perceived loss that is a subjective and personal experience. The grief theories presented in this chapter share commonalities among key concepts and assumptions, but differ in details of the description and processes. In the 1940s, psychiatrist Erich Lindemann introduced the study of grieving that provided a foundation for many later theorists. His research described the familiar symptoms of grief as somatic symptoms, fixation on the deceased, guilt, forceful reactions, and changes in established roles or behaviors. Lindemann's most noted analysis was the explanation of grief as exhibiting both psychological and physical symptoms, with the progression of grief following a subjective timeline (Satin, 1982). The following theories of grieving are not presented in chronological order but are grouped by similarities.

Kübler-Ross Grief Cycle

A psychiatrist, Elisabeth Kübler-Ross, began studying the emotional responses of people with terminal illnesses in 1969. Through her qualitative research, she developed the Grief Cycle to assist physicians in caring for terminally ill patients (2005). The theory has since evolved and has been applied to any perceived sense of loss (see Box 13.4). This theory focuses on the individual's personal and subjective experience and response, and it provides a general framework useful for assessing clients, understanding the grief process, and assisting individuals to experience grief.

> ## BOX 13.4 Research Application of Kübler-Ross's Grief Cycle
>
> Current research has expanded the application of the Kübler-Ross Grief Cycle to include a variety of causes of grieving other than the death of a loved one. For instance, one study examined the transition to retirement through the lens of the Kübler-Ross Grief Cycle. This study provides guidelines for retirement planning and preparation to assist with the transition through the stages as outlined by the grief model (Wheatley, 2013).

The Grief Cycle is explained in five unordered stages: denial, anger, bargaining, depression, and acceptance (Kübler-Ross, 1969). A person may vacillate between stages and cycle through different emotions at various times. This vacillation reflects the subjective nature of grieving, the individual's development, as well as cultural and familial influences. Denial is described as the initial shock and inability to grasp the reality. Anger is the initial acceptance of reality with misplaced blame of self, others, or spiritual sources. Bargaining is the negotiation for change and a reflection of hope to negate the problem or find a resolution. The stage of depression reflects heartbreak and fear as the individual begins to accept the circumstances. The individual may seek isolation and may cry or show other emotional responses. In the final stage of acceptance, the individual acknowledges the inevitable. Acceptance is commonly demonstrated with a calm and steady retrospective analysis (Kübler-Ross, 2005).

The Grief Cycle may be used to assist health care providers as they plan and implement care, or it may be used as a guide for patients as they progress through their experiences. It is common for people to swing between two or more stages before moving to the next. Also, an individual may become trapped in one stage and unable to transition to another stage. This is detrimental to the emotional recovery process and achieving resilience (Kübler-Ross, 2005).

Worden's Four Tasks of Mourning

Psychologist William Worden (2009) explained the grieving process as the accomplishment of four tasks aimed to establish a new equilibrium. The four tasks of mourning include accepting the reality of the loss, laboring through the pain, adjusting to a new reality, and continuing the process of living. He notes that these tasks are not accomplished in a linear fashion within a specific timeline. An individual's experience is subjective; therefore, the timeline for completion varies with the individual. As a result, a task may be revisited at a later time.

The first task, acceptance of the reality of the loss, enables the individual to understand the loss and death on a deep level. The individual comprehends the full impact and meaning of the experience. The second task is laboring through the pain of grieving. The individual must acknowledge the difficulty of this task, as well as the subjective and personal experience it represents. Some individuals may demonstrate their grief externally and feel the need to share with others, while others may internalize their grief and be private about their grief response. The third task involves a longer timeframe in which the person adjusts to the new reality. During this task, the individual adapts to internal, external, and spiritual changes. This may involve assuming new roles or needing to learn new skills. The final task highlights the continuation of the process of living. The individual will have new relationships and experiences while valuing the memories and continuing to feel connected to the deceased (Worden, 2009).

Bowlby and Parkes's Four Phases of Mourning

As Bowlby studied the attachment of humans to each other as described earlier, he naturally progressed to study the process of grieving when the separation was the result of death or loss. Parkes was a student of Bowlby, and together they developed the Four Phases of Mourning Theory. It is similar to the other theories that describe the grieving process in the context of stages, phases, or tasks. However, the four phases are based on the process of grieving: shock and numbness, yearning and searching, disorganization and despair, and recognition and recovery.

The shock and numbness phase of mourning occur immediately following the death of a loved one. It is a self-defense mechanism related to the emotional trauma. The yearning and searching phase is explained as the grieving individual experiences a void. The individual recognizes and understands his or her anticipated future has forever changed. During this phase, the individual experiences many emotions. The disorganization and despair phase is expressed in withdrawal as the individual accepts the loss. Gradually, the feelings of longing for the deceased become less intense. However, apathy, anger, and pervasive questioning may intensify. The reorganization and recovery phase is the adjustment to a new normal. The individual experiences surges in energy and interest in enjoyable activities. The loss is no longer in the forefront of the individual's mind, and the individual can reflect on positive memories, set new goals, and demonstrate new patterns (Bowlby, 1961).

Rando's Six Rs Process of Mourning

After studying responses to grief, clinical psychologist Therese Rando developed the Six Rs Process of Mourning. This theory emphasizes mourning as a time-consuming and complex process. Mourning is described as a unique, painful, and emotional experience of adjustment to the norm. While grief is an involuntary reaction to loss, mourning is an enduring and active process of adaptation to the loss. Rando describes the mourning process in three distinct phases: avoidance, confrontation, and accommodation. These three phases represent the foundation for the Six Rs Process of Mourning.

The first R is recognition of the loss and is associated with the avoidance phase. Recognition is when the individual understands the loss and the meaning of the loss. The confrontation phase consists of three additional "R" processes: react, recollect, and relinquish. React is the emotional response to the primary loss and any secondary losses such as loss of income or financial security. Recollect refers to the reflection and rumination of memories. Relinquish is when the individual begins to "move on" and accepts the world has changed. The accommodation phase consists of the two final Rs: readjust and reinvest. Readjust is a less acute phase of loss and is the process of returning to lived experiences and activities. Reinvest is the formation of new relationships and commitments. The individual accepts the change, establishes new purpose and goals, and integrates the loss into the changed life (Rando, 1993).

Continuing Bonds Theory of Grief

Klass, Silverman, and Nickman (1996) studied historical accounts of grief and the grieving process in a multitude of cultures. Through their research, they developed the Continuing Bonds Theory of Grief to explain grieving as the creation of a new evolving connection with the deceased. This requires a departure from the traditional grieving process of letting go, accepting the loss, and detaching from the deceased.

The concept of continuing bonds was popularized in the 1996 book titled *Continuing Bonds: Another View of Grief* by Klass and colleagues. The development of a bond with the deceased is viewed as a conscious, dynamic, and changing process. The individual's spiritual beliefs affect how the deceased is incorporated into the life of those who survive. Some of the ways the continuing bonds may manifest are through talking to the deceased, sensing the presence of the deceased, dreaming about the deceased, or turning to the deceased for guidance. Developing rituals and practices that incorporate the deceased such as prayer, remembrances of anniversaries, and regular memorial visitations are other examples of continuing bonds.

Having a continuing bond with the deceased does not mean that the individual is in denial and has not accepted death. It simply refers to the idea of maintaining a nonphysical connection with the deceased. The societal stigma of mental illness is often associated with the idea of having a continued bond or relationship with the deceased; however, in the Continuing Bonds Theory, the bonds with the deceased are viewed as normal and healthy. Instead of complete detachment from the deceased, the survivor has developed meaningful ways to continue the connection. The very nature of the mourner's daily life is changed by the death. The deceased is both present and absent. One cannot ignore this fact and the tension this creates in the bereavement process. The bonds shift and take new forms in time, but the connection is always there.

TABLE 13.2 Foundational Concepts of Stress and Coping Frameworks	
Stress and Coping Frameworks	**Foundational Concepts**
General Adaptation Syndrome (Selye)	Explains the physiological effect of stress on the body • Three main stages of response: alarm, resistance, and exhaustion
Psychological Adaptation (Darwin, Buss)	Based on the evolution of human behavior, also referred to as EPM • Evolutionary changes assist the individual in accommodating to the environment • Theory of Natural Selection: focused on understanding adaptation in relation to survival in a specific environment
Adaptation Model of Nursing (Roy)	Explains an individual's unique balance of coping with life stressors • Adaptation uses the four adaptive modes: physiological, self-concept, roles, and interdependence
Psychological Resilience (Garmezy, Werner)	Based on an individual's coping abilities • The ability of the individual to deal with challenges through effective coping processes • Resiliency qualities developed as a process, not an inherent trait
Tidal Model (Barker & Buchanan)	An approach to mental health care and recovery emphasizing personal empowerment, personal strengths, and power in delivering mental health care • Goal is to assist people to develop their resources and to discourage dependence
Transactional Model of Stress and Coping (Lazarus, Cohen)	Guide to analyzing coping processes, subjective perceptions of the person, the environment, and available resources • Optimal outcome is the return to functional status and emotional health
Crisis Theory (Lindemann, Caplan)	Crisis is an acute subjective event causing an imbalance and disorganization in normal coping and function • Four phases of a crisis

EPM, evolved psychological mechanism.

◉ CONCLUSION

As long as nurses care for people, psychological theories will be applicable. Whether the focus of care is maternity, emergency, orthopedic, or cardiac, the nurse must apply principles of psychological theories. Delivering a baby produces a myriad of emotions and stresses for the mother and the family. The patient in a cardiac emergency is experiencing a life-threatening event with stress, grief, and crisis concerns. Whether they are pleasant or unpleasant, health care experiences are momentous occasions, changing lives, beliefs, and self-concepts. The nurse must provide care, irrespective of the clinical setting or concern, using psychological principles to develop optimal outcomes.

Regardless of the nurse's efforts or strategies to provide physical care, the patient outcomes are directly related to the psychology of the patient. A nurse can teach, advocate, and empower a patient; however, if the patient chooses not to participate due to psychological stressors, the quality of care will be compromised. The nonparticipative patient may foster frustration and a sense of failure by the nurse. However, applying psychological theories is an essential component to understanding the patient, optimizing patient outcomes, and alleviating nurse stress and anxiety.

Psychological frameworks have endless possibilities for application in nursing care. An essential component for providing holistic care involves considering the client's psychological and mental state. The challenge is choosing which framework is most applicable to the concern or problem. It is important to keep in mind that as the patient's care evolves, the psychological factors of concern will change as well. Therefore, the application of frameworks needs to be flexible and dynamic. For ease of comparison, Tables 13.2 and 13.3 summarize the theories and major concepts described in this chapter.

TABLE 13.3 Foundational Concepts of Grief Frameworks	
Grief Theory (Theorist)	**Foundational Concepts**
Kübler-Ross Grief Cycle (Kübler-Ross)	Five unordered stages of grief: denial, anger, bargaining, depression, and acceptance May be applied to any perceived loss
Worden's Four Tasks of Mourning (Worden)	The grieving is a subjective experience Involves four nonlinear tasks: Acceptance, laboring through the pain of grief, adjusting to the new reality, and a continuation of living
Bowlby and Parkes's Four Phases of Mourning (Bowlby, Parkes)	Grieving is a subjective process Based on four phases: shock and numbness, yearning and searching, disorganization and despair, and recognition and recovery
Rando Six Rs Process of Mourning (Rando)	Mourning is a complex, unique, painful, and emotional experience of adjustment to a new norm Three phases: avoidance, confrontation, and accommodation Six processes
Continuing Bonds Theory of Grief (Klass, Silverman, and Nickman)	Grieving involves creating a new relationship with the deceased instead of the traditional concept of accepting the loss and detaching from the deceased Continuing bonds with the deceased are normal and healthy

◉ KEY POINTS

- Personality Theories are used to explain and understand the human psyche including biological, behavioral, psychodynamic, humanistic, and trait-learning theories. These theories have become the basis for designing and developing patient-specific care.

- The Theory of Analytical Psychology proposes that personality evolves through the life span toward self-realization. Carl Jung believed in the unique characteristics of the individual and the equilibrium of the conscious and unconscious psyche.

- The Trait Theory explains personality development through general and wide-ranging personal attributes. Traits are described as stable characteristics, thoughts, or behaviors with some being more dominant than others.

- The Biological Theory of personality development explains that innate personality traits and aspects of personality are present at birth. These inherited traits are often described as an individual's disposition or temperament.

- Behavioral theorists or social learning theorists believe that personality development is the result of an individual interacting with the environment.

- Humanistic theories value the individual's subjective experiences and emphasize motivation to achieve self-actualization.

- Self-Determination Theory is concerned with intrinsic motivation related to personal development. Three primary components are essential for self-growth including competence, relatedness, and autonomy.

- Bandura's Social Learning Theory considers body image an essential component of self-esteem and psychological development. Children witness adults' self-degradation related to body image insecurities and eventually learn similar behaviors.

- Self-Esteem Theory emphasizes self-confidence, self-respect, and an awareness of personal values as the essence of self-esteem and a critical factor in individual psychology. Psychological conditions such as depression and anxiety may result from lack of self-esteem and self-confidence.

- Bowlby's Attachment Theory explains the psychological connection and attachment between humans. It describes the attachment behaviors of infants and the effect of attachment on social and emotional development. There are four basic attributes of Attachment Theory: safe haven, secure base, proximity maintenance, and separation distress.

- Stress is a generic term used to explain mental, physical, or emotional burden on the body.

- Coping is a subjective response to address or alleviate stress.

- The General Adaptation Syndrome Theory describes the physiological effect of stress on the body. Learning to adapt to stress and thrive in the environment is the overall goal. However, sustained and chronic exposure to stress will eventually lead to physiological changes, disease, or eventually death.

- Psychological adaptation is based on the evolution of human behavior and is also referred to as EPM, which assists the individual in accommodating to the environment. The evolutionary changes result from current needs, historical needs, or consequences from another EPM.

- Sister Callista Roy developed the Adaptation Model of Nursing to explain an individual's unique balance of coping with life stressors. She described people as biopsychosocial beings, constantly interacting with the internal and external environment. Each individual must find a unique balance between physiological, self-concept, roles, and interdependence modes of adaptation when responding to stress.

- The Resiliency Theory focuses on the ability of the individual to deal successfully with challenges through effective coping processes.

- The Tidal Model was developed as an interprofessional approach to mental health care and recovery through personal empowerment. This model emphasizes personal strengths and adaptation of care to meet the needs of individuals by empowering them to explore meaning in their experiences.

- The Transactional Model of Stress and Coping is a guide to analyze coping processes of stress as well as available resources. The model consists of a primary and secondary appraisal.

- Lindemann described the signs of grief as somatic symptoms, fixation on the deceased, guilt, forceful reactions, and changes in established roles or behaviors. He described grief as exhibited in both psychological and physical symptoms.

- A crisis is a temporary, acute, subjective event causing an imbalance and disorganization in normal coping and function. An individual's usual modes of coping or problem solving are no longer available or effective.

- Rapoport-categorized crises are divided into three main types: developmental, role transition, or accidental.

- The four phases of a crisis involve the experience of anxiety immediately after the crisis event, escalation of anxiety, continued escalation and help-seeking behavior, and active crisis characterized by unproductive behaviors.

- Elisabeth Kübler-Ross developed the Grief Cycle Theory to explain grief as a personal and subjective experience. It provides a general framework to assess and assist individuals experiencing grief. It is explained in five unordered stages: denial, anger, bargaining, depression, and acceptance.

- Worden's Four Tasks of Mourning depicts the grieving process as the accomplishment of four tasks focused on the process of establishing a new equilibrium: acceptance, the pain of grieving, adjustment, and continuation of the living process.

- Bowlby and Parkes's Four Phases of Mourning presents the process of mourning in four phases: shock and numbness, yearning and searching, disorganization and despair, and recognition and recovery.

- The Six Rs Process of Mourning occurs in three distinct phases: avoidance, confrontation, and accommodation. These three phases represent the foundation for the Six Rs Process of Mourning: recognition, react, recollect, relinquish, readjust, and reinvest.

- Continuing Bonds Theory of Grief explains grieving as the creation of a new relationship with the deceased instead of the traditional concept of accepting the loss and detaching from the deceased.

REFERENCES

Adler, A. (1928). Characteristics of the first, second and third child. *Children*, 3(5),14–52.

Ainsworth, M. D., & Bell, S. M. (1970). Attachment, exploration, and separation: Illustrated by the behavior of one-year-olds in a strange situation. *Child Development*, 41, 49–67.

Ainsworth, M. D., Blehar, M., Waters, E. & Wall, S. (1978). *Patterns of attachment: A psychological study of the strange situation*. Hillsdale, NJ: Erlbaum.

Allport, G. W. (1937). The functional autonomy of motives. *The American Journal of Psychology, 50,* 141–156.

Azarmi, S., & Farsi, Z. (2015). Roy's adaptation model-guided education and promoting the adaptation of veterans with lower extremity amputation. *Iranian Red Crescent Medical Journal, 17*(10), e59544. Retrieved from http://ircmj.com/en/articles/59544.html

Bandura, A. (1986). *Social foundations of thought and action: A social cognitive theory.* Upper Saddle River, NJ: Prentice Hall.

Barker, P. (2000). The tidal model of mental health care: Personal caring within the chaos paradigm. *Mental Health Care, 4*(2), 59–63.

Bowlby, J. (1961). Process of mourning. *International Journal of Psychoanalysis, 42,* 317–339.

Bowlby, J. (1980). *Loss.* London, UK: Penguin.

Branden, N. (2001). *The psychology of self-esteem* (32nd anniversary ed.). San Francisco, CA: Josey-Bass.

Buchanan, P., & Barker, P. (2008). Clarifying the value base of recovery: The 10 tidal commitments. *Journal of Psychiatric and Mental Health Nursing, 15,* 93–100.

Buss, D. M. (2004). *Evolutionary psychology: The new science of the mind.* Boston, MA: Pearson.

Caplan, G. (1964). *Principles of preventative psychiatry.* New York, NY: Basic Books.

Cervone, D., & Pervin, L. (2008). *Personality: Theory and research* (10th ed.). Hoboken, NJ: Wiley.

Cohen, F. (1984). Coping. In J. D. Matarazzo, C. M. Weiss, J. A. Herd, N. E. Miller, & S. M. Weiss (Eds.), *Behavioral health: A handbook of health enhancement and disease prevention* (pp. 114–129). New York, NY: Wiley.

Cohen, S., Evans, G., Stokols, D., & Krantz, D. (2013). *Behavior, health, and environmental stress.* New York, NY: Springer.

Deci, E. D., & Ryan, R. M. (2002). *Handbook of self-determination research.* New York, NY: University of Rochester Press.

Depue, R. A., & Collins, P. F. (1999) Neurobiology of the structure of personality: Dopamine, facilitation of incentive motivation, and extraversion. *Behavioral and Brain Sciences, 22,* 491–569.

Dobratz, M. (2014). Life closure with the Roy adaptation model. *Nursing Science Quarterly, 27,* 51–56.

Folkman, S. (2013). Stress: Appraisal and coping. In M. Gellman & J. R. Turner (Eds.), *Encyclopedia of behavioral medicine* (2013 ed., pp. 1913–1915). New York, NY: Springer.

Freud, S. (1990). *The ego and the id.* New York, NY: W. W. Norton.

Garmezy, N. (1973). Competence and adaptation in adult schizophrenic patients and children at risk. In S. R. Dean (Ed.), *Schizophrenia: The first ten dean award lectures* (pp. 163–204). New York, NY: MSS Information.

Hanna, R., Crittenden, V., & Crittenden, W. (2013). Social learning theory: A multicultural study of influences on ethical behavior. *Journal of Marketing Education, 35*(1), 18–25.

Herrick, A., Stall, R., Goldhammer, H., Egan, J., & Mayer, K. (2014). Resilience as a research framework and as a cornerstone of prevention research for gay and bisexual men: Theory and evidence. *AIDS and Behavior, 18*(1), 1–9.

Jensen, T., Ellestad, A., & Dyb, B. (2013). Children and adolescents' self-reported coping strategies during the Southeast Asian Tsunami. *British Journal of Clinical Psychology, 52*(1), 92–106.

Jung, C. (2006). *The undiscovered self: The problem of the individual in modern society.* New York, NY: New American Library.

Klass, D., Silverman, P., & Nickman, S. (1996). *Continuing bonds: New understandings of grief.* New York, NY: Routledge, Taylor & Frances.

Kübler-Ross, E. (1969). *On death and dying.* New York, NY: Macmillan.

Kübler-Ross, E. (2005). *On grief and grieving: Finding the meaning of grief through the five stages of loss.* New York, NY: Simon & Schuster.

Langsley, D. G., Kaplan, D. M., & Pittman, F. (1968). *The treatment of families in crisis.* New York, NY: Grune & Stratton.

Lazarus, R. S., & Cohen, J. B. (1977). Environmental stress. In I. Altman & J. F. Wohlwill (Eds.), *Human behavior and environment* (Vol. 2, pp. 89–127). New York, NY: Springer.

Lindemann, E. (1944). Symptomology and management of acute grief. *American Journal of Psychiatry, 101,* 141–148. doi:10.1176/ajp.101.2.141

Maslow, A. (1962). *Toward a psychology of being.* Princeton, NJ: Van Nostrand.

Mischel, W. (1993). Behavioral conceptions. In W. Mischel (Ed.), *Introduction to personality* (5th ed., pp. 295–316). New York, NY: Harcourt Brace.

Rando, T. (1993). *Treatment of complicated mourning.* Champaign, IL: Research Press.

Rapoport, L. (1962). The state of crisis: Some theoretical considerations. *Social Service Review, 36*(2), 211–217.

Rogers, C. R. (1957). The necessary and sufficient conditions of therapeutic personality change. *Journal of Consulting and Clinical Psychology, 21,* 95–103.

Rosenfield, S., & Mouzon, D. (2013). Gender and mental health. In C. S. Aneshensel, J. C. Phelan, & A. Bierman (Eds.), *Handbook of the sociology of mental health* (2nd ed., pp. 277–296). New York, NY: Springer.

Roy, C. (1980). The Roy adaptation model. In J. P. Riehl & C. Roy (Eds.), *Conceptual models of nursing practice* (2nd ed., pp. 179–188). New York, NY: Appleton-Century-Croft.

Satin, D. G. (1982). Erich Lindemann: The humanist and the era of community mental health. *Proceedings of the American Philosophical Society, 126*(4), 327–346.

Selye, H. (1955, Oct 7). Stress and disease. *Science, 122,* 625–631. doi:10.1126/science.122.3171.625

Selye, H. (1956). *The stress of life.* New York, NY: McGraw-Hill.

Szabo, S., Tache, Y., & Somogyi, A. (2012). The legacy of Hans Selye and the origins of stress research: A retrospective 75 years after his landmark brief "Letter" to the editor of Nature. *Stress: The International Journal on the Biology of Stress, 15*(5), 472–478.

Tidal Model. (2015). A model of the person. Retrieved from http://www.tidel-model.com/theory

Werner, E. E. (1989). *Vulnerable but invincible: A longitudinal study of resilient children and youth.* New York, NY: McGraw-Hill.

Wheatley, M. (2013). Framework for planning a successful retirement. *Nursing Management, 20*(1), 23–25.

Winter, D., Brown, R., Goins, S., & Mason, C. (2016). *Trauma, survival and resilience in war zones.* New York, NY: Routledge.

Worden, J. W. (2009). *Grief counseling and grief therapy: A handbook for the mental health practitioner* (4th ed.). New York, NY: Springer Publishing.

Role-Related Frameworks

Rose Utley

We can't all be good at everything. This is partly the logic behind having a team in the first place, so each role can be filled with the person best suited for that role and together, every job and every strength is covered.
—Simon Sinek

I have spent many years of my life in opposition, and I rather like the role.
—Eleanor Roosevelt

 KEY TERMS

Baumrind Parenting Styles
expressive role behaviors
instrumental role behaviors
interactionist perspective
Maternal Role
   Attainment Theory
Maternal Role
   Collapse Theory

Parsons's Sick Role
role
role ambiguity
role conflict
role incongruity
role overload
role strain
role theory

Role Transition Theory
Roy's Role Function Mode
Social Role Theory
structuralist perspective
Transition Shock Model

LEARNING OBJECTIVES

1. Differentiate structuralist's and interactionist's perspectives of role and role theory.
2. Define and differentiate concepts and constructs related to role theory.
3. Describe theories and models related to role theory, caregiving, and caretaking roles.
4. Understand the significance of role concepts, constructs, and frameworks for clinical practice, education, leadership, and research.
5. Compare and contrast role theories in terms of emphasis and key concepts.

Role theory is a field of study that includes a family of terminology and conditions that impact the person's ability to function in society. Origins of role concepts and the field of role theory come from anthropology, psychology, and sociology. The concept of role is a universal phenomenon that applies to people from all cultures and all professional, familial, and or social relationships. The term *role* has diverse meanings but commonly refers to the behaviors of a person in a certain social position. Role refers to both expected and socially determined behaviors and the actual behaviors of the person (Hardy, 1978).

In nursing, the term *role* is a noun or a verb concerned with understanding the experiences, actions, responsibilities, and factors that inhibit or enhance professional development within nursing. Understanding barriers and challenges in meeting the role functions for nurse educators, clinicians, leaders, and researchers is essential for improving care delivery and advancing the profession. The concepts of role theory (i.e., role ambiguity, conflict, incongruity, strain, and overload) are helpful for understanding the professional roles; familial roles of parenting and grandparenting; and societal roles such as friend, coworker, volunteer, and neighbor, among others. Role theory is useful for examining role perceptions and functions of nurses, health care providers, patients, and caregivers; and for anticipating and/or mitigating role stress.

According to Muller and Litwin (2011), people do more than merely function within a role; they function in multiple roles and are involved in defining those roles and giving them significance, meaning, and importance. The development of the individual's self-concept is believed to be an ongoing process that occurs throughout the life span. Roles are prioritized and identified by the importance to the individual's self-concept, which evolves over time. More significant roles are given priority in resources including investment of time and energy. Therefore, "A role is a structural position that an individual holds within a social group, whereas identity is a subjective self-evaluation of this role" (Muller & Litwin, 2011, p. 110). Thus, roles become a part of the person's self-concept and identity.

◉ OVERVIEW OF ROLE PERSPECTIVES

In this chapter, the concept of role is discussed from the structuralism and the interactionist's perspectives. Then, the constructs central to role theory and the interrelationships between role constructs are described followed by a summary of role-related frameworks useful in nursing. Social Role Theory, Roy's Role Function Mode, Transition Role Theory, and Transition Shock Model are discussed. Examples of practical applications from the literature are provided for the clinician, educator, nurse leader, and researcher roles.

Social Structuralism Perspective

The social *structuralism* perspective was introduced in the 1920s and hypothesizes that roles are linked to the individual's positions in society. An individual's behavior is shaped by the social structures and systems within society. Roles exist to enable the social system to function, and therefore the nature of the relationship between an existing role within the social structure will adapt as society changes. Structuralism focuses on society, social systems, the social structure, and the person's roles within society. Society and the social systems within it shape the customs, rules, and expectations for the individual's role performance. The term *role*, defined from a structuralist perspective, is the customs, rules, and expectations associated with a person in a particular position (Banton, 1965).

Roles are what link the individual's behaviors to social structure. Structuralists are concerned with taking on a role and internalizing society's role expectations. Roles are the primary mechanism for the functioning of a social system, and they change as society and the institutions within it evolve. Behaviors of individuals acting in roles are determined by societal consensus. Sanctions in the form of social disapproval act as motivators for adherence to established role expectations and norms.

Interactionist Perspective

In contrast to the structuralist approach to role theory, the *interactionist* is concerned with meaning and explaining role behaviors. Interactionists do not deny that societal structure influences role behavior but instead emphasize that social structure alone does not predict a person's role behavior.

The interactionist approach developed in the 1930s as interest shifted from a focus on "role-taking" and societal structure to the relationships between role and the mind, one's self, groups, and society (Brookes, Davidson, Daly, & Halcomb, 2007). Authors such as Mead (1934) drew attention to the relationship between the individual's self-understanding and role taking in society. The interactionist perspective, also referred to as *symbolic interactionism*, focuses on how the individual negotiates meaning in a new role. The focus is on the individual engaged in reciprocal social connections and the "role-making" process. Self-reflective communication that focuses on the symbolic acts in one's speech and nonverbal behavior is essential to the role-making process.

ROLE CONSTRUCTS

The study of role theory incorporates many constructs (two or more concepts combined to form a new term). Most role constructs are concerned with the inner psychological experiences of the person that are influenced by social forces, both structural and interactional. The experience of role stress, role conflict, and role ambiguity denotes internal conditions stemming from the perception that individuals in particular roles may experience. These constructs come to life when certain structural forces such as customs, rules, and expectations conflict, or when interaction, communication, and connection with others do not mesh. Common role constructs, which serve as a foundation for understanding role theory, are discussed in this section.

Role Stress and Strain

Role stress is a perceived condition that results when the social environment produces demands on the individual that are difficult to meet or demands that conflict with those of other roles. Hardy (1978) also includes exposure to role obligations that are "vague, irritating, difficult, conflicting or impossible to meet" (p. 76) as sources of role stress. Therefore, role stress is due to factors external to the individual such as workload, family responsibilities, or a new career. Excessive role stress results in a subjective feeling of distress called *role strain*. Because role strain is internal, it can be mediated by cognitive coping strategies as well as by manipulation of environmental factors that are causing role stress. Role stress and the person's response to role strain are affected by communication and interactions between people, societal expectations and attitudes, and power structures. The nature of these social structures determines the degree to which the environment is perceived as stressful.

Since social structures are major contributors to developing and sustaining role stress, they also contribute to conditions that lead to role strain. *Role strain* is a subjective experience that manifests as a cognitive and affective disturbance such as, distress, anxiety, or uneasiness (Hardy, 1978). These manifestations can occur regardless of whether a change is perceived as positive or negative. The evolution of changes in family structure and family cohesion (e.g., increase in divorce and remarriage rates), combined with changing work environments, complex health care systems, and social organizations contributes to role stress and strain. As a result, the experience of role ambiguity, role conflict, role overload, and role incongruity is a common phenomenon in modern society.

Role Ambiguity

Role ambiguity exists when there is a lack of clarity about the expectations of the role. This commonly occurs in new positions or positions that are undergoing change. For example, acquiring a new role as a parent or as a professional in a new career is typically associated with uncertainty and lack of role knowledge and experience, resulting in role ambiguity. In addition to uncertainty, common features of role ambiguity include a lack of clarity, confusion, and/or a lack of agreement about the role expectations (Brookes et al., 2007; Hardy, 1978).

As noted earlier, role ambiguity may occur in either personal or professional roles. However, regardless of the type of role ambiguity, it will typically relate to one or more of the following: (a) how the work will be evaluated, (b) how the individual can advance, (c) uncertainty about the scope of responsibilities, or (d) uncertainty about the expectations of others (Handy, 1985). Lack of clarity about professional role expectations has been further classified by the source of the expectations. In nursing, as well as other professional roles, four sources of expectations fuel role ambiguity: institutional, professional–peer, public, and self-expectations (Benne, & Bennis, 1959). Regardless of the source, the effect of uncertainty, unclear expectations, and lack of role knowledge or experience contributes to role ambiguity, which also contributes to other role constructs. An example of a study of the relationship between role ambiguity and role strain in an academic setting is presented in Box 14.1.

Role Conflict, Incongruity, and Overload

Role conflict occurs when the individual assumes two or more conflicting or incompatible roles (Biddle & Thomas 1979; Brookes et al., 2007). The two roles may be contradictory or mutually exclusive. Role conflict from the coexistence of two differing roles is seen in a person who is a supervisor to his or her spouse, or a close friend. Other examples of role conflict may be subtle and internalized. A female nursing supervisor may face conflicting expectations in the roles of female, nurse, and leader. As a woman and a nurse, societal expectations such as demonstration of caring, compassion, and supportive behaviors may conflict with expectations for a leader to be firm, directive, and make hard decisions. Role conflict may cause role stress and strain.

The term *role incongruity* shares similarities to role conflict. Both can occur when the individual transitions to a new role or experiences new role expectations. Both are sources of roles stress. However, *role incongruity* occurs when the role expectations are in conflict with the individual's attitudes, values, and beliefs (Brookes et al., 2007; Hardy. 1978). Similar to role conflict, role incongruity can adversely affect role performance making it difficult for the individual to meet role expectations. The nurse's ability to understand and modify role expectations can be useful in resolving or managing conflicts that arise.

Role conflict and role overload are related, but distinct concepts have been used interchangeably in the literature. More accurately, however, *role conflict* results when pressures experienced within a given role are incompatible with fulfilling another role (Biddle & Thomas, 1979; Kelly, 1982). Role overload can lead to role conflict when the time demands of one role inhibit performance in another role. Thus, when the demands for a role exceed the resources and time available, *role overload* exists. Role conflict is likely to be a result of role overload when the individual has limited support and no alternatives to achieve satisfactory role performance. The person can carry out individual role demands effectively but cannot complete multiple expectations for a role. In role overload, the person's resources are

---

BOX 14.1 Study of Role Strain and Role Ambiguity

Cranford (2013) studied the relationship between role ambiguity and role strain experienced by first time nursing faculty from 31 public colleges and universities. Role strain and four determinants of role strain (i.e., role ambiguity, interpersonal support, instructional competency, and demographics) were measured using a 16-item Likert scale. Role ambiguity accounted for 44% of the variance in role strain, with the other factors combined accounting for only 8%.

inadequate to meet the demands of the role (Brookes et al., 2007). Role overload is a type of role stress that may be more prevalent in highly industrialized and competitive societies, or in high-level roles within businesses and corporate systems.

ROLE THEORY PERSPECTIVES

Based on our understanding of the role constructs previously discussed, a variety of perspectives related to role functioning have developed. In this section, we begin with coverage of theories and models that are concerned with role processes such as transition, shock, and adaptation. These include Role Transition Theory, Transition Shock Model, Social Role Theory, and Roy's Role Function Mode. The chapter concludes with coverage of frameworks concerned with types of roles including the sick role, caregiver role, parenting, and grandparenting.

Role Transition Model

Transition is the "passage or movements from one state, condition, or place to another" (Duchscher, 2008, p. 442). Role transition occurs when individuals move from one role to a less familiar role. The degree of similarity between the old and new role and between the old and new role expectations are major determinants of role stress experienced during the transition process. Role Transition Theory is especially relevant for novice nurses who are leaving the world of academia and beginning their clinical nursing practice, or changing from one area of practice to another.

Duchscher (2008) describes the stages of Role Transition Theory for new graduate nurses as encompassing three phases of movement from initial orientation to the end of the first year. The model was developed using a grounded theory approach to clarify and understand the graduate nurse's journey of becoming characterized by progressing through the stages of doing, being, and knowing. Initially, and for first 3 months, the new nurse is immersed in the "doing stage." The doing stage involves the processes of learning, performing, concealing the lack of confidence and knowledge, adjusting, and accommodating. As a result, the new nurse experiences shock as the realities and demands of the work environment challenge previous student experiences. During this initial "doing" phase, the new nurse faces the discrepancies between classroom experiences and the real-life practice of nursing as a career. This first stage is characterized by strong and fluctuating emotions as graduates work through the processes of discovering, learning, performing, concealing, adjusting, and accommodating. The challenge is for the new nurse to assimilate into a new environment that emphasizes providing collaborative-based care.

After the doing stage, the new graduate nurse transitions to the "being stage" around the fourth and fifth month. The transition is marked by a consistent and rapid advancement in the nurse's thinking, knowledge level, and skill competency. The new nurse engages in searching, doubting, and in examining and questioning behaviors. Around the fifth to seventh month, the new nurse may experience a crisis due to a lack of self-confidence or worry about failing to meet personal expectations and those of patients and coworkers. Moving through this crisis serves to develop the nurse's practice and provides a sense of recommitment to the profession, which sees the nurse through the next several months of transition.

The final stage of the graduate nurse's role transition begins around the eighth month and is generally completed by the end of the first year of employment. Referred to as the "knowing" stage, it is characterized by a change in thinking and changes in the sources of stress and support. The new graduate nurse is no longer focused on his or her individual capabilities, performance, and responsibilities. Instead, concerns shift to dealing with the broader health care system. Thus, the factors contributing role stress change from the nurse's ability to cope with his or her new role, to dealing with stresses related to the system. During this final stage, the new graduate nurse also commonly experiences a shift in sources of professional support from nonnursing family and friends to coworkers.

The role transition experience for new graduate nurses involves making major adjustments to the changes in both personal and professional roles. Duchscher summarized the role transition process for new graduates as a journey that "was by no means linear or prescriptive nor always strictly progressive, [yet] it was evolutionary and ultimately transformative for all participants" (Duchscher, 2008, p. 444).

Transition Shock Model

The concept of transition shock was developed from Duchscher's grounded theory study of new graduate nurses as they move from the familiar role of a student to the role of a professional nurse (Duchscher, 2008, 2009). The Transition Shock Model that emerged describes and explains the transition of new graduate nurses during the first stage of role transition (Duchscher, 2009). The model is based on the work of Kramer who coined the term "reality shock" to describe the dissonance between school-based learning and the reality of the work world. The Transition Shock Model incorporates multiple elements including cultural shock, transition theory, reality shock, role adaptation, growth and development, and change theory.

In the role transition process, the new nurse moves through three types of changes: (a) developmental and professional, (b) intellectual and emotive, and (c) changes in skill and role relationships (Duchscher, 2008, 2009). Each area involves changes in experience, meanings, and expectations. Four factors influence the intensity and duration of transition shock including roles, responsibilities, relationships, and knowledge. The new nurse's personal and professional adjustments are intensely experienced during the first 1 to 4 months postorientation, referred to as *transition shock*. According to Duchscher (2009), *transition shock* is the most "immediate, acute and dramatic stage in the process of professional role adaptation for the new nurse" (p. 1111). For the new graduate nurse, the contrast between the relationships, roles, responsibilities, knowledge, and performance expectations within the student environment to those required in professional nursing practice may result in cognitive and affective experiences of loss, doubt, confusion, and disorientation. Duchscher encourages teaching students about the Transition Shock Theory and incorporating preparatory academic and clinical experiences that will decrease the intensity of the transition shock experience.

Social Role Theory

Social Role Theory focuses on the relationships and interactions between individuals, groups, societies, and the economic and social systems in which people live and work (Dulin, 2007). Social Role Theory is concerned largely with the intersection between roles and social concepts such as age, gender, ethnicity, occupation, and social class. Each individual occupies certain positions in society, has relationships with others, and holds expectations about certain social roles. The term *social role* is viewed as expected behaviors, including rights and obligations of a person who holds a given position in society. A distinction is made between the status or position of the person and his or her role, with the role being the enactment of behaviors relevant to the position.

According to Murray (1998), "Social Role Theory provides a general framework for analyzing the psychological processes associated with the transition from one role to another" (p. 106). Social roles involve a reciprocal relationship, for example, to assume the parent role there must be a child. And with these reciprocal roles come expectations (Deasy, 1964). The Social Role Theory provides a linkage between the individual and society and provides a framework for looking at the individual's functioning in a social role.

Eagly, a social psychologist, looked at the reciprocal roles assumed by males and females and developed a social role theory of gender differences (Eagly, 1987; Eagly, Wood, & Diekman, 2000). Her theory explains how the physical differences between men and women led to a division of labor in society and influenced role development. Eagly and colleagues based the division of social roles on Bakan's (1966) concepts of agentic and communal qualities. Accordingly, most beliefs about the differences between men and women can be divided into communal and agentic dimensions. Agentic qualities are characterized by self-assertion, self-expansion, and mastery behaviors and tend to be attributed to males more than females, whereas selflessness, concern for others, and a desire to connect with others characterize communal qualities attributed primarily to females more than males.

Social Role Theory has been used to study a range of phenomena including aggression, helping behaviors, stereotypes, leadership styles, parenting, ethical decision making, athletic performance, and emotional vulnerability (Dulin, 2007). Dulin notes that most research supports the underlying idea that males and females act according to the social norms that have resulted from a division of labor at work and in the home. See Box 14.2 for a study of gender stereotypes based on Social Role Theory.

Roy's Role Function Mode

Roy's Adaptation Model, discussed in Chapter 9, offers a holistic perspective on human adaptation to the environment that occurs through the physiologic, self-concept, interdependence, and role function adaptive modes. Each adaptive mode provides a means by which we can observe a person's adaptation (San Mateo, Roy, & Andrews, 1999). In this chapter, the focus is on the role function adaptive mode, which comprises behaviors associated with role performance and adaptation of the human system.

Roy defined role as a set of expectations concerning how a person in one position acts toward others in reciprocal role relationships. She defines role transition as the "process of assuming and developing a new role" (Roy & Andrews, 1991, p. 364). The process of role transition is reflected through expressive and instrumental role behaviors. *Expressive role behaviors* are the subjective aspects of role performance, specifically one's feelings and attitudes associated with role performance. *Instrumental role behaviors* are observable, objective, role activities performed by the individual.

Roy's concepts of role transition and the role function mode of adaptation have been used to uncover role adaptation processes experienced by frail elders and their family caregivers (Shyu, 2000). In this study, Shyu identified the specific processes of role adaptation experienced between caregiver and care receiver as they transitioned from the hospital to home (Box 14.3).

BOX 14.2 A Study of Gender Stereotypes Using Social Role Theory

Diekman, Goodfriend, and Goodwin (2004) studied the nature of gender stereotypes in working women using Social Role Theory. They conducted two related studies to explore the relationships among perceived power and social roles of men and women, and gender stereotypes. The first study examined participants' beliefs about the power of men and women in the future. The second study examined the perceived gains or losses in power in men and women. In Study 1, participants defined power as having control in occupational, political, and economic realms. In Study 2, participants perceived women as gaining power as they shift from traditional to nontraditional (i.e., male dominated) professional roles. However, a shift in men's roles to include more nontraditional (i.e., female dominated) professional roles was not associated with perceived decreases in men's power. The authors noted that women were perceived to make gains in individual and relational power more so than economic, political, or occupational power.

BOX 14.3 Role Adaptation in Caregiving and Care Receiving

Shyu (2000) conducted a grounded theory study to explore the role adaptation of care-givers and frail elderly who were discharged from the hospital to home. Through the use of interviews with caregivers and care receivers, she uncovered the core process coined as *role tuning*. Role tuning describes the process used by caregivers and care receivers to achieve a harmonious pattern of caregiving and care receiving. Role tuning was seen as an adaptive process, influenced by three stages: First, the engaging phase, characterized by uncertainty during the preparation for caregiving. The second phase, role negotiation, occurred immediately after discharge when the caregiver and care receiver returned to a familiar environment yet assumed unfamiliar roles. The final phase, role settling, was characterized by achieving a stable pattern of caregiver and care receiver interaction. The changing nature of role tuning and the movement of the dyad through the three phases of role tuning are supported by Roy's concept of role transition and role function mode of adaptation.

ROLE FRAMEWORKS RELATED TO CAREGIVING AND CARETAKING

Caregiving and caretaking are assumed to be inherent in the roles of nurses and parents. As life expectancy increases, caregiving for aging parents and relatives often becomes a reality. Though the intensity and duration of caregiving vary greatly, the experience places pro-portional stress and caregiver burden on the care providers. Adding the caregiver role to a person's existing complement of social roles requires renegotiating priorities, dealing with increased energy expenditures, and coping with the physical and psychological strains on the health of the caregiver (Raina et al., 2004).

Factors that mediate caregiver stress, strain, and burden include the intensity of care required, the duration of caregiving, other demands on the caregiver, resources available, and the personal characteristics of the caregiver such as hardiness and resilience. Additional factors include the characteristics of the care recipient, the relationship with the care recipi-ent, and the history of interaction between the care recipient and caregiver. These factors all play out in the individual's existing social, cultural, and economic environment to create a unique context for caregiving. Social support models of stress suggest that social support buffers the person's appraisal of life events. Social support through formal and informal support groups is believed to reduce the stress response and facilitate coping with adverse events (Cho, 2007). Culture plays a role in mediating caregiver burden by influencing the caregiving expectations. The economic environment of the care recipient and caregiver affects the resources available and can increase or decrease caregiver stress, strain, and bur-den. In this section, the role frameworks related to patients, family caregiving, parenting, and grandparenting roles are highlighted.

Parsons's Sick Role Theory

Talcott Parsons, a medical sociologist, proposed that illness affects the total person by limiting the person's ability to fulfill social roles. "Illness is a state of disturbance in the normal functioning of the total human individual, including both the states of the organ-ism as a biological system and of his [*sic*] personal and social adjustments" (Parsons, 1951, p. 143). Parsons viewed health as a prerequisite for society and illness as a "with-drawal behavior" that adversely affects the person's self-esteem (Parsons, 1964). Sickness not only affects the individual and his or her family but can also be dysfunctional for the society as a whole.

Parsons coined the term *sick role* to refer to an individual's illness expectation. He described the sick role as consisting of a series of rights, obligations, and expectancies that can be categorized as role relationships, reactions to one's illness, and behavioral beliefs. The person who is ill has the right to be excluded from normal role expectations and has the right to receive care. This exemption from normal roles, however, depends on the nature and severity of the illness. The more severe the illness, the greater is the exemption from fulfilling social roles.

Assuming the sick role comes also with obligations. The individual should want to be well and should seek qualified medical care. Blame for the illness does not lay solely with the individual. Recovery or cure is seen as requiring outside intervention beyond personal will power. Expectancies for the person who assumes the sick role are to seek help, to strive to get well, and to not remain in the sick role longer than social expectations allow. Therefore, those who are ill are encouraged to resume normal social roles and functions when able.

Assumptions underlying the sick role are that being sick is not a deliberate action, nor a choice of the individual. The sick person is not able to take care of himself or herself and needs to be relieved of normal role expectations. Also, the person in the sick role should desire to resume presickness roles. Parsons emphasized that sick individuals do not simply remove themselves from social roles, but instead they substitute the sick role for normal roles.

Caregiving Stress Process Model

By its very nature, the caregiving experience is continually changing and evolving. The Caregiving Stress Process Model developed by Pearlin, Mullen, Semple, and Skaff (1990) is focused on the informal processes that occur in the caregiver role and the impact of those stressors and processes on the caregiver's health. Pearlin's model identifies primary and secondary stressors and factors that moderate those stressors. Primary stressors are those directly related to the individual and his or her caregiving needs. These could include physiological processes associated with the care receiver's condition such as memory loss, wound care, and hygiene needs. The secondary stressors arise from demands created by meeting the care receiver's needs, for example, loss of sleep, loss of socialization, or loss of income due to full-time caregiving demands. Factors that moderate the effect of other stressors, such as the caregiver's self-efficacy, coping skills, social and financial support, are additional considerations.

The outcomes of caregiving stress will manifest as degrees of well-being and potential changes in physical and mental health. Also, the caregiver's role is interrelated with other social roles. If caregiving stressors produce role overload, they may impact the caregiver's performance in other roles such as employee, parent, and friend. The moderating factors alone or in combination can help us to lessen the negative impact of caregiving role stress.

Conceptual Model of Caregiving Process

A multidimensional model of caregiving was developed by Raina et al. (2004) to describe and explain the factors contributing to caregiver role processes used in providing long-term care to a disabled child. The process model was conceptualized as a systems model organized by five constructs: (a) background and context, (b) child characteristics, (c) caregiver strain, (d) intrapsychic and coping/supportive factors, and (e) health outcomes.

Factors related to each construct were identified based on the research literature (Raina et al., 2004). The first construct, background and context, provides input to the system and includes the setting in which caregiving takes place and the social and economic characteristics of the family. Research on the second construct, child characteristics, identified the severity of disability as impacting the caregiver's health. The child's motor and cognitive impairment, dependency in activities of daily living, and behavioral problems were found to be key factors associated with caregiver health. Next, the constructs of caregiver strain, intrapsychic factors such as self-perception, and coping factors all interact to affect caregiver health outcomes. The three coping factors identified from research literature are: family function, social support, and stress management; psychological and physical health were the two health outcomes identified.

Raina et al. (2004) developed the model to explain the adaptation of parent caregivers to caring for their child with a disability. Research suggests there are significant differences in how caregivers adapt to caregiving demands. Many studies have explored the relationship between caregiving and health outcomes of the caregivers. However, most have focused on the stress related to caregiving demands without considering the contextual stressors that influence the caregiver's adaptation and health outcome. They note that the complex nature of stress processes must be identified. In addition, contextual factors, which influence the caregiver's role adaptation, must be considered, even if not directly related to caregiving. Thus, to gain a more comprehensive picture of caregiver's role, this model attempts to recognize the stressors occurring in the broader social context.

Baumrind's Parenting Styles

Based on a long-term study of parents, Baumrind (1966, 1967) identified three types of parenting styles based on a two-dimensional continuum. Parenting styles were categorized according to the degree of demandingness and degree of responsiveness. The continuum classifies parents who are high in demandingness and responsiveness as *authoritative*; those high in responsiveness but low in demandingness as *permissive*, and those high in demandingness but low in responsiveness are referred to as *authoritarian*.

Each parenting style is characterized by common behaviors and expectations. The authoritarian parent enforces rules of behaviors and has high expectations regarding behavior. Those with the authoritarian style hold a high degree of control in shaping and influencing the child's behavior and attitudes. They value obedience, order, and tradition. Control is achieved by punishment and restricting the child's autonomy. In contrast, the permissive parenting style demonstrates affirming and nonpunitive behaviors and encourages the free will of the child. They impose few rules and value the autonomy of the child. As a result, they often include the child in decision making.

The authoritative style is a mix between the authoritarian and permissive styles. They tend to display assertive communication and set clear expectations, yet they temper this by considering the child's perspective. Verbal give and take is encouraged, and the authoritative parent may share with the child the reasoning behind decisions made and may seek to understand the child's objections. They can strike a balance between allowing autonomy while maintaining parental control. Baumrind sees the authoritative style as most desired.

Later, two additional parental styles were added, the negligent style by Maccoby and Martin (1983) and the harmonious by Baumrind (1971). The negligent style describes parents who are emotionally detached and uninvolved. Even with the addition of this fourth style, not all parenting styles were reflected. Researchers found a small number of parents were highly responsive yet more moderate in demandingness. They did not use overt discipline, yet were able to maintain control of their children. This style was called *harmonious* (Baumrind, 1971). Greenspan (2006) argued the harmonious style that demonstrated a high degree of warmth, moderate control, and high tolerance should replace the authoritative style as the preferred parenting style.

Responsible Fatherhood Model

Based on a review of the literature on fathering, Doherty, Kouneski, and Erickson (1998) developed a conceptual model that describes influences on responsible fathering. Central to the model is the triad relationship between the father, mother, and child. Each comes to

the relationship with factors that influence the relationship. Father factors include role identification, knowledge, skills and commitment, psychological well-being, relationship with
his father, and external factors such as the type of employment and residential status. Child
factors include developmental status, age, gender, and temperament; behavioral difficulties;
and attitude toward the father. Factors related to the mother include her attitude and expectations of the father's role, support of the father, and employment characteristics.

In addition to the factors, each individual brings to the triad co-parental relationship factors, and contextual factors are in operation (Doherty et al., 1998). Co-parental relationship
factors include external conditions such as marital status, dual versus single wage earner,
and custodial arrangement. Internal factors that represent the quality of the relationship
include commitment, cooperation, mutual support, and conflict. Contextual factors involve
institutional, employment, and economic conditions; race or ethnicity, resources, challenges;
cultural expectations; and social support.

This model focuses on concepts that contribute to and detract from the father-child relationship and the father's ability to assume an active role in the child's life, regardless of
whether the father lives with the child. The model depicts four domains of responsible
fathering as identified in the literature: paternity, presence, economic support, and involvement with the child. A key finding reflected in this model is that fathering is uniquely sensitive to contextual influences (Doherty et al., 1998).

Maternal Role Attainment Theory

In 1961, Rubin developed a theory on maternal role adjustment that described the mother as
progressing through taking in, taking hold, and letting go stages after delivery. Each stage
is characterized by dependent, dependent-independent, and interdependent behaviors,
respectively (Rubin, 1967). Later, Mercer, a pediatric nurse, expanded the model to look at
the process of becoming a mother (Mercer, 1995, 2004). Mercer's Role Attainment Theory
describes how the new mother develops her maternal identity and bonds with her child.
Maternal role attainment is a process that begins with psychological preparation for the role
and extends from prepregnancy through the first year after delivery. Motherhood is viewed
as a developmental process that involves interaction with the infant. The process results in
maternal–child bonding and culminates in "becoming a mother." Mercer initially borrowed
the four stages of role acquisition theory proposed by Thornton and Nardi (1975) to explain
the process. The four distinct phases in the process are: anticipation, formal, informal, and
personal stages. These stages were renamed in 2004 as: (a) commitment, attachment, and
preparation; (b) acquaintance, learning, and physical restoration; (c) moving towards a new
normal; and (d) achievement of maternal identity.

The first stage begins before conception and continues up to the birth of the child. It
involves psychosocial preparation for the role and adapting to the physiological changes
of pregnancy. The second stage encompasses the period immediately after birth up to the
time the child is brought home. In this stage, the focus is on modeling learned behaviors,
following family norms, and conforming to common social practices. During the first 4
months, the mother progresses to stage three and settles into a new norm. She develops
her maternal identity and becomes increasingly comfortable with her decision making
and mothering skills. Around the fourth month, the mother enters the fourth stage characterized by increased confidence in the role of motherhood and has fully bonded with
her child.

According to Mercer (2004), the mother progresses sequentially through these stages at
her own pace. During these stages, the mother develops her maternal identity in conjunction
with attaching and bonding with the child. Mother–infant bonding is viewed as crucial to the
child's growth and development of a sense of mastery, identity, and self-worth. The nurse's
understanding of the process of material role attainment can foster the maternal–child

bonding process and impact how a mother perceives motherhood and ultimately attains the maternal role.

Maternal Postpartum Role Collapse Theory

The Maternal Postpartum Role Collapse Theory is rooted in traditional role theory concepts and symbolic interactionism philosophy. The theory emerged during a grounded theory study of postpartum depression in African American women (Amankwaa, 2005). Three key constructs of the theory are: role stress, role strain, and role collapse. Role stress is an antecedent for developing role strain and role collapse. In the context of motherhood, role stress is defined as "the worry and concern of mothers as they experienced life situations during the postpartum period" (Amankwaa, 2005, p. 30). Social structural conditions create a deficit in resources such as finances, health, support systems, education, and produce role stress and strain. Role strain is conceptually defined as the subjective emotional reaction to the stressful postpartum experience. Signs of role strain may include social withdrawal and/or decreased productivity.

Postpartum Role Collapse Theory was derived from mothers' reports of their inability to function effectively during the postpartum period. The trajectory of the theory begins with the experience of role stress which results in role strain. When role strain is sustained, the new mother experiences role disintegration. There are two potential outcomes of role disintegration: one is positive adaptation, referred to as *role reorganization*; the other is role collapse. The experience of role collapse is characterized by depression and the inability of the new mother to function during the postpartum period. It is attributed to the increasing demands and pressures experienced by a new mother. When role disintegration occurs the new mother may obtain assistance and experience role reorganization; however, if assistance is inadequate, the new mother is at risk for experiencing role collapse.

Neugarten and Weinstein's Types of Grandparents

In 1964, gerontologists Neugarten and Weinstein identified five types of grandparents: the formal, fun seeker, surrogate, reservoir of family wisdom, and the distant figure. Familiarity with these types provides a useful perspective and understanding of the type of involvement and connection grandparents provide. The formal grandparent fulfills typical expectations by maintaining contact, providing supportive services, and showing an interest in the child. These grandparents achieve balance when it comes to the degree of involvement. The fun seeker is predominantly involved in providing leisure, play, and entertaining the child. The surrogate style plays a major role in caretaking for the child. The reservoir of family wisdom style is involved in giving advice and acts as an authority for the family. The fifth style is the distant figure who has limited contact and interacts with the child primarily on special occasions.

Cherlin and Furstenberg's Five Styles of Grandparenting

Similarly, Cherlin and Furstenberg (1985, 1992) classified grandparenting into five styles: the detached, passive, supportive, influential, and authoritative. Both the detached and passive grandparents have little interaction with their grandchildren. However, the difference between the two types is the frequency of interaction. Detached grandparents frequently interact, whereas the passive grandparents see the grandchildren infrequently. Grandparents who assume a supportive role have supportive interactions with the parents and are involved in running errands or completing chores for the parents of their grandchildren. The authoritative type interacts in a similar manner. However, these parents tend to demonstrate parent-like behaviors involving discipline, communication, rules, and giving advice. Finally, the influential type refers to those who demonstrate both supportive and authoritative dimensions.

TABLE 14.1 Comparison of Role Frameworks

Theory/Model	Emphasis	Major Concepts
Role Transition Model	Difference between old and new roles and expectations Three types of changes (developmental/professional; intellectual/emotive; and skills/role relationships)	Three stages of transition: doing, being, and knowing
Transition Shock Model	Explains first stage of role transition model	Cultural shock, transition theory, reality shock, role adaptation, growth and development, and change
Social Role Theory	Psychological processes associated with role transition Rights and obligations of persons holding a given position	The intersection between roles and social concepts of age, gender, ethnicity, occupation, and social class
Roy's Role Function Mode	Adaptation to roles	Role transition and adaptation expressed through instrumental and expressive behaviors
Parsons's Sick Role Theory	Fulfilling social roles Sick role consists of rights, obligations, and expectancies	Withdrawal behavior Illness expectations
Caregiving Stress Model	Informal processes occurring during caregiving role	Primary and secondary stressors
Conceptual Model of Caregiving Process	Focus on long-term care of disabled child Multidimensional factors contribute to caregiving role processes	Five constructs: background/context, characteristics of the child, caregiver strain, intrapsychic and coping/supportive factors, and health outcomes
Baumrind's Parenting Styles	Parenting styles based on two-dimensional continuum of demandingness and responsiveness	Four styles: permissive, neglectful, authoritarian, and authoritative
Responsible Fathering	Triad relationship between mother, father, and child and factors that influence the relationships	Four domains: paternity, presence, economic support, and involvement
Maternal Role Attainment	Developmental process involves developing maternal identity and bonding with child	Four stages: (a) commitment, attachment, and preparation; (b) acquaintance, learning, and physical restoration stage; (c) moving toward a new normal; and (d) achievement of maternal identity

(*continued*)

TABLE 14.1 Comparison of Role Frameworks (continued)		
Theory/Model	**Emphasis**	**Major Concepts**
Maternal Postpartum Role Collapse Theory	The experience of role stress postpartum and the outcomes of role disintegration	Role stress, role strain, role disintegration, and role collapse
Neugarten and Weinstein's Grandparenting Types	Types of grandparenting based on nature of interaction with the grandchild	Grandparenting types: formal, fun seeker, surrogate, a reservoir of family wisdom, and distant
Cherlin and Furstenberg's Grandparenting Styles	Styles of grandparenting based on the nature of interaction with the grandchild	Grandparenting styles: detached, passive, supportive, influential, and authoritative

In both classifications, the grandparent's impact can stem from direct, indirect, or a combination of actions or influences. Direct influences result from direct contact and face-to-face interaction. Indirect influences may be in the form of providing financial assistance or through influencing the parent's behavior. These direct and indirect influences, coupled with changes in the nuclear family structure due to divorce or social services interventions, often place grandparents in a more central role than in the past. Interest in studying grandparenting roles is growing due to the impact of the grandparent's longer and healthier life spans. Thus, grandparents of today are able to assume more active and central roles in their children's and grandchildren's lives for a longer time span than ever before.

CONCLUSION

The concepts discussed in this chapter depict a complex interrelated dynamic and evolving system. In Table 14.1, the emphasis and major concepts of the role frameworks discussed in this chapter are summarized and provide a structure for drawing comparisons. Role theory, as a field of study, can be understood from a structuralist position in which roles are linked to one's position in society or to interactionism that is concerned with understanding and explaining the meaning of the roles assumed. This conceptual system, called *role theory*, adds to our understanding of role development, role adaptation, and the effects of negative role constructs such as role ambiguity, role incongruity, role stress, role conflict, and role overload. These constructs, in turn, play a part in how effectively we carry out our personal, familial, and professional roles and our degree of role satisfaction.

KEY POINTS

- Role theory may be conceptualized from a structuralist view, which emphasizes one's position in society, or from an interactionist perspective, which is concerned with exploring and understanding the meaning of specific roles.
- Role constructs identify sources of struggle and processes experienced as a result of functioning within multiple social roles.
- The Role Transition Model focuses on the processes experienced due to reality shock.

- The role transition process in nursing involves three types of changes: developmental/professional, intellectual/emotive, and changes in skills and role relationships.
- Factors that influence the intensity and duration of transition shock include roles, relationships, responsibilities, and knowledge.
- Social Role Theory always involves reciprocal relationships and expectations.
- Roy's role function adaptation mode is one of four modes central to adaptation.
- The sick role comprises the expectations ill persons hold about their role functioning.
- Caregiver role stress is mediated by multiple factors including characteristics of the care recipient, relationship to the care recipient, history, and context.
- Baumrind's Parenting Styles are derived from a two-dimensional continuum of demandingness and responsiveness.
- The Responsible Fatherhood Model identifies four domains as influencing the fatherhood role: paternity, presence, economic support, and involvement.
- Mercer's Maternal Role Attainment Theory identifies four sequential stages of maternal role attainment that begins at preconception and ends up to a year after the child is home.
- Maternal Role Collapse Theory describes the negative outcome experienced because of continual maternal role stress, strain, and overload.
- Neugarten and Weinstein identify five types of grandparent roles: (a) formal, (b) fun seeker, (c) surrogate, (d) reservoir of family wisdom, and (e) distant figure.
- Cherlin and Furstenberg classify the five types of grandparenting styles as (a) detached, (b) passive, (c) supportive, (d) influential, and (e) authoritative.

REFERENCES

Amankwaa, L. C. (2005). Maternal postpartum role collapse as a theory of postpartum depression. *The Qualitative Report, 10*(1), 21–38.

Bakan, D. (1966). *The duality of human existence: An essay on psychology and religion.* Chicago, IL: Rand McNally.

Banton, M. (1965). *Roles: An introduction to the study of social relations.* New York, NY: Basic Books.

Baumrind, D. (1966). Effects of authoritative parental control on child behavior. *Child Development, 37*(4), 887–907.

Baumrind, D. (1967). Child care practices anteceding three patterns of preschool behavior. *Genetic Psychology Monographs, 75*(10), 43–88.

Baumrind, D. (1971). Harmonious parents and their preschool children. *Developmental Psychology, 4*, 99–102.

Benne, K. D., & Bennis, W. (1959). Role confusion and conflict in nursing: The role of the professional nurse. *The American Journal of Nursing, 59*(2), 196–198.

Biddle, B., & Thomas, E. (1979). *Role theory: Concepts and research.* Huntington, NY: Robert E. Krieger.

Brookes, K., Davidson, P., Daly, J., & Halcomb, E. (2007). Role theory: A framework to investigate the community nurse role in contemporary health care systems. *Contemporary Nurse, 25*(1–2), 146–155.

Cherlin, A., & Furstenberg, F. (1985). Styles and strategies of grandparenting. In V. L. Bengtson & J. F. Robertson (Eds.), *Grandparenthood* (pp. 97–116). Beverly Hills, CA: Sage.

Cherlin, A., & Furstenberg, F. (1992). Styles of grandparenting. In A. Cherlin & F. Furstenberg (Eds.), *The new American grandparent, a place in the family, a life apart* (pp. 52–81). Cambridge, MA: Harvard University Press.

Cho, E. (2007). A proposed theoretical framework addressing the effects of informal caregivers on the health-related outcomes of elderly recipients in home health care. *Asian Nursing Research, 1*(1), 23–34.

Cranford, J. S. (2013). Bridging the gap: Clinical practice nursing and the effect of role strain on successful role transition and intent to stay in academia. *International Journal of Nursing Education Scholarship, 10*(1), 1–7.

Deasy, L. (1964). *Social role theory: Its component parts, and some applications.* Washington, DC: The Catholic University of America Press.

Diekman, A. B., Goodfriend, W., & Goodwin, S. (2004). Dynamic stereotypes of power: Perceived change and stability in gender hierarchies. *Sex Roles, 50*(3/4), 201–215.

Doherty, W., Kouneski, E., & Erickson, M. (1998). Responsible fathering: An overview and conceptual framework. *Journal of Marriage and Family, 60*(2), 277–293. doi:10.2307/353848

Duchscher, J. E. B. (2008). A process of becoming: The stages of new nursing graduate professional role transition. *The Journal of Continuing Education in Nursing, 39*(10), 441–450.

Duchscher, J. E. B. (2009). Transition shock: The initial stage of role adaptation for newly graduated registered nurses. *Journal of Advanced Nursing, 65*(5), 1103–1113.

Dulin, A. M. (2007). A lesson on social role theory: An example of human behavior in the social environment theory. *Advances in Social Work, 8*(1), 104–112.

Eagly, A. H. (1987). *Sex differences in social behavior: A social role interpretation.* Hillsdale, NJ: Erlbaum.

Eagly, A. H., Wood, W., & Diekman, A. (2000). Social role theory of sex differences and similarities: A current perspective. In T. Eckes & H. Trautner (Eds.), *The development of social psychology of gender* (pp. 123–174). New York, NY: Psychology Press, Taylor & Francis.

Greenspan, S. (2006). Rethinking "harmonious parenting" using a three-factor discipline model. *Child Care in Practice, 12*(1), 5–12.

Handy, C. (1985). *Understanding organizations.* London, UK: Penguin Books.

Hardy, M. E. (1978). Role stress and role strain. In M. E. Hardy & M. E. Conway (Eds.), *Role theory perspectives for health professionals* (pp. 73–109). New York, NY: Appleton-Century-Crofts.

Kelly, J. (1982). Role theory as a model for human interaction: Its implications for nursing education. *The Australian Nurses Journal, 12*(1), 42–43, 51.

Maccoby, E., & Martin, J. (1983). Socialization in the context of the family: Parent child interaction. In P. H. Mussen (Series Ed.) & E. M. Hetherington (Vol Ed.), *Handbook of child psychology: Socialization, personality, and social development* (Vol. 4, pp. 1–101). New York, NY: Wiley.

Mead, G. H. (1934). In C. W. Morris (Ed.), *Mind, self, and society from the perspective of a social behaviorist.* Chicago, IL: University of Chicago.

Mercer, R. T. (1995). *Becoming a mother: Research on maternal identity from Rubin to the present.* New York, NY: Springer Publishing.

Mercer, R. T. (2004). Becoming a mother vs role attainment. *Journal of Nursing Scholarship, 36*(3), 226–232.

Muller, Z., & Litwin, H. (2011). Grandparenting and well-being: How important is grandparent-role centrality? *European Journal of Ageing, 8*(2), 109–118.

Murray, T. A. (1998). Using role theory concepts to understand transitions from hospital-based nursing practice to home care nursing. *Journal of Continuing Education in Nursing, 29*(3), 105–111.

Neugarten, B., & Weinstein, K. (1964). The changing American grandparent. *Journal of Marriage and Family, 26*(2), 199–204.

Parsons, T. (1951). *The social system.* New York, NY: Free Press.

Parsons, T. (1964). *Social structure and personality.* Glencoe, IL: Free Press.

Pearlin, L., Mullen, J., Semple, S., & Skaff, M. (1990). Caregiving and the stress process: An overview of concepts and their measures. *The Gerontologist, 30*(5), 583–594.

Raina, P., O'Donnell, M., Schwellnus, H., Rosenbaum, P., King, G., Brehaut, J., . . . Wood, E. (2004). Caregiving process and caregiver burden: Conceptual models to guide research and practice. *BMC Pediatrics, 4*(1), 1–13. doi:10.1186/1471-2431-4-1

Roy, C., & Andrews, H. A. (1991). *The Roy adaptation model: The definitive statement.* San Mateo, CA: Appleton & Lange.

Roy, C., & Andrews, H. A. (1999). *The Roy adaptation model* (2nd ed.). Stamford, CT: Appleton & Lange.

Rubin, R. (1961). Basic maternal behavior. *Nursing Outlook, 9,* 683–686.

Rubin, R. (1967). Attainment of the maternal role: Part I. Processes. *Nursing Research, 16*(3), 237–245.

Shyu, Y. (2000). Role tuning between caregiver and care receiver during discharge transition: An illustration of role function mode in Roy's adaptation theory. *Nursing Science Quarterly, 13*(4), 323–331.

Thornton, R., & Nardi, P. M. (1975). The dynamics of role acquisition. *American Journal of Sociology, 80*(4), 870–885.

Frameworks for Communities, Populations, and Organizational Systems

We all belong to the universe; we all receive from it and give to it; we are all parts of the whole.
—Jean Vanier, *Community and Growth* (p. 11)

Part III explores frameworks related to the needs, issues, functions, and structures of communities, populations, and organizations. Chapter 15 is organized around the economics that supports the large units of society. Chapters 16 through 18 look specifically at frameworks through which nurses may view the organizations and communities themselves and exercise leadership to promote change. Chapter 19 reviews frameworks for evaluation whereby organizations and communities strive to attain and maintain excellence, especially where the health of persons and community is at stake. The segment concludes with Chapter 20, frameworks that give perspective to the variety of sociocultural strengths and stressors resulting from the multifaceted and multicultural nature of health care. We hope this section conveys the interconnectedness and the importance of the roles that healthy communities and organizations play in the overall health of nurses and their patients.

Economic Frameworks

Kristina Henry

Where you live should not determine whether you live, or whether you die.
—Bono

There are people in the world so hungry, that God cannot appear to them except in the form of bread.
—Gandhi

 KEY TERMS

Critical Social Theory	macroeconomics	Patterson Cultural-Structure
Dependency Theory	Mead's Nonworking Poor	Model
economic analysis	microeconomics	Personal Theory of Poverty
economics	Murray's Underclass	Structural Theory of Poverty

LEARNING OBJECTIVES

1. Describe economic frameworks in terms of basic premises, assumptions, processes, and goals as applied to nursing and the health care environment.

2. Compare and contrast economic frameworks as applied to nursing and the health care environment.

3. Analyze economic frameworks as applicable to nursing processes, health care, and sociocultural environment.

The study of economics is complex, multifaceted, and based on a variety of perspectives, social structures, and human behaviors. Economic frameworks, based on anthropological and sociological science, are used to analyze the distribution of wealth and poverty within societies and cultures as related to human behaviors. These frameworks are used to explore and examine economic concepts and perspectives and rationalize decisions for the distribution of societal resources. Economic frameworks are not quantitative or qualitative in nature, but rather broad and conceptual. They are based on assumptions to guide or forecast. Therefore, economic frameworks are frequently used in politics for supporting or arguing critical issues and establishing public policy.

⬤ ECONOMIC CONCEPTS

As health care providers, we do not often think about the economic impact of our actions or the relationship of economics to the health care environment. However, as we explore economic frameworks in this chapter, it is vital to understand some key concepts and basic definitions. *Economics* is a broad term used to explain the factors affecting goods and services, including production, distribution, and consumption. It is also a social science exploring behaviors and interactions related to structure and process. *Economic analysis* is the process of critically examining current and existing conditions, as well as advocating for moral and ethical considerations of what should be. *Microeconomics* is the study of a specific economic unit such as a business or household and buyers or sellers. *Macroeconomics* is the study of grand economic concerns such as unemployment or inflation. These concepts are described as broad and generic with variance depending on application and interpretation (Backhouse & Medema, 2009).

Economic analysis is not applied solely in the business and finance realm; it is used in a variety of diverse social themes including health care, government, crime, education, law, and the environment. This type of analysis takes into account any entity using commodities for income and expenses with potential benefits and losses (Backhouse & Medema, 2009). For instance, in health care, patients are billed for time and expertise of care providers. This impacts the future health and well-being of the population, economic productivity, and the future of the economy as a whole.

Microeconomics explores the specific units constituting an economic market. The specific unit can be a private or public entity with a tangible product or service, such as a hospital or clinic. The goal in a free market is to have an equal supply and demand. However, due to many influencing factors, achieving equilibrium is a challenge (Howitt, 1987). For example, limited resources will influence cost and accessibility resulting in unaffordable care for many. In health care, inequitable distribution or access of care creates a moral and ethical dilemma.

Macroeconomics is a broad and comprehensive view of the economic system used to examine market interactions. The application of macroeconomics is for the purpose of fiscal decisions and policy development. It looks at long-term projections and system-wide changes resulting from the microeconomic units. An example of the application of macroeconomics in health care is the analysis of the Affordable Care Act on unemployment or hiring practices. As health care continues to change, economic analysis is critical for organizational success and for meeting societal health care needs (Howitt, 1987).

⬤ POVERTY FRAMEWORKS

Poverty is an economic concept, as well as an anthropological and sociological concept. The overlap and interdependence of these concepts related to poverty lead to a multifaceted analysis; thus, separately studying the concepts can be a challenge. In underdeveloped countries, poverty is often deeply rooted and overwhelming in the societal structure and function. This all-consuming poverty stems from a lack of governmental support and structure, as well as a lack of resources, industry, and funding. It is a cyclical culture, stunting growth and development for the nation. Poverty in developing countries is often attributed to political and social powers. However, in the United States and other developed countries, poverty is attributed to two basic theories: personal or structural. The *Personal Theory of Poverty* is a result of personal traits and failings (Small, Harding, & Lamont, 2010), whereas the *Structural Theory of Poverty* is founded on the failings of the economic and social structures (Rank, Yoon, & Herschl, 2003).

These theories are based on contrasting premises, thus leading to considerable debate among economists. This debate frequently occurs in the political realm with the need for policy development and passage. Politicians who align with the personal theory seek to limit governmental assistance and believe assistance restricts personal responsibility for support and financial development, thus creating a cycle of poverty. This is considered a conservative perspective. Politicians who align with the structural theory recognize the role of social and economic structures in promoting and creating poverty. They seek to provide governmental assistance to improve the circumstances of those in poverty as they seek financial independence. This is considered a liberal perspective (Bradshaw, 2006; Jordan, 2004).

Poverty frameworks cannot be attributed to any particular researcher or study. During biblical times, poverty theory was identified as disparity resulting from penance from god. Poverty frameworks have been widely discussed and studied throughout history from the perspective of the dominant social issues or concerns of the time (Bradshaw, 2006).

Personal Theory of Poverty

According to the Personal Theory, poverty is a result of personal characteristics such as laziness, lack of education, irresponsibility, or other inferior attributes. The individual fails to climb out of poverty due to lack of initiative, ambition, or motivation. Impulsive decision making and behaviors and minimal long-term planning are common factors. Poverty is justified because of failure to perform and unwillingness or opposition to societal opportunities for success or compensation (Rank et al., 2003).

The Personal Theory is based on the assumption that the same people live in poverty from year to year, and that no one ever leaves a state of poverty. Policies fostering this theory are designed to assist the individual to improve circumstances resulting in poverty and assist them to improve their quality of life (Bradshaw, 2006). Research has supported the relevance and application of the personal theory to poverty analysis. See Box 15.1 for an example of the application of personal theory to research.

Structural Theory of Poverty

Structural theory blames the system and focuses on poverty as the direct result of specific social and structural failings that favor one societal group over another. Gender, social class, age, and race are all examples of societal groupings. Lack of employment, low minimum wage standards, and lack of affordable childcare, health care, or housing are all contributing factors (Rank et al., 2003). When household income is too low, or adequate paying jobs are not available, poverty rates will increase.

An example of a structural cause of poverty is seen in the disproportionately high number of single women in poverty compared to men, which is due in part to men receiving greater compensation than women for the same job (Rank et al., 2003). Patriarchal structures, which empower men and devalue women, contribute to economic disparity between men and women. Thus, nations offering the most resources and support to their populations have the least amount of poverty (Rank et al., 2003). Policies addressing structural theory focus on altering the defective structure to reduce or eliminate poverty.

BOX 15.1 Research Application of the Personal Theory of Poverty

A research study supporting the Personal Theory of Poverty found those living in poverty had higher rates of cigarette smoking. The results indicated a direct relationship between smoking and income; as income increases smoking prevalence decreases. This study represents the existence of values, behaviors, and decision making associated with poverty (Small, Harding, & Lamont, 2010).

People who work in minimum wage jobs struggle to raise a family and are unable to advance in social class. The cost of child care, health care, education, and other living expenses create barriers that are extremely difficult to conquer. These societal structures create a cycle of poverty, which is overwhelming and incapacitating. From the structural perspective, personal attributes such as work ethic or intelligence have a negligible effect on improving poverty.

Patterson's Cultural-Structure Theory

Cultural sociologist, Orlando Patterson fused personal and structural theory to analyze and address poverty. He believed these theories were interrelated and interdependent, and one theory could not be all-inclusive for such a profound social concern such as poverty. Structural factors affect individuals and form the culture in which they live and ultimately impact individuals' choices and behaviors. Patterson (2000) views behaviors perpetuating poverty, such as criminal activity, women as single parents, and substance abuse, as adaptive behaviors to the culture or living environment. Culture and living environment are created by societal structures, thus creating a link between the personal and structural theories of poverty.

Patterson has developed and applied his theory of poverty through the study of African American history in the United States. He explains poverty as a result or outcome of the relationship between societal structure and learned behaviors. This relationship forms a dynamic, interactive, and adaptive culture of poverty (2000).

In his study of poverty in urban African Americans in the United States, Patterson describes a mass of impoverished and disengaged young people who have developed a violent and caustic way of life (Patterson, 2015). This way of life has been promoted by racial profiling and forceful law-enforcement practices. Patterson uses his theory to explain recent events involving urban African Americans and police brutality, whereas others primarily blame racism (see Box 15.2 for an example of Patterson's Structural Theory of Poverty).

There is much debate between personal and structural theories as to the primary causes of poverty. Historically, theorists have described the personal and structural perspectives as competing theories. However, a more recent analysis supports a synthesis of both theories (Jordan, 2004). From this perspective, poverty is described and analyzed as an interrelated and interdependent concept from *both* theories. This analysis explores poverty through the dynamic nature of culture *and* structural elements instead of the rigid and unchanging perspectives used in the past. Poverty is reinforced by a complex compilation of personal and structural factors (Bradshaw, 2006). Recent research applies the combined personal and structural theories to develop community-based programs to address poverty (Box 15.3).

BOX 15.2 Research Application of Patterson's Structural Theory of Poverty

Patterson explains the recent unrest in the United States between urban African Americans and police as an example of the application of his theory (Patterson, 2015). Although they are in the minority, the norms and behaviors of urban culture are generationally learned and present an aggressive, disrespectful, and threatening image. This image is supported by conditions of poverty such as long-term unemployment, single parenting, and substance abuse. Patterson (2015) notes that many of the police involved in the events being studied were also African Americans; therefore, factors other than racism must also be in operation.

> ### BOX 15.3 Research Application of Personal and Structural Theory
>
> The concept of personal and structural theory synthesis has been applied in community-based efforts to address poverty. Addressing poverty, through both the personal and structural perspective, has established an evidence-based approach that empowers the people in the community. Through interpersonal community relationships and established community organizations, people are provided assistance and support. The trust and shared values among the community members create a sense of shared purpose and empowerment that ultimately benefits the entire community as they strive to decrease poverty (Bradshaw, 2006).

⊙ CULTURAL FACTORS OF POVERTY

Theorists describe poverty as a mindset or culture (Grondona, 2000; Lindsay, 2000). Poverty is based on cultural factors used to assess the culture for possible poverty gauges. Nations are described as poverty prone or poverty resistant based on mental models or value-based decision making. Both Grondona and Lindsay define poverty as a result of decisions and actions based on cultural values. For example, values such as trust, empowerment, safety, and innovation will be supported in a developed country. In a nation where poverty, suppression, control, grandiose goals, passivity, and unstable governments dominate the value system, poverty will perpetuate without changes in culture and values of the population.

Social and anthropological perspectives of poverty are often described and explained as the culture of poverty. The culture of poverty does not differentiate between developed or underdeveloped countries but uses a broad view to explain poverty as a form of perpetuated socialization and behavior. This creates a subculture of dependent individuals unable to escape poverty. Thus, the culture of poverty is founded on specific fundamental characteristics including powerlessness, personal unworthiness, dependency, and marginality. Essentially, individuals living in the culture of poverty feel forgotten, alienated, and extremely vulnerable (Lewis, 1998).

Environmental factors, behaviors, and personal characteristics of the poor interact and reinforce poverty and dependence. Research has identified and demonstrated this theory through the study of teen pregnancy, drug abuse, and increasing divorce rates (Rodgers, 2000). Attitudes and behaviors are passed from one generation to the next and result in an established culture of poverty. Without adaptation to the environment, behaviors, and personal characteristics, the culture persists. Poverty generates a limited perspective and the development of specific behaviors. Children raised in this environment are conditioned, and thus poverty is perpetuated to the next generation (Jordan, 2004). Research has validated these cultural principles of generational poverty (Box 15.4).

Murray's Underclass

In 1984, political scientist and sociologist Charles Murray termed *underclass* to describe and represent a social class resulting from generational poverty. Murray believed that generations pass critical behaviors resulting in low income and the perpetuation of poverty from one generation to the next. Individuals composing the underclass have been further described as deficient in the skills or behaviors needed to find work in a developed economy. Because of the lack of training, skills, or behaviors, the underclass is perpetually unemployed and unstable, thus dependent on governmental assistance for sustenance. The underclass is frequently viewed as unproductive members of society who are unwilling or unable to work.

BOX 15.4 Research Application of Principles of Generational Poverty

A long-term study that began as an investigation of mental disorder prevalence in the Great Smokey Mountains yielded great economic and social data as well (Akee, Simeonova, Costello, & Copeland, 2015). Ultimately, the researchers discovered a direct correlation between increased income and the development of positive characteristics. The added income also lowered the incidence of behavioral and emotional disorders. This research demonstrates the effect of income and poverty on the development of children, including their ability to improve their circumstances.

In a capitalistic society, those who are prosperous view the poor social class as stagnated and a burden to society (Murray, 1984).

In 1999, Murray applied personal theory concepts to explain the persistent poverty of the underclass. Their deviant criminal actions, children born to single mothers, unemployment, and dependency on governmental assistance is attributed to their own lack of initiative and irresponsibility. The underclass does not bear the responsibility of alleviating their poverty status. Murray cites the increase in incarcerated populations as a direct result of the growth of the underclass.

To address the disproportionate ratio of African Americans in the underclass population, Murray expanded his research (1999). He notes an increase in African American male unemployment rates and an increase in illegitimate births as compared to Caucasians. Murray noted that in 1982, 58% of African American children were born to single women and that percentage increased to 69% in 1997. This data supports his explanation of predetermined generational poverty (Murray, 1999).

Murray's research is the basis for his book titled *Losing Ground: American Social Policy, 1950–1980* based on the study of the urban African American culture in the United States. His research emphasized governmental assistance programs as contributing to and perpetuating poverty. He describes governmental assistance as an incentive or reward, as it encourages people to remain unemployed and encourages single mothers to have children. As a result, governmental assistance discourages long-term solutions to generational poverty (Murray, 1984). Therefore, this theoretical perspective promotes the limitations of governmental assistance programs.

Mead's Nonworking Poor

Lawrence Mead, a political science professor, believes that the government has a responsibility and duty to prevent pervasive and long-term poverty. He believes poverty is the result of societal disorder and not caused by a lack of personal opportunity. He claims that governmental assistance is too permissive. It devalues self-sufficiency and independence as unmotivating and unempowering, thus creating and sustaining a defeated culture (1992).

Mead (1992) claims that the failure of voluntary solutions, such as training and incentive programs, to overcome poverty demonstrates the veracity of his analysis. Mead supports public policy that enforces values, including implementation at institutions such as homeless shelters and schools. He believes that the only solution to poverty is for the poor to increase their efforts; governmental aid is not the solution.

The Nonworking Poor Theory supports empowering individuals to help themselves and promotes a work ethic standard. Mead supports the requirement of work and fulfilling other obligations for receiving governmental assistance. Through the enforcement of values, such as promoting a work ethic and abiding by laws, the individual may receive governmental assistance when needed. Mead (1992) believed that this method of conditional assistance would promote a long-term solution to poverty. This theory was the basis for welfare reform in the United States, thus supporting conditional assistance and not perpetuating a state of entitlement.

Critical Social Theory

The Critical Social Theory is a general sociological philosophy used to analyze and address health care disparities and inequalities. It is based on the works of Karl Marx and Sigmund Freud and later expanded by theorists from the Frankfurt School (Geuss, 1981). It involves the study of people using critical analysis and interpretation of society based on external social, political, cultural, symbolic, and economic factors for the purpose of change (Charmaz, 1995). This theory focuses on the social perspective, relationships, and norms within a given society in the context of providing relevant and rational solutions, thus promoting societal change.

One example of Critical Social Theory is the differences between people in various socioeconomic classes. As patient advocates, it is imperative to identify health care disparities due to socioeconomic status. For instance, if the prevalence of nutrition deficiencies is identified as greater in people of lower socioeconomic status, it narrows the focus and enables the researcher to identify a specific population and disparity. This provides the basis for a direct approach and the ability to develop specific solutions rather than trying to generalize solutions that may or may not be applicable or relevant. The application of this theory demonstrates efficiency by allowing health care providers to prioritize allocation of resources to the most vulnerable populations and not waste resources when not needed.

Historically, low socioeconomic status has been attributed to barriers in health care such as lack of access, lack of preventative care, and provider bias. To address these barriers, according to the Critical Social Theory, nurses would analyze societal factors (external social, political, cultural, symbolic, and economic) for the purpose of identifying solutions and promoting change. The foundation of Critical Social Theory is based on the discovery of social inequality and oppression through analysis to advocate for justice and concentrate on solutions. As social and health disparities are a universal challenge for nurses, analysis and application of the Critical Social Theory are being extended to nurse educators and academic institutions as well (Box 15.5).

Dependency Theory

The Dependency Theory originated by economists Hans Singer and Raul Prebisch (Vernengo, 2004). Similar to the Critical Social Theory, Dependency Theory was developed to explain the result of asymmetrical wealth distribution in capitalistic society. Capitalism is based on the following principles: private ownership, competitive market, and maximization of profits. People are able to accumulate wealth in exchange for products or services. Through these capitalistic principles, developing countries transition to cash crops from sustainable

---

BOX 15.5 Research Application of Critical Social Theory

Health care disparities present a universal challenge for nurses. This study examines nursing academia and curricula related to the Critical Social Theory (Rozendo, Salas, & Cameron, 2016). Nursing is based on advocacy and safety of patients. Therefore, educational preparation must support the identification of challenges and practical interventions in providing care for vulnerable populations. The findings of this study indicate nursing education supports World Health Organization recommendations.

TABLE 15.1 Comparison of Economic Frameworks

Theory/Concept	Theorists	Key Concepts
Personal Theory of Poverty	Small, Harding, and Lamont	Poverty is justified as the result of personal characteristics: laziness, lack of education, lack of initiative, ambition, or motivation.
Structural Theory of Poverty	Rank, Yoon, and Herschl	Blames the system; poverty is the result of social and structural failings that favor one societal group over another: gender, social class, age, race.
Cultural-Structure	Orlando Patterson	Personal and Structure Theory are interrelated and interdependent.
Underclass	Charles Murray	The underclass results from generational poverty. Frequently viewed as unproductive members of society who are unwilling or unable to work.
Nonworking Poor	Lawrence Mead	Supports the requirement of work and other obligations (conditions) for receiving governmental assistance. Conditions prohibit a state of entitlement.
Critical Social Theory	Karl Marx and Sigmund Freud	A philosophy used to analyze and address health care disparities and inequalities. The study of people using critical analysis. Interpretation of society is based on external social, political, cultural, symbolic, and economic factors.
Dependency Theory	Hans Singer and Raul Prebisch	Explains the result of asymmetrical wealth distribution in capitalistic society. Developing countries are subservient to the modern or advanced society.

farming. Thus, a division of labor and an unequal relationship develops between the countries. The developing country (which is producing the cash crops) is essentially subservient to the more modern or advanced society. This domination creates a dependent culture in the developing country (Frank, 1966).

Change is supported, but it occurs to the benefit only of the dominant culture. To ensure long-term maintenance and stability, the dominant culture supports change in the developing sector only if it ultimately supports the dominant culture. This leaves the developing sector powerless to affect change across cultures or society. As a result, the division of power and resources forms two separate, coexisting, yet unequal economies (Frank, 1966).

There are many consequences to economic inequality, such as effects on mortality and public health. Mortality and public health are directly correlated to the availability of resources. As available services and social programs are dependent on the capital provided by the dominant sector, it stands to reason the subservient culture would have less access and fewer resources for health care. The theory suggests that the distance from the center of power directly influences the quality of life (Frank, 1996). The further removed from the source of power and influence, the greater the disparity in health care.

The manufacturing relationship Asia has with the industrialized cultures of the world is a prime example of the Dependency Theory. The capital from external countries, such as the United States, is directly responsible for influencing specialization and industrialization in Asia. Asia depends on the sale of goods and services to the United States and other developed countries for its livelihood. Thus diversification and overall economic growth are limited. The outcome is a financial dependency on the industrialized cultures for sustainability.

⦿ CONCLUSION

This chapter focuses on economic concepts and frameworks based on anthropological and sociological concepts, such as poverty. On a broad scale, these concepts and frameworks are used to analyze the distribution of wealth and poverty within society, including the rationalization of societal resource distribution. These same concepts may also guide or forecast the distribution of health care resources and policies from a broad societal perspective, as well as provide specific applications to health care systems or units.

In today's economic climate, it is essential for health care systems to maximize profits while improving access and quality of health care. The current climate of reimbursement tied to accountability and quality makes an economic analysis of income and expenses crucial for sustainability. However, this is not an isolated or independent concept. There are many variables to consider. Any economic decisions should be analyzed based on moral and ethical principles as well. The basic concepts and premises of the frameworks discussed in this chapter are outlined in Table 15.1.

⦿ KEY POINTS

- Economics is a broad term used to explain all factors affecting goods and services, including production, distribution, and consumption.

- Economic analysis is the process of critically examining current and existing conditions, as well as advocating for moral and ethical considerations of what should be.

- Microeconomics is the study of a specific economic unit such as a business or household and buyers or sellers.

- Macroeconomics is the study of grand economic concerns such as unemployment or inflation.

- The Personal Theory of Poverty is associated primarily with developed countries and is based on poverty as a result of personal traits and failings.

- The Structural Theory of Poverty is associated primarily with underdeveloped countries and is founded on the failings of the economic and social structures.

- Charles Murray coined the term *underclass* to describe a social class resulting from generational poverty (i.e., enduring poverty from one generation to the next).

- For underdeveloped countries, Grondona and Lindsay defined poverty as a result of decisions and actions based on cultural values.

- The culture of poverty is founded on the concepts of powerlessness, personal unworthiness, dependency, and marginality.

- Lawrence Mead supports the requirement of work and fulfilling other obligations for receiving governmental assistance. Mead believed that conditional assistance promoted a long-term solution to poverty.

- The Critical Social Theory is the study of people using critical analysis and interpretation of society based on external social, political, cultural, symbolic, and economic factors for the purpose of change. It focuses on the social perspective, relationships, and norms within a given society.

- Patterson explains poverty as a result or outcome of the relationship between societal structure and learned behaviors.

- The Dependency Theory explains the result of asymmetrical wealth distribution in capitalistic society. Developing countries transition to cash crops from sustainable farming; the subsequent relationship is unequal in which the developing country is essentially subservient to the more modern or advanced society.

REFERENCES

Akee, R., Simeonova, E., Costello, E., & Copeland, W. (2015). *How does household income affect child personality traits and behaviors?* (Working Paper 21562). Cambridge, MA: National Bureau of Economic Research.

Backhouse, R., & Medema, S. (2009). Retrospectives on the definition of economics. *Journal of Economic Perspectives, 23*(1), 221–233.

Bradshaw, T. (2006). *Theories of poverty and anti-poverty programs in community development* (Rural Poverty Research Center. Working Paper No. 06-05). Columbia: University of Missouri. Retrieved from https://www.questia.com/library/journal/1G1-240703119/theories-of-poverty-and-anti-poverty-programs-in-community

Charmaz, K. (1995). Between positivism and postmodernism: Implications for methods. *Studies in Symbolic Interaction, 17*, 43–72.

Frank, G. (1966). *The development of underdevelopment.* Boston, MA: New England Free Press.

Geuss, R. (1981). *The idea of a critical theory.* Cambridge, UK: Cambridge University Press.

Grondona, M. (2000). A cultural typology of economic development. In L. E. Harrison & S. P. Huntington (Eds.), *Culture matters* (pp. 44–55). New York, NY: Basic Books.

Howitt, P. M. (1987). Macroeconomics: Relations with microeconomics. In P. M. Howitt (Ed.), *The new palgrave: A dictionary of economics* (pp. 1–5). London, UK and New York, NY: Macmillan and Stockton.

Jordan, G. (2004, Spring). The causes of poverty cultural vs. structural: Can there be a synthesis? *Perspectives in Public Affairs, 18*–34. Retrieved from http://www.asu.edu/mpa/Jordan.pdf

Lewis, O. (1998). The culture of poverty. *Society, 35*(2), 7–9.

Lindsay, S. (2000). Culture, mental models, and national prosperity. In L. E. Harrison & S. P. Huntington (Eds.), *Culture matters* (pp. 282–295). New York, NY: Basic Books.

Mead, L. (1992). *The new politics of poverty: The non-working poor in America.* New York, NY: Basic Books.

Murray, C. (1984). *Losing ground: American social policy, 1950–1980.* New York, NY: Basic Books.

Murray, C. (1999). *The underclass revisited.* Washington, DC: AEI Press.

Patterson, O. (2000). Taking culture seriously: A framework and Afro-American illustration. In L. E. Harrison & S. P. Huntington (Eds.), *Culture matters* (pp. 202–218). New York, NY: Basic Books.

Patterson, O. (2015, May 9). The real problem with America's inner cities. *The New York Times,* p. SR6.

Rank, M., Yoon, H., & Hirschl, T. (2003). American poverty as a structural failing: Evidence and arguments. *Journal of Sociology and Social Welfare, 30*(4), 3–29.

Rodgers, H. (2000). *American poverty in a new era of reform.* New York: M. E. Sharpe.

Rozendo, C., Salas, A., & Cameron, B. (2016). A critical review of social and health inequalities in the nursing curriculum. *Nurse Education Today, 50,* 62–71. doi:10.1016/j.nedt.2016.12.006

Small, M. L., Harding, D. J., & Lamont, M. (2010, May). Reconsidering culture and poverty. *The Annals of the American Academy of Political and Social Science, 629,* 6–27.

Vanier, J. (1989). *Community and growth.* Mahwah, NJ: Paulist Press.

Vernengo, M. (2004). *Technology, finance and dependency: Latin American radical political economy in retrospect.* Salt Lake City: University of Utah Department of Economics. Retrieved from http://www.economia.unam.mx/cegademex/DOCS/matias_vernengo1.pdf

Community and Population Health Frameworks

Lucretia Smith

Neighborhoods and communities are complex organisms that will be resilient only if they are healthy along a number of interrelated dimensions, much as a human body cannot be healthy without adequate air, water, rest, and food.
—Ben Bernanke

KEY TERMS

Canadian Model of
  Community Health
  Nursing
communities
community health nurse
Community Mobilization
  and Community
  Organization and
  Community
  Building

Integrative Model for Holistic
  Community Health Nursing
Integrated Model of
  Population Health and
  Health Promotion
Milio's framework of
  prevention
multiple interventions
  for community health
  framework

Omaha system
population health
  populations
Population-Based Public
  Health Nursing
  Interventions Model
public health nurse
Public Health Nursing Model
White's construct for public
  health nursing

LEARNING OBJECTIVES

1. Describe community health and community nursing frameworks in terms of history, concepts, and uses.
2. Describe public/population health and related frameworks in terms of history, concepts, and uses.
3. Compare and contrast definitions and uses of the terms person, community, and nursing in community and public/population health frameworks.
4. Analyze research evidence and nursing utilization of community-based frameworks.
5. Compare characteristics of community health and population health frameworks.

As an introduction to this section, an overview of the terms community, public, and population health nursing is presented. As with many terms in nursing, there is not uniform agreement, and there is overlap. American Public Health Association, Public Health Nursing

Section (2013) defines public health nursing as the "practice of promoting and protecting the health of populations using knowledge from nursing, social, and public health sciences" ... [which] "focuses on improving population health by emphasizing prevention, and attending to multiple determinants of health" (p. 1). The term *community health nurse* (CHN) was initially used to define nurses who worked in scattered settings outside of health care institutions (Clark, 2015). Today, community health nursing is defined as "a population-focused, community-oriented approach aimed at health promotion of an entire population, and prevention of disease, disability and premature death in a population" (World Health Organization [WHO] Regional Office for South-East Asia, 2010, p. 7).

Kuss, Proulx-Girouard, Lovitt, Katz, and Kennelly (1997) distinguished between the roles of the CHN and *public health nurse* (PHN) based on the client and setting. The PHN sees the public, the larger population as the client, whereas the CHN sees individuals, families, and small groups as the client. For the CHN, the community (which is a subcategory of the population), is the setting for clinical practice. Clark (2015) also offers another distinction that is helpful. Communities are differentiated on their size and internal connections. *Communities* are smaller segments of a population, composed of individuals or groups who share common interests, interact with one another, and function collectively. *Populations* include groups of individuals who may or may not interact with one another. They may be residents of a specific geographic area such as a neighborhood, state, region, or country, or they may be described as larger aggregates or subgroups that share a common characteristic such as a medical diagnosis. *Population health* is a focus of the PHN in which the client is the population, and the interventions are population based and systems level rather than focused on the individuals within the population.

⊙ OVERVIEW OF COMMUNITY AND PUBLIC HEALTH FRAMEWORKS

Concepts relevant to community and public health nursing, such as aggregates, epidemiology, and population focus, tend to be included in many nursing frameworks previously presented. Although the frameworks containing these relevant concepts were not specifically intended for community health, they are germane to its practice. These frameworks have been explored in earlier chapters, but will be briefly highlighted here due to their relevance to community health.

Examples of such multipurpose frameworks are those of Florence Nightingale with her emphasis on environmental assessment and intervention, Betty Neuman's conceptualization of the person system integrated within broader systems, and Rosenstock and colleague's Health Belief Model (Chapter 9). Perhaps the oldest serious look at community nursing was through the work of Florence Nightingale whose concern was with the patient's environment. Her framework, now generally referred to as Nightingale's Environmental Theory, contains concepts of cleanliness, the health of houses, and healthy food availability (Nightingale, 1860/1969). Attention to these concepts is foundational in the practice of community nursing. Neuman's Systems Model, discussed in more detail in Chapter 11, was originally a model for nurses working in the community mental health setting (Neuman, 1996). This model is easily suited to work with groups of people and communities within the broader environmental system. The Health Belief Model, initially developed in the 1950s, continues to be used in modern-day public health settings (Skinner, Tiro, & Champion, 2015). It focuses on the client's perceptions of susceptibility, severity, benefits barriers, action cues, and performance efficacy, which predict the likelihood that clients will utilize services and products offered in community and public health arenas. The Health Belief Model is especially useful for guiding assessment and intervention (see Chapter 9, for further explanation of this theory).

Other nursing frameworks that support community health and public health nursing are discussed in some depth in other chapters in this book. See Pender's Health Promotion Model (Chapter 9), Roy's Adaptation Model (Chapters 9 and 14), King's Theory of Goal Attainment (Chapters 9 and 10), and Orem's Self-Care Deficit Theory (Chapter 11). These frameworks can easily be applied to nursing practice in the care of individuals as well as groups.

COMMUNITY HEALTH FRAMEWORKS

In this chapter, additional frameworks specific to community and public health nursing practice are reviewed. These frameworks were created specifically for use by health care professionals, usually nurses in community health settings. Many deal with certain geographic areas or specific populations. Each contains concepts applicable to the health of groups of people.

Milio's Framework of Prevention

In 1976, Milio proposed the Framework of Prevention, which contains six propositions that revolve around health decisions, specifically how the individual, or group of individuals, may be influenced to make better health decisions. The first proposition notes the health status of populations is the result of lack (or excess of) health resources. Lack of adequate nutrition, safe drinking water, and excessive pollution are examples. The second proposition is populations have a limited selection of health habits. These choices are related to the actual and perceived options available, beliefs and expectations developed and refined over time by socialization, formal learning experiences, and immediate experiences (Milio, 1976).

The third proposition regards organizational behavior. Specifically, the options available to individuals and the public's awareness of those options are influenced by the organizations. Thus, the range of choices available to the individual is determined by the decisions and policies established by businesses, governmental, and nongovernmental organizations. Fourth, the choices of individuals and populations at any given time concerning potentially health-promoting or health-damaging selections are directly affected by their resources (Milio, 1976). For example, if access to care, insurance coverage, or financial resources are limited, the individual's ability to engage in health-promoting activities will be limited.

Fifth, social change is the result of a change in the choice of health behaviors by a significant number of people in the population. This change is accomplished by increasing the public's awareness of health options and the benefits of participating. Finally, health education can have little or no effect on the health of individuals and populations unless new or newly perceived health options are available (Milio, 1976). Thus, more than education about healthy choices is needed; access and affordability issues must be addressed.

Vallgårda (2012) argued that the Framework of Prevention results in the manipulation of behavior and aims to change behavior without full understanding by the population involved, which is not ethical. Also, Vallgårda maintained that the idea people do not know what is best for them, or what their preferences are, is objectionable in a free society. Milio (1976) addressed this issue in her original work, stating, "current policy and allocative decisions clearly constrain personal choice-making, even if not so perceived by many people. The Framework for Prevention suggests strategies that will enhance the freedom to choose, making it readily possible for individuals and groups who now have difficult options to create healthful lifestyles" (p. 438).

Community Energy Theory

Carl Helvie, over a period of 15 years, developed the Community Energy Theory with the completed framework published in 1998 (Helvie & Nichols, 1998). The theory is heavily influenced by Organizational System Frameworks (see Chapter 17) and the work of Rogers and King (see Chapter 9). The major concepts include humans, environment, health, and nursing. Underlying these concepts is the concept of energy, which is a changing field over time. Energy is affected by internal exchanges (e.g., local resource exchange) and external exchanges of resources outside the community. According to Helvie, the human energy system (in this case, the community of humans) has the following characteristics:

- Is an open system
- Exists in an environment that is also energy
- Has the ability to exchange energy with the environment (both internal and external)
- Has changing needs that vary by time and situation
- Has the ability to adapt holistically to energy exchanges and achieve balance (Helvie & Nichols, 1998)

The ability to achieve balance or adapt determines the level of health. Adaptation or the movement toward illness or health on the energy continuum requires assistance from others. The PHN assists individuals to maintain or regain balance in the adaptation to energy exchanges.

The term *energy* as used in the Community Energy Theory can be "bound" in the subsystems of the community such as neighborhoods. Energy can also be kinetic or the energy of motion while carrying out a role or interacting with another in the community. Potential energy "refers to all of the knowledge, skills, flexible patterns, attitudes, and values of all personnel in community organizations, as well as of the community population who are recipients of services" (Helvie & Nichols, 1998, p. 29).

The internal exchange of energy occurs between the internal environment and the subsystems such as the environment's sanitation and the educational subsystem, or between subsystems, such as the economic and educational subsystems. External energy exchange happens between the whole community and other communities or the state or nation, or between subsystems of the community and the state or nation. Any of these exchanges may require adaptation that may be temporary or may require a change in the community. When there is poor adaptation (entropy or lack of energy to adapt and grow), intervention is needed.

In the Community Energy Theory, nurses act in the community using the energy model to follow the nursing process, that is, they begin by assessing the balance of energy exchanges. Then, planning and intervention are prioritized in terms of energy, with the goal to maintain or regain an appropriate balance of energies.

The Integrative Model for Holistic Community Health Nursing

The impetus for the Integrative Model for Holistic Community Health Nursing came from the need for a model that dealt with the holistic nature of humans outside the acute care setting (Laffrey & Kulbok, 1999). The Integrative Model is concerned with the conflict between holistic nursing of individuals within the community and having the entire community as a client. The model was proposed to highlight the many levels of care and collaboration involved in providing continuity of care, to assist nurses in clarifying their role in the community, and to establish collaboration among nurses and between nurses and other professionals.

The Integrative Model rests on six assumptions and three types of care. Assumptions describe the interacting concepts and systems as integrated, inseparable, with the targets of care viewed as part of a whole system. The interventions involve assumptions that recognize the effect of care on the whole, maximize health potential through interventions, and use a team approach. The types of care are depicted as illness care, illness/disease prevention, and at the core, health promotion. These types of care can be directed to the client, family, aggregate or group, community, and eventually to the whole of society.

As practice model, the Integrative Model for Holistic Community Health Nursing encourages care at multiple client levels, from individuals and their families to global communities. Although it emphasizes health promotion, the interventions around illness care and prevention are also relevant to the role of a CHN. One especially strong thread is the emphasis on population care as communication between nurses at all levels of care and in all foci (Laffrey & Kulbok, 1999).

Canadian Model of Community Health Nursing

The Canadian Model of Community Health Nursing was originally developed in 2003 to support nurses' control over the delivery of nursing care and the environment in which care is delivered (Community Health Nurses of Canada [CHNC], 2011). The current model, published in 2011, built on the original by refining the concepts and components. The CHNC (2011) defines the current model as, "A professional practice model that includes the structure, process, and values that support nurses' control over the delivery of nursing care and the environment in which care is delivered" (p. 9).

There are 13 components of the Canadian Model that represent the focus, scope, and influencing factors in community health nursing. The focus is on the client, CHN, code of ethics, values, principles, and social and environmental determinants of health. The scope includes community health nursing standards, delivery structure, delivery processes, and discipline-specific competencies. Influencing factors include governmental support, management practices, professional relationships and partnerships, professional regulatory standards, and theoretical foundations.

The paradigm underlying the components of the model includes person, health, nursing, environment, and social justice as central to the role of community health nursing. The Canadian community nurse standards of practice include health promotion, prevention, health protection, health maintenance, restoration and palliation, professional relationships, capacity building, access and equity, professional responsibility, and accountability. These standards are directly related to the competencies in specific community heath areas and are pictured as a subset of nursing with overlapping standards/competencies for those supervised by nurses. The standards along with the paradigm underlie the work nurses undertake using the components of the model.

Community Mobilization, Community Organization, and Community Building

The concepts of community mobilization, organization, and building form the basis of several frameworks and models that are relevant to health and cultural changes within communities. In the late 1800s, social workers called their efforts to coordinate services for new immigrants to the United States "community organization." In 1921, Lindeman wrote a treatise on the importance of struggling for release from outside controls and defined a new relationship between the community and larger units such as counties and nations. This concept of community organization was utilized by African Americans during the post-reconstruction period, by the populist movement of the 1930s, and by the labor movement in the 1940s. Its applicability to health for the community worldwide is evident with the WHO adopting the "healthy communities" approach to health promotion (Wallerstein, Minkler, Carter-Edwards, Avila, & Sánchez, 2015). An underlying theme for each of the communities involved in change was empowerment, or the challenge of having "power over" to become "power with" (Lippman et al., 2013; Wallerstein et al., 2015). This paradigm led to frameworks that were primarily aimed at inclusion of the community in the direction and ownership of its health.

Community engagement or community building models operate from five key concepts: community capacity, empowerment, critical consciousness, participation and relevance, and health equity. Wallerstein et al. (2015) proposed a model for the evaluation of frameworks (or programs) claiming to include community, or use community engagement. This model evaluates frameworks using three scales: strength versus needs-based, consensus versus conflict management, and collaboration versus advocate. They suggest that legitimate community building can occur anywhere within the three scales; however, the evaluation of the framework's placement within each scale should be consistent with the needs and strengths of the community itself.

An example of a disease and culture-specific community engagement model was published by Lippman et al. (2013). This model spoke specifically to South African community mobilization for the specific needs of those with HIV/AIDS. As a result of the synthesis of literature and practice realities, six community mobilization domains applicable to the culture of South Africa were identified. These domains are: shared concerns, critical consciousness, organizational structures/networks, leadership (individual and institutional), collective activities/actions, and social cohesion.

One example of the cultural differences in South Africa relative to community mobilization was "organizations/networks, while essential, operated differently than originally hypothesized—not through formal organizations, but through diffuse family networks" (Lippman et al., 2013, p. 1). Although adaptation of the domains to South African culture was needed, the domains did provide a structure useful to guide researchers and health care providers in the community mobilization process.

Multiple Interventions for Community Health Framework

In the mid-1980s, community and public health shifted from defining health and wellness in terms of single risks and single interventions to recognizing the influences of multiple factors and the need for complex and multileveled interventions (Edwards, Mill, & Kothari, 2004). The result has been a push for complex models and interventions, which have proliferated rapidly. However, many did not incorporate a comprehensive framework for testing, organizing, and sharing knowledge.

The Multiple Intervention Program Framework for Researchers was created to fill the gap. The framework can be visualized in a four-stage circle of progression. The first stage describes the socio-ecological features of the problem; the second identifies intervention options; the third is focused on optimizing the potential impact. The final stage is the monitoring and evaluation of program impact, spin-offs, and sustainability, which may help identify a new problem or provide input into the previous stage to help optimize the impact (Edwards et al., 2004).

Since the early 1970s, models and interventions have been based largely on the socio-ecological perspective of health. They encompass the idea that the relationship between humans and their environment is reciprocal and that humans in environments can be described at several levels: the individual, family, organization, community, and population. According to Edwards et al. (2004):

> Determinants may be "nested," so the strength of determinants at one level of the socio-ecological system will enhance or suppress how determinants interact at another level. Therefore, it is essential to consider not only the "layers" of determinants but also their interactions ... Those delivering health promotion programs are embracing the complexity of multiple intervention program design. It is time for researchers to do the same. (p. 45)

Some examples of increasing complex nursing models were reviewed and analyzed by Bigbee and Issel (2012). See Box 16.1 for more information.

> **BOX 16.1 Use of Conceptual Models for Community Health Nursing**
>
> As a result of the need for a stronger theoretic base for community nursing, Bigbee and Issel (2012) reviewed existing models and recommended rigorous testing and analysis that could be guided by the Multiple Interventions for Community Health Framework. The Community-as-partner model is based on Neuman's health system in conjunction with the nursing process and proposes eight subsystems along with lines of defense. The Dimensions Model of Community Health (or the Epidemiologic Prevention Process) uses the nursing process and public health prevention levels along with the determinants of health and dimensions of nursing. The Association of State and Territorial Directors of Nursing proposed a model using the nursing process, core public health functions, and essential services. It was later subsumed by the Quad Council (Quad Council, 2011) as a framework for competency evaluation in PHNs. The Public Health Nursing Population-focused Practice Model focuses on strategies and outcomes in several levels of care using the Intervention Wheel. The Los Angeles County Health Department proposed a model also using the Intervention Wheel, which was based on the nursing process and addressed health indicators. The Comprehensive Multi-Level Nursing Practice Model emphasizes interventions of personal preventive nursing, organized indigenous caregiving, and community empowerment using the PHN model and community-based action research.
>
> PHN, public health nurse.

FRAMEWORKS FOR PUBLIC AND POPULATION HEALTH

White's Construct for Public Health Nursing

In 1982, Marla Salmon White, a professor at the University of Minnesota, published a Construct for Public Health Nursing in response to the controversy regarding the definitions, education, practice, and domains of public health nursing. White contended the confusion in terminology was derailing public health. She believed defining the role, or form, of public health nursing should follow rather than lead the function of PHNs because the function will be more amenable to rapidly changing social needs than prescribed roles. The Construct for Public Health lies squarely on the premise that the greatest good is the greatest good for the greatest number (White).

The Construct for Public Health Nursing begins with three practice priorities: (a) prevention, (b) protection, and (c) promotion. There are three interventions necessary to achieve those priorities: education, engineering, and enforcement. The scope of public health nursing practice is broad and includes everything from individual nursing to global politics. White contends such a scope represents both the context and the commitment of this area of practice. According to the Construct for Public Health, the determinants of health as classified by *Healthy People* and published in 1979, affect and are affected by public health nursing. The nursing process (assessment, diagnosis, planning, implementation, and evaluation) and the valuing process (being committed to the health of the public) are the essential dynamics of the model.

According to Bigbee and Issel (2012), the Construct for Public Health is a conceptual model that contains determinants of health, the nursing process, the valuing process, and the PHN's scope of practice. They note the model has not been empirically documented nor tested and critique it for lack of inclusion of a theory base and failure to use the nursing metaparadigm. They also note the model does not address prevention levels, essential services, standards, or functions. However, the model identifies four categories of intervention: (a) human/biological; (b) environmental; (c) medical; technological and organizational; and (d) social, which can be useful for analyzing intervention structures and processes. Furthermore, the model describes the scope of prevention as ranging from individual, to family, community, and global care, giving practitioners a firm base for an increasingly complex and muliticultural practice envirnoment (White, 1982).

Population-Based Public Health Nursing Interventions Model

In 1994, the public health nursing section of the Minnesota Department of Health proposed a public health intervention model aimed at providing consistent nursing care with the use of evidence-based methods. The model was refined by nursing experts and practicing nurses to include a list of 17 public health interventions meant to organize the scope of practice for PHNs (Keller et al., 1998).

The Population-Based Public Health Nursing Interventions Model, also called the Minnesota Wheel, is practice-based and conceived as a spoked wheel with four concentric circles. The outer circle contains the 17 interventions (Box 16.2). The next three concentric circles depict population-based actions at the systems, community, and finally the individual level.

The model rests on several assumptions. The first assumption is interventions are based on analysis and evaluation of the health status of the community and the populations with risk. The second assumption is all levels of intervention (individual, community, and systems) will be used to address a problem. Third, the core public health functions, assessment policies, and quality improvement goals are addressed. The fourth assumption is the nursing process underlies all interventions, and fifth, the model is not used exclusively by nursing but supports all efforts to promote and protect public health.

The Public Health Interventions Model was revised and reintroduced as the Intervention Wheel as a result of a systematic critique funded by a federal Nursing Special Projects Grant (Keller, Strohschein, Lia-Hoagberg, & Schaffer, 2004b). As a result, several of the definitions were expanded and clarified. The critique verified the 17 interventions that encompassed the breadth, scope, and depth of public health roles without significant overlap. Evidence-based changes made in the model included re-leveling the case finding intervention, so it appears only at the individual/family level. There was also evidence that although each intervention was a discrete function, there was interdependence and simultaneous use. Using that evidence, the interventions on the wheel were rearranged from alphabetical to categorical to reflect those relationships (as noted in Box 16.2). Also, the expert consensus was to include policy enforcement as part of policy development, supporting their opinion that without enforcement, policy development was not effective. Other modifications included integrating provider education into health teaching, changing *delegated medical care* to *delegated functions*, and expanding "disease investigation" to "disease and other health event investigation."

Data generated by Keller et al. (2004b) not only supported the validity of the Public Health Interventions Model but supplied multiple best practice suggestions and exemplars of effective community health practice. For example, using the disease investigation intervention at the "population-based, systems-focused action level," a PHN collaborated with the state health department and the federal vaccine program to address cases of rubella in a migrant population. Outreach workers and private providers were trained to provide referrals to public health and a satellite vaccine-provider site for the migrant population was developed (Keller, Strohschein, Lia-Hoagberg, & Schaffer, 2004a).

The Public Health Nursing Model

The Public Health Nursing Model was published in 1997 to clarify and explain the roles and practice of PHNs (Kuss et al., 1997). They use the symbol of a tree as a graphic representation of the model, which is grounded in the concept of empowerment and is based on five assumptions. The first assumption is public health nursing is a synthesis of nursing and public health sciences. Second, the focus of public health nursing involves the larger population and its interactions. Next, public health nursing practice addresses the large contexts of the

---

BOX 16.2 Interventions for the Population-Based Public Health Nursing Interventions Model

Original Alphabetical List	Revised Categorical List
Advocacy	*Group 1*
Case Finding	Investigation
Case Management	Outreach
Coalition Building	Screening
Community Organization	Case Finding
Consultation	*Group 2*
Counseling	Referral/Follow-Up
Delegated Functions	Case Management
Disease/Event Investigation	Delegated Functions
Health Collaboration	*Group 3*
Outreach	Health Teaching
Policy Development	Counseling
Referral/Follow-up	Consultation
Screening	*Group 4*
Social Marketing	Collaboration
Surveillance	Coalition Building
Teaching	Community Organizing
	Group 5
	Advocacy
	Social Marketing
	Policy Development
	Enforcement

Sources: Keller et al. (1998, 2004).

---

population. The fourth assumption is human involvement with the environment is inevitable, and finally, members of a population make decisions that affect the health of the population.

Explicit concepts of the Public Health Nursing Model include:

- History/education
- Public health nursing roles/health functions
- Community empowerment
- Public health nursing service target
- Outcomes of protection, promotion, prevention, and access
- Environmental forces

The model also addresses four implicit concepts that are not depicted in the model's graphic. These are: caring, nursing process, interdisciplinary collaboration, and community partnership. Kuss et al. see these implicit concepts as incorporated into all levels of the tree model. See Kuss et al. (1997) for a graphic of the Public Health Nursing Model.

This model is suggested for practice and research because it proposes clarification of population-focused nursing roles and could be individualized for a recipient of care while focusing on the community as client. The Public Health Nursing Model can be effectively used as a framework for the development of health policy as it encourages participation from all stakeholders in the process of both policy creation and the implementation of the core functions of public health.

Integrated Model of Population Health and Health Promotion

The Integrated Model of Population Health and Health Promotion is also of Canadian origin as it serves as the official model for the Public Health Agency of Canada. The purpose of the model was to demonstrate how a population health approach may be implemented by influencing a range of health determinants and using health promotion strategies (Hamilton & Bhatti, 1996).

The Integrated Model is visualized as a cube (see the Public Health Agency of Canada website for a graphic model). The front of the cube lists the 12 determinants of health: income and social status, social support network, education, working conditions, physical environments, biology and genetics, personal health practices and coping skills, healthy child development, and health services. The sides of the cube contain the five strategies of health promotion. These strategies are: strengthening community action, building healthy public policy, creating supportive environments, developing personal skills, and reorienting health services. The top of the cube shows the levels of intervention as individual, family, community, system, and society.

The model is built on the following seven values and assumptions. First, comprehensive action will be taken on all determinants of health using evidence-based practice. Second, collaboration is the best way for organizations to analyze, plan, and act on the full range of possible actions. The third assumption points out the importance of multiple well-coordinated entry points to planning and implementation. Fourth, society as a whole is responsible for the health of its members despite the fact that certain groups have higher problem rates. Furthermore, the solution to those problems lies in changing the values and structures of that society. The fifth assumption is that health comprises an individual's lifestyle, social, and physical environment. Sixth, opportunities to meet physical, mental, social, and spiritual needs are necessary for optimal health. These include opportunities for justice, equity, respect, and caring as opposed to status and power. Finally, meaningful participation of the members of the society is necessary to achieve a comprehensive mix of policy and programs that will influence health decisions.

Omaha System Taxonomy

The Omaha System is an evidence-based taxonomy that provides a system for storing, organizing, and sharing clinical data (Martin, 2005). In the 1970s, the Visiting Nurses Association of Omaha, Nebraska, revised home health and public health records to use a problem orientation. From the outset, the reorganization was intended for computer use. The Division of Nursing, U.S. Department of Health and Human Services (DHHS), between 1975 and 1986, funded research to refine the system and validate its reliability, validity, and usefulness (Omaha System, 2016).

The taxonomy contains three categories or schemes. The first is the problem classification scheme or client assessment. This scheme suggests four domains: environmental, psychosocial, physiological, and health related for the assessment of the client. The second, or intervention scheme, contains four categories of action (teaching/guidance/counseling, treatments/procedures, case management, and surveillance). It also includes 75 targets or objects of action such as "anatomy/physiology" or "stress management." The third scheme is the Problem Rating Scale for Outcomes, which measures the range of severity for the concepts of knowledge, behaviors, and status. *Knowledge* is defined as what the client knows, *behavior as what the client does*, and *status* as the number and severity of the client's signs and symptoms or predicament. Each concept represents a continuum for examining problem-specific client ratings. Using the Problem Rating Scale for Outcomes along with the problem classification and intervention schemes provides a problem-solving model useful for educators, clinicians, administrators, and researchers (Omaha System, 2016).

Although the system is a result of public health nursing efforts, multiple health professional roles and systems use the model. Despite its beginnings, Kerr et al. (2016) declare the use of the system at the community level is still in its infancy. This statement led Kerr to test a community health use of the system across cultures (see Box 16.3).

 ## CONCLUSION

Many frameworks in multiple health care arenas are suited to guide research about, and care for, the community as client. The growth in the number of frameworks and the gradual shift from a provider and problem focus to a community and strength focus can be traced in the history of community and public health nursing. The frameworks presented here represent some of that numerical growth and focus shift. Specifically, these frameworks address the issues, challenges, and advantages of caring for a population either in place of or in addition to the individual client. See Tables 16.1 and 16.2 for a brief comparison of the frameworks presented in this chapter.

BOX 16.3 Use of the Omaha System in Assessing Communities

Using the research question, what is the feasibility of using the Omaha System to Capture Community level data and consistently describe community observations in international settings? Kerr et al. (2016) designed an empiric study. Nursing students from five countries used the Omaha System's taxonomy, with consistent terminology to describe 284 communities. Findings included the use of all 11 of the selected problems in every country and the use of each sign/symptom in at least three countries. The results supported the use of the system for community level observation and further emphasized its use as an electronic means of naming and sharing community data between countries.

TABLE 16.1 Characteristics of Community Health Frameworks

Framework	Selected Characteristics
Milio's Framework of Prevention	Making good health easier and bad health more difficult will increase a community's health
Community Energy Theory	Balance of energy and adaptation to exchange determines level of community health
Integrative Model for Holistic Community Health Nursing	Arrows highlighting differences/similarities between community as context and community as client
Canadian Model of Community Health Nursing	Focus is the client, community health nurse, code of ethics, values, principles, and social and environmental determinants of health Influencing factors include government, management, relationships and partnerships, regulatory standards, and theoretical foundations
Community Mobilization, Community Organization and Community Building	A series of models with a history of empowering the community to choose health
Multiple Interventions for Community Health	A research framework for the testing and evaluation of increasingly complex models

TABLE 16.2 Characteristics of Population-Focused Frameworks

Framework	Selected Characteristics
Salmon White's Construct for Public Health	Nursing actions must achieve the best outcome for the greatest number of people
Population-Based Public Health Nursing Interventions Model	Intervention Wheel with best practice use in levels of care (from system to individual)
Public Health Nursing Model	Illustrated as a tree rooted in community empowerment
Integrated Model of Population Health and Health Promotion	Concerned with addressing all determinants of health both in assessment and intervention
Omaha System Taxonomy	Taxonomic (now electronic) system for the storage, use, and sharing of public health data

● KEY POINTS

- Nursing theorists such as Nightingale, Neuman, Roy, King, Orem, and Pender, in addition to the Health Belief Model developed by Rosenberg and colleagues, can be used to address community health.

- Milio's Framework of Prevention is based on six propositions that underlie the practice of population-based care: (a) health is influenced by deficits or excesses, (b) behaviors are habitual selections from limited choices; (c) organizations determine the range of choices available; (d) individual choice is affected by personal and societal resources; (e) social change results in shifts in choice making; and (f) effective health education requires new or newly perceived options.

- White's Construct for Public Health Nursing identifies three practice priorities: (a) prevention, (b) protection, and (c) promotion, and three interventions needed to achieve those priorities: education, engineering, and enforcement.

- Community Energy Theory is based on Rogers's and King's work and sees health as the balance of and adaptation to the exchange of energies.

- The Public Health Nursing Model uses a graphic of a tree to illustrate the roles and practice of PHNs with an emphasis on community empowerment.

- The Population-Based Public Health Nursing Interventions Model, also known as the Minnesota Wheel, contains 17 interventions and underlying practice assumptions.

- The Omaha System is a taxonomy of assessment, interventions, and outcomes, which began as a method of organizing and communicating health information.

- The Canadian Model of Community Health Nursing is based on the community nurse standards of practice. Competencies for community health nursing are drawn directly from the model.

- The Integrated Model of Population Health and Health Promotion used the Canadian Model of Community Health Nursing and broadened the assumptions and scope by adding health determinants and underlying values.

- Community Mobilization and Community Organization and Community Building are sets of concepts used both formally and informally to address social problems. Problem-specific models are drawn from the concepts to guide the resolution of the identified problem.

- The Multiple Interventions for Community Health Framework was created to organize the multiple complexity models developed in response to specific community health problems. It is intended to push research into complexity thinking as it tests the models.

REFERENCES

American Public Health Association, Public Health Nursing Section. (2013). *The definition and practice of public health nursing: A statement of the public health nursing section.* Washington, DC: Author.

Bigbee, J. L., & Issel, L. M. (2012). Conceptual models for population-focused public health nursing interventions and outcomes: The state of the art. *Public Health Nursing, 29*(4), 370–379.

Clark, M. J. (2015). *Population and community health.* Upper Saddle River, NJ: Pearson.

Community Health Nurses of Canada. (2011). *Canadian community health nursing: Professional practice model & standards of practice.* Toronto, ON, Canada: Author.

Edwards, N., Mill, J., & Kothari, A. R. (2004). Multiple intervention research programs in community health. *The Canadian Journal of Nursing Research, 36*(1), 40–54.

Hamilton, N., & Bhatti, T. (1996). *Population health promotion: An integrated model of population health and health promotion.* Ottawa, ON, Canada: Health Promotion Development Division. Retrieved from http://www.phac-aspc.gc.ca/ph-sp/php-psp/index-eng.php#toc

Helvie, C. O., & Nichols, B. S. (1998). Reconceptualization of community health nursing clinicals for undergraduate students. *Public Health Nursing, 15*(1), 60–64.

Keller, L. O., Strohschein, S., Lia-Hoagberg, B., & Schaffer, M. (1998). Population-based public health nursing interventions: A model from practice. *Public Health Nursing, 15*(3), 207–215.

Keller, L. O., Strohschein, S., Lia-Hoagberg, B., & Schaffer, M. A. (2004a). Population-based public health interventions: Innovations in practice, teaching, and management. Part II. *Public Health Nursing, 21*(5), 469–487.

Keller, L. O., Strohschein, S., Lia-Hoagberg, B., & Schaffer, M. A. (2004b). Population-based public health interventions: Practice-based and evidence-supported. Part I. *Public Health Nursing, 21*(5), 453–468.

Kerr, M. J., Flaten, C., Honey, M. L., Gargantua-Aguila, S. del R., Nahcivan, N. O., Martin, K. S., & Monsen, K. A. (2016). Feasibility of using the Omaha system for community-level observations. *Public Health Nursing, 33*(3), 256–263.

Kuss, T., Proulx-Girouard, L., Lovitt, S., Katz, C. B., & Kennelly, P. (1997). A public health nursing model. *Public Health Nursing, 14*(2), 81–91.

Laffrey, S. C., & Kulbok, P. A. (1999). An integrative model for holistic community health nursing. *Journal of Holistic Nursing, 17*(1), 88–103.

Lindeman, E. (1921). *The community: An introduction to the study of community leadership and organization.* New York, NY: Association Press.

Lippman, S. A., Maman, S., MacPhail, C., Twine, R., Peacock, D., Kahn, K., & Pettifor, A. (2013). Conceptualizing community mobilization for HIV prevention: Implications for HIV prevention programming in the African context. *PLOS ONE, 8*(10), e78208. doi:10.1371/journal.pone.0078208

Martin, K. S. (2005). *The Omaha system: A key to practice, documentation, and information management* (Reprinted 2nd ed.). Omaha, NE: Health Connections Press.

Milio, N. (1976). A framework for prevention: Changing health-damaging to health-generating life patterns. *American Journal of Public Health, 66*(5), 435–439.

Neuman, B. (1996). The Neuman systems model in research and practice. *Nursing Science Quarterly, 9*(2), 67–70.

Nightingale, F. (1860/1969). *Notes on nursing: What it is and what it is not.* New York, NY: Dover.

Omaha System. (2016). Solving the clinical data-information puzzle: Omaha system overview. Retrieved from http://www.omahasystem.org/overview.html

Quad Council. (2011). Quad council competencies for public health nurses. Retrieved from http://www .resourcenter.net/images/ACHNE/Files/QuadCouncilCompetenciesForPublicHealthNurses_ Summer2011.pdf

Skinner, C. S., Tiro, J., & Champion, V. L. (2015). The health belief model. In K. Glanz, B. K. Rimer, & K. Viswanath (Eds.), *Health behavior and health education: Theory, research, and practice* (pp. 75–94). San Francisco, CA: Jossey-Bass.

Vallgårda, S. (2012). Nudge: A new and better way to improve health? *Health Policy, 104*(2), 200–203.

Wallerstein, N., Minkler, M., Carter-Edwards, L., Avila, M., & Sánchez, V. (2015). Improving health through community engagement, community organization, and community building. In K. Glanz, B. K. Rimer, & K. Viswanath (Eds.), *Health behavior and health education: Theory research, and practice* (5th ed., pp. 277–300). San Francisco, CA: Jossey-Bass.

World Health Organization Regional Office for South-East Asia. (2010). *A framework for community health nursing education.* Geneva, Switzerland: Author.

Organizational System Frameworks

Kristina Henry

To do things differently, we must see things differently. When we see things we haven't noticed before, we can ask questions we didn't know to ask before.
—John Kelsch, former corporate director of quality, Xerox Corporation

⬤ KEY TERMS

Bolman and Deal's four frames	Complex Adaptive System	Microsystem Model
Chaos Theory	Critical Systems Thinking Theory	Open Systems Theory
Closed Systems Theory	General Systems Theory	organizational system

⬤ LEARNING OBJECTIVES

1. Explore the basic concepts of organizational system frameworks.
2. Analyze the applicability of organizational system frameworks to health care organizational systems.
3. Review evidence-based utilization of organizational system frameworks.
4. Compare and contrast basic concepts and premises of organizational system frameworks.

Organizational system frameworks are based on organizational structure and processes related to analyzing and synthesizing the complex nature of organizational systems. The basis of an *organizational system* is the coordination of a multitude of entities working toward common purposes. Organizing these interrelated entities and their individual perspectives is a challenge and may lead to barriers to success. The frameworks and concepts identified in this chapter are diverse and represent methods to analyze the organizational structure and processes to maximize outcomes.

The humanistic and cultural components of organizational leadership, such as management and change, are not isolated in practice from organizational structure and practices. These concepts must be coordinated and are dependent on each other for organizational function. However, for purposes of managing chaos, organizational leadership, management, and change are addressed in Chapter 18.

⬤ ORGANIZATIONAL FRAMEWORKS

Organizational frameworks are used to describe and understand the organizational processes or structure. The concepts of process and structure explain the interrelated aspects of organizations needed to lead and manage organizations successfully. These concepts are essential for grasping the organizational purpose, goals, and needs; and for the selection and application of appropriate leadership and management frameworks.

General Systems Theory

The General Systems Theory (GST) was first described by Ludwig von Bertalanffy in the first half of the 20th century to describe common concepts characteristic of a system. GST incorporates a broad, universal set of frameworks that may be applied to any system to clarify goals and processes for accomplishment. The GST originated from a biological perspective of living organisms. Therefore, a system is described as a complex and chaotic entity of multiple interdependent parts, functions, and relationships that are both internal and external to the system. Using various scientific and multidisciplinary approaches, GST examines a system as a whole unit (von Bertalanffy, 1968).

GST acknowledges the system is composed of a relationship of many parts, thus leading to a complicated and disorderly entity. However, it supports a comprehensive and holistic approach including teamwork and collaboration for a collective process. Each component of the system must be studied, including the internal and external environment. Methods may involve both quantitative and qualitative techniques for investigation and inquiry, in addition to theoretical concepts from a variety of disciplines.

The primary application of this theory is to study and analyze the interdependent components of the system to optimize productivity. For instance, if a company is experiencing delayed distribution, each component that is involved in the distribution would be evaluated to determine the cause. Once the cause is established, potential solutions are reviewed. In health care, an example of application of GST would be risk or safety analysis. If a patient experiences a medication error, all departments, processes, and care providers involved would be analyzed to pinpoint the cause. For example, the direct cause could be related to the location of the medication in the distribution system, the medication label, or the allergy documentation system. All of the interdependent systems linked to the administration of medications must be assessed and evaluated.

Critical Systems Thinking Theory

Critical Systems Thinking Theory has evolved from the basic premise of the GST (Flood & Jackson, 1991). Building on the broad view of organizations, the Critical Systems Thinking Theory expounds on five elements for system analysis: critical awareness, social awareness, complementarism at the methodology level, complementarism at the theory level, and human emancipation. The content of this theory is similar to the GST; however, the Critical Systems Thinking Theory gives more detail and direction for critical analysis and direct application. Using each of the five elements to analyze the system gives a thorough assessment and evaluation of the system, including the social context and perspective.

The first concept, critical awareness, involves an analysis and evaluation of the principles, strengths, and weaknesses throughout the system. The next concept, social awareness, is the analysis and evaluation of the organizational culture. The effect and influence of the organizational culture on the system are a primary component. Complementarism at the methodology level involves the assessment and analysis of a multitude of tasks and methods. Complementarism at the theory level is advocating for a multitude of theories to support and explain system existence. Human emancipation is the human resource process of development to improve the quality of life for individuals, families, and communities interacting within and with the system.

A multitude of system frameworks exist. However, the Critical Systems Thinking Theory advocates for a direct and thorough examination of the system and theoretical application specific to the needs, goals, and culture of the system. The analysis of diverse frameworks and systems provides varied perspectives and enforces deeper understanding, thus promotes selection and application of the most relevant frameworks.

Open Systems Theory

The Open Systems Theory for organizational systems dispels the notion that organizations are closed and isolated entities. It describes organizational systems as manipulated by and reliant on the associated environment. All aspects of the environment affect the system: political, economic, cultural, and educational. As the environment experiences shifts or changes, the organizational system must adapt to sustain and thrive. This dependency on the environment creates an essential relationship of collaboration and cooperation (Scott, 2002).

As with several other theories, the Open Systems Theory describes the organizational system as consisting of interdependent subsystems. The subsystems may be differentiated by department or task-based organizational design. However, the subsystems are not all equivalent, nor are they all essential. If one subsystem fails, it does not mean the organizational system will fail as well (Katz & Kahn, 1978).

Open Systems Theory provides a way to analyze a health care system, as all health care systems rely on the external environment for sustainability. Political, economic, cultural, and educational influences impact the operational standards for patient care and, ultimately reimbursement and funding. Politically, as legislation changes, reimbursement processes and standards of operations must adapt. Economically, the health care system is affected if it serves predominantly uninsured or underinsured versus Medicare and insured patients (i.e., if the organization is not for profit or for profit). Culturally, the health care system's base of operation is directed by its mission and values, which can be influenced by liberal or conservative views. Educationally, a system with an environment of high educational level will demonstrate more complex skills and knowledge, whereas a system with an environment of low education will produce a simple and rudimentary organizational system. The function of the entire health care system is dependent on the environment, thus supporting the Open Systems Theory.

Closed Systems Theory

The Closed Systems Theory describes organizational environments shut off from outside political, cultural, and technological influences. The organization in a closed system is self-regulating and operates with little consideration for any external considerations. The organizational process and structure are based on internal managers, technology, and goals while ignoring the impact of governmental regulations, supply and distribution, or economic policies. For this reason, the closed system has been criticized for lack of adaptability to environmental influences, thus limiting long-term organizational sustainability (Daft, 2001).

Examples of closed systems include production lines or innovative development departments. Both examples are devoid of meetings with or information from other departments. In the production line, outside influences undermine efficiency and quality as it is described as interference. Closed systems models are described as mechanistic and are used to maximize efficiency. In the innovative development department, outside interaction and influence pose a risk to any new and original progress (Daft, 2001).

Complex Adaptive Systems

Complex Adaptive Systems (CAS) are complicated and dynamic operating systems with multiple processes and teams. The CAS comprises many independent entities and stakeholders with potentially conflicting goals and regulations. It is an interdisciplinary process involving adaptation, coordination, collaboration, and cooperation on all levels of the system. Key factors of the CAS are resiliency and flexibility for sustainability as the CAS adapts and evolves (Olson & Eoyang, 2001).

Each level of the system has an independent perspective and function, yet it is connected to the entire system and interacts dynamically with the system. This relationship means that changes in one level will affect other levels of the system regardless of whether there are defined boundaries or the system is open. For this reason, communication and risk management processes must be efficient, detailed, and comprehensive. As there is no locus of control, the result is often chaotic and unpredictable. There is a constant state of evolution and adaptability based on influences from the CAS history. A state of equilibrium is nonexistent in a CAS, which by its nature is unpredictable (Olson & Eoyang, 2001).

Health care systems comprising acute care facilities and community clinics are considered CASs as are academic institutions. The changes in the health care culture in the United States, including policy and reimbursement, have resulted in the necessity for organizations to be adaptable and flexible for survival. Every organization faces challenges and barriers. However, only systems able to adapt and overcome will achieve success and longevity. CASs must recognize their unpredictable complexity and develop processes to address uncertainty and enhance productivity to achieve goals (Sturmberg, O'Halloran, & Martin, 2013).

The CAS model has been widely used in research and applied to health care systems since the mid-1990s. It has been applied to specific organizational processes such as clinical pathways, management, and medication errors (Arndt & Bigelow, 2000; Begun, Zimmerman, & Dooley, 2003). Organizational leadership and management analysis based on the CAS model have been widely used (McDaniel, Driebe, & Lanham, 2013; Zimmerman, Lindberg, & Plsek, 2001). A study by Bircher and Kuruvilla (2014) describes a health model based on CAS principles (see Box 17.1). Another study by McDaniel et al. (2013) explored health care organizations and systems using the CAS model (see Box 17.2).

The CAS model is also used to analyze and understand failures and disasters. In health care, this would translate to "never events." Organizations dissect the events and occurrences that led to the ultimate failure. Using the CAS model, organizations are able to identify and examine the complexity of the situation, including interactions, interdependencies, and conditions responsible for the event. This process involves investigating the complex course or "drift into failure," including all the complex components (Dekker, 2011).

Chaos Theory

Similar to the CAS theory, the Chaos Theory describes organizational systems as open, nonlinear, and dynamic entities influenced by forces of disorder precipitated by either the system itself or the environment. As the system and the environment evolve and adapt, the inability to predict outcomes or random events creates challenges. The challenge of managing unexpected outcomes or events is the foundation of the Chaos Theory. Systems able to expect the unexpected are more stable, sustainable, and successful (Levy, 1994).

Risk and innovation are necessary for organizational system survival. However, these concepts define chaos and instability. The Chaos Theory is used to analyze experimentation in the organizational system to manage the process and create a balance of initiative and experience. A system comprising constant change and turmoil is counterproductive and destructive. But a chaotic system is not powerless. It successfully balances the chaos and instability of change with the stability of experience and wisdom (Levy, 1994).

BOX 17.1 Complex Adaptive System: Developing Plan of Care

The Meikirch Model of Health was designed to emphasize the need for collaboration among social entities and resources (health, socioeconomic, and environmental) to improve and achieve health goals. This coordination of resources and efforts is based on CAS principles. Health is a complex concept affected by many components: the individual, family, community, government, caregivers, businesses, and many other interconnected entities, efforts, and resources. As viewed through the CAS model, health goals and promotion could be better achieved with coordination of these complex resources and efforts (Bircher & Kuruvilla, 2014).

BOX 17.2 Complex Adaptive System: Health Care Analysis

This study examines health care organizations and systems based on the CAS model (McDaniel, Driebe, & Lanham, 2013). Over the last decade, health care has experienced many changes and challenges, including technological advances and information systems. An analysis using the CAS model emphasizes diverse perspectives, thus supporting meaningful understanding of the various relationships and interdependent components. The CAS analysis of health care leads to the development of innovative, effective, and efficient management strategies (McDaniel et al., 2013).

A common analogy used to explain Chaos Theory is the "butterfly effect." Essentially, the butterfly effect acknowledges that a butterfly flapping its wings in Asia can impact the weather in North America. More simply, forces of nature that affect weather in one part of the world will impact weather across the globe. Applying this idea to organizations means that even small changes in one department or unit will ultimately impact other units and the organization as a whole (Wheatley, 2001).

Health care organizations are inherently chaotic entities. There are multiple units, departments, patients, families, health care providers, and staff all with different perspectives and priorities. Successful organizations account for the unknown and the disorder that comes with these diverse perspectives and priorities. Leaders within the organization acknowledge the chaotic environment and incorporate this into the strategic plan. Chaos management may be accomplished by fostering autonomy and empowerment and creativity and innovation while maintaining organizational expectations. Leadership and management strategies are used to manage chaos and have clear boundaries and expectations.

Bolman and Deal's Four Frames

Bolman and Deal (2003) developed the Four Frame Model to examine and understand the increasing complexity of organizations. This model synthesizes social and behavioral sciences with management and political principles to develop a comprehensive view of organizations using four frames: structural, human resource, political, and symbolic. Viewing the organization through each of the four frames creates a whole perspective and more in-depth understanding of the organization. Leaders have strengths and weaknesses in specific frames and tend to focus on situations through specific frames. According to the model, when dealing with challenges it is beneficial to reframe and view the situation from a different perspective.

The structural frame is based on the organization and arrangement of the institution. This view focuses on the organization through organizational charts, hierarchies, and job descriptions, as well as formal policies and procedures. The structural frame defines and establishes unified goals, direction, and purpose of the organization.

The human resource frame highlights the people and relationships that compose the organization. The focus is on professional and individual training and development, including suitability within an organization. The people are the foundation of the organization. This frame is based on feelings, emotions, or bias.

The political frame emphasizes authority, power, and competition for limited resources. Competing interests and values lead to the necessity to manage conflict: network, negotiate, compromise, and influence. The political goal of organizational leaders is to establish an appropriate balance of effective management with creative innovation. This frame is based on balancing political influence and power for organizational success.

The symbolic frame is based on finding a sense of meaning and significance. This frame depicts the soul and passion of the organization in the context of organizational culture. The symbolic frame is reflected in ceremonies, traditions, and rituals. Graduation and retirement ceremonies reflect meaning and purpose in the symbolic frame. Examples of additional concepts relevant to Bolman and Deal's four frames are provided in Table 17.1.

In summary, people tend to lean toward a certain frame based on their interests and personalities. Using the Four Frame Model to view the change or conflict through a different frame may alter one's perspective and thus facilitate communication. For example, if a person's focus is primarily a structural frame, choosing to view the situation through the political, human resource, or symbolic frame may improve understanding (Bolman & Deal, 2003). Because all organizational change involves some degree of conflict, the Four Frames Model may be helpful in broadening perspectives, facilitating communication, and managing conflict.

Microsystem Model

The Dartmouth Institute developed the Microsystem Academy as an innovative process improvement model, which deconstructs a health care system into workable units called *clinical microsystems*. The clinical microsystems are the patient-centered units of the health care system. This model emphasizes the importance of the direct level of care, and thus empowers those stakeholders at the bedside (Nelson et al., 2002).

Once the microsystems are identified, the mesosystem and macrosystem levels are recognized and analyzed. All levels of the system are studied independently and in relation to their effect on the other levels. The microsystem is defined as the smallest interdependent unit. In health care, this may be the emergency department or lab department. The mesosystem is a middle-level organizational unit, such as a same-day surgery center or a facility

TABLE 17.1 Examples of Concepts Relevant to Bolman and Deal's Four Frames

Structural	Human Resource	Political	Symbolic
Organizational charts	People	Power and authority	Culture
Policies and procedures	Biases and feelings	Competition for resources	Meaning and spirit
Coordination of efforts	Skills and development	Management and leadership	Ceremony
Technology	Training	Influence	Rituals
Roles	Maximize human potential	Conflict	Stories and myths
Rules		Negotiation	

Source: Bolman and Deal (2003).

TABLE 17.2 Examples of Factors Relevant to the Microsystem Model

Microsystem	Mesosystem	Macrosystem
Clinical practice setting Daily huddles, team meetings, staff meetings Best practice Practice benchmarks Active engagement Coaching	Support and facilitate Resources Develop performance measures Link daily work to results Set goals and expectations Advocacy Address barriers Facilitate communication and coordination	Develop vision and mission Manager and leadership development Regular feedback Liaison with external forces Design system measures and goals Develop budgets and resources Accountability

Source: Nelson et al. (2002).

TABLE 17.3 Comparison of Organizational System Frameworks' Premises

Theory	Basic Premise
General Systems Theory	Describes a system as a complex and chaotic entity of multiple interdependent parts, functions, and relationships (internal and external)
Critical Systems Thinking Theory	Five elements for system analysis: critical awareness, social awareness, methodology complementarism, theory complementarism, and human emancipation
Open System	Organizational systems manipulated by and reliant on the associated environment All aspects of the environment affect the system: political, economic, cultural, and educational
Closed System	Organizational environment is shut off from outside influences, is self-regulating and operates with little consideration for external influences
Complex Adaptive System	Includes independent entities and stakeholders with potentially conflicting goals and regulations Involves adaptation, coordination, collaboration, and cooperation on all system levels
Chaos Theory	Open, nonlinear, and dynamic entities influenced by forces of disorder; inability to predict outcomes or random events creates challenges
Microsystem Model	Process improvement model that deconstructs a health care system into workable units: microsystem, mesosystem, and macrosystem
Bolman and Deal's Four Frames	A comprehensive view of organizations using four frames: structural, human resource, political, and symbolic

in a health care system. The macrosystem is the larger influencing systems, which includes external stakeholders and governmental regulations.

Changes made at all levels impact the other levels in the microsystem model. For instance, if the budget is cut or there are decreases in reimbursement at the macrosystem level, then the microsystem level may expect to see changes in staffing or other methods to decrease expenditures. The mesosystem level would facilitate the communication between the microsystem and macrosystem, as well as advocate for both. Some of the factors relevant to the Microsystem Model are shown in Table 17.2.

⬤ CONCLUSION

This chapter represents theories, methods, and models to analyze organizational structures and processes. The complex and chaotic nature of organizations, especially in health care, requires the use of tools and guides to assist with organizational analysis and evaluation. The key to success and sustainability is to emphasize organizational strengths while addressing organizational weaknesses. Emphasizing strengths and addressing weaknesses leads to a coordinated organizational approach with everyone working toward common goals and objectives. Without organizational system frameworks, organizational chaos would be unmanageable and would lead to a disorganized and unwieldy process. Table 17.3 compares organization system frameworks presented in this chapter.

⬤ KEY POINTS

- The basis of an organizational system is the coordination of a multitude of entities working toward common purposes.
- The GST originated from a biological perspective of living organisms. It describes a system as a complex and chaotic entity of multiple interdependent parts, functions, and relationships that are both internal and external to the system.
- The Critical Systems Thinking Theory expounds on five elements for system analysis: critical awareness, social awareness, complementarism at the methodology level, complementarism at the theory level, and human emancipation. Using each of the five elements to analyze the system will give a thorough assessment and evaluation of the system, including social context and perspective.
- The Open Systems Theory describes organizational systems as manipulated by and reliant on the associated environment. All aspects of the environment affect the system: political, economic, cultural, and educational. As environment experiences shift or change, the organizational system must adapt to sustain and thrive.
- The Closed Systems Theory describes organizational environments that are shut off from outside influences and function solely within the organization. The organization is self-regulating and operates with little consideration for any external considerations.
- CASs comprise of many independent entities and stakeholders with potentially conflicting goals and regulations. It is an interdisciplinary process involving adaptation, coordination, collaboration, and cooperation on all levels of the system.
- The Chaos Theory describes organizational systems as open, nonlinear, and dynamic entities influenced by forces of disorder precipitated by either the system itself or the environment. As the system and the environment evolve and adapt, the inability to predict outcomes or random events creates challenges. The challenge of managing unexpected outcomes or events is the foundation of the Chaos Theory.

- Bolman and Deal's Four Frames Model synthesizes social and behavioral sciences with management and political principles to develop a comprehensive view of organizations using four frames: structural, human resource, political, and symbolic. Viewing the organization through each of the four frames creates a whole perspective and provides more in-depth understanding of the organization.

- The Microsystem Model is a process improvement model that deconstructs a health care system into workable units the microsystem, mesosystem, and macrosystem.

REFERENCES

Arndt, M., & Bigelow, B. (2000). Commentary: The potential of chaos theory and complexity theory for health services management. *Health Care Management Review, 25*(1), 35–38.

Begun, J., Zimmerman, B., & Dooley, K. (2003). Health care organizations as complex adaptive systems. In S. M. Mick & M. Wyttenbach (Eds.), *Advances in health care organization theory* (pp. 253–288). San Francisco, CA: Jossey-Bass.

Bircher, J., & Kuruvilla, S. (2014). Defining health by addressing individual, social, and environmental determinants: New opportunities for health care and public health. *Journal of Public Health Policy, 35*(3), 363–386.

Bolman, L., & Deal, T. (2003). *Reframing organizations: Artistry, choice, and leadership* (3rd ed.). San Francisco, CA: Jossey-Bass.

Daft, R. (2001). *Organization theory and design* (7th ed.). Florence, KY: South-Western College Publishing.

Dekker, S. (2011). *Drift into failure: From hunting broken components to understanding complex systems.* Surrey, England: Ashgate Publishing.

Flood, R. L., & Jackson, M. C. (Eds.). (1991). *Critical systems thinking: Directed readings.* New York, NY: Wiley.

Katz, D., & Kahn, R. (1978). *The social psychology of organizations* (2nd ed.). New York, NY: Wiley.

Levy, D. (1994). Chaos theory and strategy: Theory, applications, and managerial implications. *Strategic Management Journal, 15,* 167–178.

McDaniel, R. R., Driebe, D. J., & Lanham, H. J. (2013). Health care organizations as complex systems: New perspectives on design and management. *Advances in Health Care Management, 15,* 3–26.

Nelson, E. C., Batalden, P. B., Huber, T. P., Mohr, J. J., Godfrey, M. M., Headrick, L. A., & Wasson, J. H. (2002). Microsystems in health care: Part 1. Learning from high-performing front-line clinical units. *The Joint Commission Journal on Quality Improvement, 28*(9), 472–493.

Olson, E., & Eoyang, G. (2001). *Facilitating organization change.* San Francisco, CA: Jossey-Bass.

Scott, W. R. (2002). *Organizations: Rational, natural, and open systems.* Upper Saddle River, NJ: Prentice Hall.

Sturmberg, J., O'Halloran, D., & Martin, C. (2013). Healthcare reform: The need for a complex adaptive systems approach. In J. P. Sturmberg & C. M. Martin (Eds.), *Handbook of systems and complexity in health* (pp. 827–853). New York, NY: Springer.

von Bertalanffy, L. (1968). *General system theory: Essays on its foundation and development.* New York, NY: George Braziller.

Wheatley, M. (2001). *Leadership and the new science: Discovering order in a chaotic world.* San Francisco, CA: Berrett-Koehler.

Zimmerman, B., Lindberg, C., & Plsek, P. (2001). *Edgeware: Insights from complexity science for health care leaders.* Irving, TX: Veterans Health Administration.

Leadership Frameworks for Organizational Systems

Kristina Henry

Vision without action is merely a dream. Action without vision passes the time. Vision and action can change the world.
—Joel Barker

KEY TERMS

Apprenticeship Model of Mentoring
autocratic leadership
bureaucracy theory
communication
Contingency and Situational Leadership Theory
democratic leader
Difficult Conversations
emotional intelligence
Five-Phase Mentoring Relationship Model

GROW Model
Havelock's Theory of Change
Hudson's Five-Factor Mentoring Model
Imposter Phenomena Theory
Lewin's Change Theory
logic models
management
Model of Caring Mentorship for Nursing

Quantum leadership theory
Rogers's diffusion of innovation
Scientific Management Theory
Theory of Servant Leadership
Tipping Point Theory
Transactional Leadership Theory
Transformational Leadership Theory
Transitional Theory

LEARNING OBJECTIVES

1. Explore development and application of organizational system leadership frameworks to health care organizations and systems.
2. Analyze organizational system leadership frameworks related to complex organizational health care systems.
3. Describe the attributes and assumptions of organizational system leadership frameworks and their applicability to health care organizations and systems.
4. Compare and contrast organizational system leadership frameworks as applied to health care organizations and systems.

The vision, mission, values, and culture of an organizational system are based on the leadership of the organization and support the goals of the organization. Organizational leadership mirrors the complexity and chaos that is inherent in organizational systems. Organizational systems leadership is a fluid and dynamic process requiring adaptation and flexibility as the needs of the organizational system and all of its entities work together. The organizational system leader must be aware of external influences, such as community or political pressures, as well as internal influences of organizational goals and culture.

This chapter reviews frameworks related to organizational systems leadership, which includes leadership, management, organizational change, communication, and mentoring frameworks. To support organizational systems, both leadership and change concepts are represented to maximize successful leadership in organizational and system change initiatives. The following frameworks are easily adaptable and generalizable to diverse organizations and systems, which address a range of topics, projects, and populations.

● LEADERSHIP FRAMEWORKS

In this section, classic and modern leadership concepts, theories, and models are reviewed. Each offers a unique perspective, focus, and definition of leadership. As a whole, these frameworks provide insight into the complex and dynamic nature of leadership, the development of leader attributes, the development of the leadership role, and the development of interpersonal relationships with mentees and subordinates.

The use of leadership frameworks is vital to the development and maintenance of organizational systems. Selection of leadership frameworks is dependent on the culture, needs, and strategic planning of each organization or system. This section focuses on organizational leadership frameworks used to guide visionary organizational processes such as change and communication. *Management* is a necessary component of leadership related to project completion and specific accomplishment of tasks. Management is frequently associated with organizational systems leadership; therefore, several management frameworks are also included in this section.

Democratic Leadership

> *The strongest democracies flourish from frequent and lively debate, but they endure when people of every background and belief find a way to set aside smaller differences in service of a greater purpose.*
> —Barack Obama

Democracy originated in ancient Greek times. Citizens fulfilled governmental roles, congregated as a legislative body, and held elections. They were granted voting authority and the authority to speak, establish laws, and make decisions regarding governance. A primary premise of democracy is freedom and the right to participate in governance (Dahl, Shapiro, & Cheibub, 2003). Through the centuries, democracy has evolved and been defined or applied in a variety of formats, from Britain to the Netherlands, as well as the United States. This chapter focuses on relating and applying the general theoretical concept of democracy to leadership characteristics and roles.

A *democratic leader* guides a group toward common goals by engaging the group members and encouraging participation. All members of the group are involved and encouraged to contribute. Once all information is gathered, and group members have supplied their input, the democratic leader is responsible for analysis and final decision making. The democratic leader empowers others to participate and contribute and recognizes the value of others' knowledge, skills, and abilities. The collaboration of members of the group should emphasize the strengths of the individual members and result in a comprehensive effort (Woods, 2010). This democratic method maximizes efficiency and effectiveness of the group.

Engaging the group members toward a common goal and utilizing the attributes of the individual members to achieve the goal are the hallmarks of the democratic leader.

Creating and sustaining a culture of participation and engagement as characterized by the democratic leadership style are time-consuming and challenging. Thus, the democratic leadership style is not useful or appropriate in all situations. For example, in health care, many situations are emergent and time is critical and therefore are not conducive to the democratic style of leadership. For instance, when a patient is experiencing a cardiac arrest, the patient cannot wait for all members of the health care team to have input. Time is crucial, and the patient cannot wait for care while the democratic leader considers the contributions of all members before rendering a decision. The application of democratic leadership to this situation would be detrimental to patient outcomes. However, a democratic culture is evident in shared governance models of health care organizations, thus creating supportive cultures for nursing input and interprofessional collaboration.

Autocratic Leadership

Those who abhor democracy would rarely immigrate to an authoritarian state if they have to.
—Joe Chung

The autocratic leadership style is based on total authority and control. In an autocratic culture, the leader is powerful and dominates the other group members or subordinates, much like a dictator. The autocratic leader supervises and oversees the group dictating all actions and decisions. The autocratic leader assumes sole responsibility for decision making (Lewin, Lippitt, & White, 1939).

This style of leadership was prevalent before the evolution and progression of democracy. Since the democratic movement, the autocratic style of leadership has acquired a negative connotation as it discourages member participation, individuality, and empowerment. Thus, the autocratic style of leadership may result in a negative culture and low morale (Lewin et al., 1939). Therefore, autocratic leadership is unpopular and frequently avoided in modern application. The control and lack of group member contribution are limiting and diminish creativity. The autocratic leader does not delegate based on expertise, but retains control and domination. Subordinates are motivated by rewards or fear, punishment, and retribution. Recent research has supported these premises based on staff satisfaction (see Box 18.1).

Despite inherent weaknesses and criticisms, there are situations in which autocratic leadership is beneficial. In health care, many situations require control and autocratic decision making for efficient and effective care delivery. Emergency situations call for rapid,

---

BOX 18.1 Research Application of Democratic Versus Autocratic Leadership Style

Researchers compared self-reported leadership styles of nurse managers with the perceptions of the staff nurses and analyzed results based on the job satisfaction of the staff nurses. The results indicated a significant variance in the perceptions of the nurse manager and the staff nurses regarding the leadership style of the nurse manager. Overall, a positive correlation was discovered between democratic leadership style and staff nurse job satisfaction. Conversely, a negative correlation was discovered between autocratic leadership style and staff nurse job satisfaction. This study demonstrates the significant effect of nurse manager leadership styles on job satisfaction of staff nurses (Daniel, Bhardwaj, & Arora, 2015).

experienced, and skillful management. There is no time for group collaboration or individual member input; one person must take the lead. Thus, autocratic leadership application would be the best choice in urgent, time-sensitive situations.

Laissez-Faire Leadership

Surround yourself with the best people you can find, delegate authority, and don't interfere as long as the policy you've decided upon is being carried out.
—Ronald Reagan

The concept of laissez-faire leadership originated as early as the 1600s by the French. This style of leadership is based on faith and trust. These leaders see others as autonomous and empowered. Individuals are given minimal direction by the leader and instead work toward common goals using their personal knowledge, skills, and abilities. As long as goals are met, and work is satisfactory, the laissez-faire leader provides minimal interference (Lewin et al., 1939). The leader relies on the team to work independently without strict oversight or direction by the leader or manager. The leader or manager delegates day-to-day decision making and task accomplishment to members of the group; however, strategic planning is still performed at the leadership level. This style of leadership is often reflected in organizations relying on creativity and innovation, such as advertising or research development.

In health care, the laissez-faire style of leadership is used to problem-solve patient care concerns or unit-based patient satisfaction initiatives. It empowers the bedside nurse to make decisions at the point of care, improves patient outcomes, and satisfaction. For instance, if a patient desires a specific diet or has specific needs regarding visiting hours, the nurse is empowered to address the patient's desires with an appropriate solution using critical thinking and creativity.

The laissez-faire leader is an expert at delegation and fosters empowerment with the use of rewards and positive affirmations. However, the laissez-faire leader is responsible for providing constructive feedback and intervening when necessary. The freedom allotted to the group is directly related to the level of skill and experience of the group members. The more knowledgeable and skillful the group is, the more freedom and latitude the leader can allow. The laissez-faire leader is ultimately responsible for success and goal accomplishment, so he or she must be confident in the ability of the team.

Laissez-faire leadership is exemplified in health care education through the accreditation bodies. For example, the Commission on Collegiate Nursing Education (CCNE) is a national accreditation agency for baccalaureate, graduate, and residency nursing programs whose purpose is to ascertain quality, integrity, effectiveness, and accountability of nursing education programs. The CCNE outlines regulatory standards for nursing programs; however, it does not dictate how to accomplish the standards. The CCNE standards are broad and general. Each program determines how to meet the standards and demonstrate program values.

The laissez-faire leadership style would not be effective in all situations. As in the example provided earlier of the patient who is experiencing a cardiac arrest or another medical emergency, it would not be an appropriate time to foster creativity and allow group members to work independently. Although it is important to delegate in this situation, this medical emergency calls for strict oversight of all members of the health care team.

Servant Leadership

The Theory of Servant Leadership was first described by Robert Greenleaf in 1970 (2015). He explained servant leaders have the conscious desire to put others' needs and priorities first. The servant leader is a member of the community or organization in which he or she leads, and the leader shares power and authority with the community or organization. The leader is humble, values, and trusts others. Greenleaf believed if organizations adopted a servant leadership model, and put the needs of the most vulnerable first, it could alter society.

Greenleaf explained the servant leadership model through ten basic principles: listening, empathy, healing, awareness, persuasion, conceptualization, foresight, stewardship, commitment to the growth of people, and building community (see Table 18.1). The servant leader must use active listening skills and be an expert at verbal and nonverbal communication strategies. The second principle describes the display of empathy through the acceptance and recognition of the unique attributes and intentions of others. Third is the healing of self and others in a holistic manner. Fourth is the ability to discover self and others through awareness and mindfulness. The principle of persuasion is the ability to convince without the use of authority and move toward consensus. Conceptualization is the sixth principle, which describes the ability to balance visionary and daily management tasks and responsibilities. Foresight is the seventh principle explained as intuition and the ability to grasp historical and future implications. The eighth principle is stewardship and the focus on the greater good of society to care for the vulnerable. The ninth principle is the commitment to the holistic growth and development of the population and team members. The tenth and final principle is the aptitude of the leader to build community spirit and form a cooperative organizational culture. These principles reflect the underlying values and beliefs held by servant leaders.

TABLE 18.1 Servant Leadership Principles

Principle	Description
Listening	Must strive to communicate with others through listening to individuals, the group, and self. They employ active listening skills to analyze all communication including verbal and nonverbal.
Empathy	Understanding and empathizing with others are vital for a servant leader. Accepting and recognizing the unique characteristics and intentions of others.
Healing	Potential to restore self and others in a holistic approach.
Awareness	Awareness of self and others for purposes of discovery.
Persuasion	Persuasion, not authority, is the primary method to convince others and build consensus.
Conceptualization	Ability to balance visionary and day-to-day management.
Foresight	Intuition and the ability to understand historical and future implications.
Stewardship	Focus on the greater good of society to care for those more vulnerable.
Commitment to the Growth of People	Committed to the holistic person: personal, professional, and spiritual development of every person.
Building Community	Seek to build community spirit within organizations as a major influence for individuals.

Source: Greenleaf (2015).

In health care and educational settings, the aspects of servant leadership are often exhibited. In clinical nursing practice, a service component is often an expectation for progressing up the clinical ladder. Employees may receive rewards for demonstrating leadership in volunteer and service activities. Likewise, institutions of higher learning such as schools of nursing may encourage and recognize leadership in community service through promotion and tenure processes. These examples demonstrate the value placed on servant leadership within health care and educational organizations.

Contingency and Situational Leadership

Contingency and situational leaders use a variety of leadership styles. The Contingency and Situational Leadership style was introduced in the 1970s and revised through the years by behavioral scientist, Paul Hersey, and management consultant, Ken Blanchard. The leadership style employed is dependent on many variables, including the situation or event, as well as the knowledge, skills, and abilities of those involved. The leader must determine which style is most appropriate in the specific environment or situation and which style will be most effective with the people involved (Hersey, 1985; Hersey & Blanchard, 1977). An underlying premise of the theory is one leadership style will not be effective all the time. Therefore situational leaders must be adaptable.

This theory is based on three main ideas: leadership style, maturity level, and competency–commitment of the individual or team. *Leadership style* is defined as the amount of direction the leader must give for tasks and communication. This is categorized into four styles labeled S1–S4. *Maturity level* is used to describe the individual or group being led and is organized into four levels labeled M1–M4. *Competency–commitment* describes the motivation and capability and is assigned a designation of D1–D4 (Hersey, 1985; Hersey & Blanchard, 1977). The various combinations of contingency leadership styles based on these categories are depicted in Table 18.2.

The S1 leadership style is described as "telling," which involves one-way communication. The leader dictates or informs the group of all necessary information. S2 depicts two-way communication referred to as *selling*. The leader supports the group and seeks group buy-in. In the S3 style, shared decision making is common. The leader provides less task support and more communication or behavioral support. Delegation characterizes the S4 style. The leader monitors progress, but the group determines task responsibility and decision making.

TABLE 18.2 Types of Situational or Contingency Leadership

Situational Leadership	Basic Principle	Maturity Level	Basic Principle	Development Level	Basic Principle
S1	Telling	M1	Unable	D1	Low competence, high commitment
S2	Selling	M2	Unable but eager	D2	Low competence, low commitment
S3	Participating	M3	Able but unwilling	D3	High competence, low or variable commitment
S4	Delegating	M4	Adept and secure	D4	High competence, high commitment

Sources: Hersey (1985); Hersey and Blanchard (1977).

The four maturity levels depict the group or the individual's characteristics and abilities. When the group or individual does not possess the knowledge or skills required to complete the assigned task, they are at the M1 level. These individuals are typically unwilling or unable to take responsibility for completing a task or assignment. The M2 level describes the beginner who is eager and willing, but lacks the knowledge or skills to complete the task. At the third level, M3, the individual or group lacks the confidence or willingness to take responsibility despite the ability and experience to do so. M4 describes the expert who is experienced and confident in his or her knowledge and abilities and is willing and able to assume responsibility.

None of the contingency–situational leadership styles are considered superior to the others because each is useful in certain situations. Thus, the leader must recognize the opportune time for utilization of each style. Likewise, the maturity level is specific to the tasks or duties required. An experienced group member may be classified as an M1 when asked to complete a task or responsibility that is outside his or her scope (Hersey, 1985; Hersey & Blanchard, 1977).

Hersey and Blanchard (1977) address the importance of leaders empowering the team and team members. Empowerment and development of the team create committed and motivated members. They describe a direct correlation between the level of empowerment and expectations as related to the performance and motivation of the team and its members. A leader with high expectations and support will develop a team and team members who are competent, independent, and motivated (Hersey, 1985; Hersey & Blanchard, 1977). These actions represent dynamic and continual developmental. As the tasks and responsibilities change, the leadership, maturity, and development approach must be adapted.

Transformational Leadership

Transformational leadership is a relationship theory based on role modeling to empower others and instill ownership through the use of positive attention and optimism. Transformational leaders can accomplish the shared vision by mobilizing individuals to work toward a common goal. The transformational leader establishes and sustains relationships through emphasizing and building on the individuals' strengths. They motivate and inspire others by praising their abilities and accomplishments. By creating a culture of commendation based on the attributes of others, the transformational leader can accomplish organizational goals while developing the strengths of the individual and the team. This relationship is mutually perceived as rewarding and constructive (Bass & Riggio, 2014).

The concept of transformational leadership involves positive empowerment of others, which inspires them to take meaningful action. The leader's charisma motivates others to work toward the common cause. These leaders are visionaries who share their enthusiasm and desire. They are able to motivate others through infectious excitement reflected in their personal spirit. This leadership style is most effective while implementing extreme or unpopular change, as the transformational leader will have established trust of the stakeholders involved.

Research has identified five primary character traits of transformational leaders: extraversion, neuroticism, openness to experience, agreeableness, and conscientiousness. Extraversion relates to the inspirational aspects of transformational leaders. Extroverts have a social and gregarious personality. Neuroticism is described as the individual's tendency to be keen and focused about goal accomplishment. Openness to experience explains the transformational leader's emotional responsiveness and visionary leadership skills. It is reflected in the expression of creativity and sensitivity to others' perspectives, needs, and goals. Agreeableness is an innate concern and consideration for others characterized by a charismatic, well-liked, and influential individual. Conscientiousness is the strength of one's work ethic and desire to accomplish broad goals.

The transformational leader focuses on connecting to and stimulating those involved in the change process. The leader must act as a mentor and coach to facilitate change by developing all members of the team. A common error for the transformational leader is to deviate from his or her focus on developing the team members and instead focus on short-term goals, data-driven responses, or become fixated on power and authority.

The transformational leader is genuine, authentic, and persuasive. There have been many examples of transformational leaders throughout history. Martin Luther King had a vision for equality, appealing to moral and ethical ideals of others, thus inspiring others for the common good. Florence Nightingale was a transformational leader for nursing and continues to influence health care in the modern world. With the emphasis on analysis of research and the implementation of evidence-based care, nurses have the opportunity to be transformational leaders in health care. The rapid developments in health care evidence, legislation, and policy create a ripe culture for the opportunities and challenges of transformational leadership.

Transactional Leadership Theory

The focus of transactional leadership is to maintain the current environment. It is not based on change, improvement, or progress, but rather maintenance of the system. Through the use of rewards and punishments, the transactional leader can maintain the current condition. Transactional leadership uses a structured process in which the subordinate is compensated for doing the work as prescribed by the leader (Krogh, Nonaka, & Rechsteiner, 2011).

The transactional leader has formal authority and closely monitors the work of subordinates, providing guidance and clarification as needed. A structured, planned, and orderly approach is used. For this reason, transactional leadership may limit creativity, innovation, and motivation. In transactional leadership, the primary responsibility of the subordinate is to follow the transactional leader. This leadership style is embedded in rules to coordinate complex organizations or projects. The use of this style of leadership is often successful in large, diverse, international corporations or military structure (Fitzsimons, James, & Denyer, 2011).

To maintain routine and performance standards, the transactional leader relies on performance reviews. Quality and performance are clearly outlined and defined, with strict regulations for reward and punishment contingent on performance. Through positive and negative reinforcement, the individual develops efficient performance. This leadership style is focused on short-term goal accomplishment while establishing an organized and structured system for repetitive tasks and practicality. Studies have compared the effect of transactional leadership style and the laissez-faire leadership style on staff motivation and organizational productivity (see Box 18.2).

In health care, this style may be used in immunization clinics and military treatment facilities. Transactional leadership is beneficial to these health care facilities as they function using fixed

---

BOX 18.2 Research Application Transactional Versus Laissez Faire Leadership Style

Researchers compared staff motivation levels and organizational productivity in businesses utilizing transactional leadership and laissez faire leadership. The study examined employee perceptions and morale. Overall, the results indicated laissez-faire leadership did not have a positive effect on morale or motivation. The study concluded that morale and motivation were directly related to organizational productivity. Thus, laissez faire leadership had a negative impact on organizational productivity (Chaudhry & Javed, 2012).

methods and specific standards with minimal deviation. Both facilities are focused on maximizing efficiency and organization, yet do not rely on creativity or changing market conditions.

Quantum Leadership Theory

Nurses Tim Porter-O'Grady and Kathy Malloch developed the theory of Quantum Leadership to address organizational concepts of complexity and chaos. This theory views the lack of order as a positive organizational attribute. The theory is based on 10 principles to guide leaders to skillfully lead and manage organizations. The following 10 principles constitute the basic construct of the Quantum Leadership Theory (Porter-O'Grady & Malloch, 2014).

1. Wholes are made of parts
2. Adding value to one part adds value to the whole
3. All health care is local
4. Simple systems make up complex systems
5. Diversity is a necessity of life
6. Error is essential to creation
7. Systems thrive when all of their functions intersect and interact
8. Equilibrium and disequilibrium are in constant tension
9. Change is created from the center outward
10. Revolution results from the aggregation of local changes (Porter-O'Grady & Malloch, 2014, pp. 49–87)

The principles are described in the context of leader characteristics, behaviors, and personality qualities. The leader must have the ability to build and sustain relationships. It is critical for the leader to be empathetic and genuine, analyzing perspectives from all angles. Self-awareness of personal strengths and weaknesses assists the leader to optimize capabilities (Porter-O'Grady & Malloch, 2014).

The quantum leader is visionary with the ability to view the organization from a broad scope, as well as break the organization into smaller units of function. Through strategic planning, coordination, and risk taking, the leader must coordinate all efforts from the most minute to the most global. This ability enables the leader to analyze potential threats and opportunities continually. As complex organizations are composed of many smaller units, each unit's function is vital to the overall goals and objectives of the organization. The quantum leader is responsible for assessing the function of each unit of the organization as well as the organization as a whole. This process supports innovative thinking and creativity (Porter-O'Grady & Malloch, 2014).

In a complex and chaotic environment, a quantum leader builds and sustains teams. The leader recognizes the value of team members and empowerment as well as the value of utilizing the strengths of the individual team members. By empowering and developing others, the leader can monitor progress and measure goals. This culture of flexibility and empowerment fosters relationships and mutual respect and creates a positive environment that contributes to open communication, innovation, and creativity for organizational growth and success (Porter-O'Grady & Malloch, 2014).

Imposter Phenomena Theory

The Imposter Phenomena is a psychological theory exhibited by leaders and high achievers who believe their professional success is attributed to luck and chance. Originally coined by clinical psychologists Clance and Imes (1978), the term refers to high-achieving individuals who are unable to internalize their accomplishments. As a result, they maintain a fear of their true nature being exposed. They are unable to take credit for their accomplishments and live in fear of being exposed as a sham. Regardless of consistent proof of their abilities and skills, leaders demonstrating imposter phenomena believe they do not warrant the praise or success bestowed on them. The leader who exhibits imposter phenomena believes his or her knowledge or abilities have been inflated beyond reality. Although the majority of studies have identified the Imposter Phenomena in primarily high-achieving women, men have also been found to experience the phenomenon (Clance & Imes, 1978; Vergauwe, Wille, Feys, De Fruyt, & Anseel, 2015).

Research has identified specific behaviors associated with the Imposter Phenomena including hardwork, feelings of fraud, charisma, and lack of confidence. High-achieving leaders display hard work and persistence. The imposter does not believe personal success has been earned, which drives the imposter to work harder and achieve success. The fear of being discovered motivates them to focus on details and may lead to stress and anxiety. Feelings of fraud lead the imposter to overcompliance with supervisors or mentors. Fear of being discovered as a fraud prevents imposters from being fully genuine and honest. Instead, they tell people what they want to hear. The imposter relies on charisma and personality to augment abilities and skills. Commendations and admiration from others are based solely on personality, not knowledge, skills, or abilities. Lack of confidence or displays of confidence is a result of believing oneself is undeserving (Clance & Imes, 1978; Vergauwe et al., 2015).

Leaders prone to the imposter phenomena are at risk for extreme anxiety and depression. Their tendencies for hard work and self-doubt may lead to over-rumination on mistakes or negative feedback. The lack of confidence limits creativity and the ability to take risks. Evidence-based approaches to address Imposter Phenomena are based on supportive communication strategies.

As the Imposter Phenomena is prevalent, communicating feelings of inadequacy with other leaders is essential for peer support. Supporting other leaders and sharing feelings and experiences eases the burden. Support may be accomplished through a mentorship program, having a mentor, and or mentoring others. Other successful strategies involve sharing positive feedback as well as journaling strengths and accomplishments. Developing and sustaining a supportive network are critical to prevent, as well as address, the Imposter Syndrome (Clance & Imes, 1978; Vergauwe et al., 2015).

The leadership frameworks discussed in this section depict a variety of perspectives and emphasize a range of factors internal and external to the organization. Some leadership frameworks emphasize the traits of the leader, relationships between the leader and others, and the leader's actions. Other frameworks consider the context and environment in which the leader functions. In Table 18.3, the basic concepts of the leadership frameworks presented in this section have been highlighted for ease of comparison.

◉ MANAGEMENT FRAMEWORKS

Although leadership frameworks explain and guide the vision and strategy for organizational goal achievement, management frameworks have focused on day-to-day functions and tasks required for organizational function and efficiency. Leadership is not attached to a position of authority, as is management (Grossman & Valiga, 2013). Thus, it can be said that leaders *could* be managers and managers *should* be leaders. As is evident in this chapter, leadership and management frameworks and roles are typically explained independently, but often they intersect, overlap, and merge.

Management focuses on supervising and monitoring others to accomplish goals and continuously improve. The manager is responsible for creating and sustaining an effective

TABLE 18.3 Comparison of Leadership Frameworks	
Leadership Theory	**Basic Concepts**
Democratic leadership	Guides a group toward common goals by engaging the group members and encouraging member participation. All members of the group are involved and encouraged to contribute.
Autocratic leadership	Based on total authority and control. In an autocratic culture, the leader is powerful and dominates the other group members or subordinates; dictates.
Laissez faire leadership	Based on faith and trust. People are autonomous and empowered to make decisions and work toward a common goal using their personal knowledge, skills, and abilities with minimal interference.
Servant leadership (Greenleaf)	The conscious desire to put others first, including their needs and priorities. Generally, is a member of the community or organization in which he or she leads and shares power and authority with the community or organization.
Contingency and situational leadership (Hersey and Blanchard)	The leadership style employed is dependent on many variables, including the situation or event, as well as the knowledge, skills, and abilities of those involved. One leadership style will not be effective all the time.
Transformational leadership	A relationship theory based on role modeling to empower others and instill ownership through the use of positive attention and optimism.
Transactional leadership	Focus is to maintain the current environment, not based on change, improvement, or progress, but rather to maintain using rewards and punishments.
Quantum leadership (Porter-O'Grady and Malloch)	Based on 10 principles to guide organization leaders to lead and manage the complicated disorderly nature of organizations. Views the disorganization and lack of order as a positive organizational attribute.
Imposter phenomena	A psychological theory exhibited by leaders and high achievers who believe their professional success is attributed to luck and chance. Believes personal knowledge or abilities are inflated beyond reality.

and efficient work environment, including coordinating the efforts of others. Therefore, the functions of a manager include organizing, budgeting, staffing, and planning. Due to the nature of the responsibilities, managers must be critical thinkers and expert problem solvers (Koontz & Heinz, 1990).

Frameworks of management have continuously evolved to reflect societal influences and developing markets. After World War II, management frameworks focused on principles of the industrial revolution and mass production. However, as a society and industry developed, management frameworks focused more on the human resources and relationships. Today, management frameworks concentrate on the chaotic and complex structure of organizations (Olum, 2004). Modern management frameworks reflect similar characteristics as the leadership frameworks previously discussed. This overlap causes confusion resulting in the interchangeable use of the terms *management* and *leadership*. This chapter distinguishes leadership and management frameworks as separate yet related functions that share common characteristics.

Scientific Management Theory

The Scientific Management Theory is one of the first established theories of management studied by Taylor (1911), a mechanical engineer and management consultant. The theory is based on concepts valued during the industrial revolution: mass production and standardization (Table 18.4). Thus, the focus of this theory is the systematic and efficient use of labor. It requires analysis of the complexity of tasks to optimize efficiency. Several outcomes stem from the application of this theory including workers being compensated based on productivity (Scheiber, 2012) and a workforce less reliant on skilled craftsman.

This mode of management requires controlled management techniques. Although advocating for a positive working environment, Taylor believed in strict management and oversight of the workers. Scientific Management Theory emphasizes the process and productivity of work to improve outcomes. Therefore, there is minimal consideration of the human resource and relationship aspects of management. When individual accomplishments or skills are not recognized, people feel devalued and unappreciated for their contributions. Thus morale is diminished. The Scientific Management Theory has been blamed for creating a monotonous work environment and alienating the workforce.

Bureaucracy Theory

Max Weber developed the Bureaucracy Theory to explain efficiency in a dynamic and complex workforce. He believed a regulated and structured approach would result in a more efficient environment and minimize waste. As industry shifted to a more complex and technological focus, Bureaucracy Theory was used to explain administrative principles of management (see Table 18.4). Rules and regulations provide structure for complex organizations. It provides a hierarchical and organized approach to addressing quality, cost control, and workforce concerns (Weber, 1968).

The modern design of Bureaucracy Theory includes three levels of management: executive, middle, and supervisory. These levels are depicted in health care organizations such as hospitals, clinics, and health care systems. The executive management level consists of chief operating officers and the board of directors who are responsible for strategic planning, including fiscal planning and goal setting. Middle management is responsible for carrying out the mission and goals set forth by the executive level. It is also responsible for the supervisors and unit level goals, including budgets. In turn, the supervisors are accountable for

TABLE 18.4 Comparison of Basic Concepts of Management Theories	
Theory (Theorist)	**Basic Concepts**
Scientific Management Theory (Taylor)	Focus on systematic and efficient use of labor. Requires controlled and strict management techniques.
Bureaucracy Theory (Weber)	Administrative principles of management, such as rules and regulations. A hierarchical approach based on three levels: executive management, middle management, and supervisors.

the day-to-day activities, including guiding and directing workers at the point of contact. In a hospital setting, the supervisor would be the unit charge nurse.

The Bureaucracy Theory is beneficial for large and complex organizations. It promotes the division of goals into distinct and manageable tasks. In addition, the role of each member of the organization is clear with defined duties and expectations. This division of roles and tasks promotes a streamlined process.

CHANGE FRAMEWORKS

In health care leadership, change is a common topic for theory or model application. Change presents challenges and barriers to all health care organizations. By its nature, change can be evolutionary or revolutionary; it can be fluid or abrupt, planned or unplanned, as well as positive or negative. In the inherently chaotic and complex health care environment, nurses and patients must have energy and incentive to effect change. Stakeholders need to recognize the impact and influences of change on all other entities involved and communicate and empower each other to adapt and be resilient. The process of change presents an immense responsibility, coupled with a multitude of challenges.

Regardless of practice specialty, nurses need to be experts at managing the change process. The nurse's caring and compassionate attributes combined with the ability to thrive in a demanding and complex health care environment positions the nurse to lead change initiatives to meet the health care needs of individuals, communities, organizations, and systems. From bedside care to organizational leadership, from institutional policies to healthcare policy, change is constant and continuous. Nurses have moved beyond merely accepting change to leading and managing change.

The change processes presented in this chapter focus on organizational change. Comparison of the basic concepts of these frameworks is highlighted in Table 18.5. For change frameworks relevant to behavioral change of the individual, please see Chapter 4. The reader may find some of the behavioral change frameworks are also useful in systems leadership and may be generalizable to situations involving organizational change.

Lewin's Change Theory

In 1951, Kurt Lewin developed a well-known and commonly used change theory. He described three dynamic stages of change: unfreezing, moving (or change), and refreezing. The unfreezing stage involves the change preparation, including problem analysis and stakeholder identification. The moving stage consists of the acceptance of the need for change and implementation of the change process. Stakeholder buy-in and participation are essential for successful implementation. The refreezing stage is the final integration of the change in which it becomes the cultural norm for the organization. These stages are fluid and dynamic, not distinct categories with specific timelines for completion (Lewin, 1951).

Lewin (1951) identified the presence of driving and resisting forces in the change process. Driving forces are change agents who empower and motivate others to implement and embrace change or modification. Resisting forces are those people or circumstances that oppose the modification. For change to successfully occur, the driving forces must outweigh the resistant forces and lead and control change process. Lewin's Change Theory is explained in greater detail in Chapter 4.

Havelock's Theory of Change

Havelock (1973) expanded on Lewin's Change Theory to address realistic challenges and barriers to the change process. Havelock's Theory of Change is based on change being initiated and implemented by an outside entity or change agent. The change agent is

TABLE 18.5 Comparison of Organizational Change Frameworks	
Change Theory	**Basic Concepts**
Lewin's Change Theory	Three dynamic stages of change: unfreezing, moving, and refreezing.
Havelock's Theory of Change	Based on change being initiated and implemented by an outside entity or change agent.
Rogers's Diffusion of Innovation	Used to guide long-term change processes. For instance, when a proposed change in practice is not initially adopted; however, later is accepted as a standard of practice.
Transitional Theory	Relates to the humanistic response, experience, and perceptions associated with change.
Tipping Point (Gladwell)	Describes change as sudden and dramatic versus a gradual or evolutionary process.
Logic Models	A visual representation of the change process, a tool used to evaluate the progress of resource and activity coordination.

responsible for establishing a relationship with the organization, assessing the need for change, and implementing the change. Once the change process has been completed, the change agent detaches from the organization and the organization is expected to sustain the change.

Havelock emphasizes building a relationship with the organization or system as a prerequisite for change. Once a relationship is established, the change agent becomes familiar with the organization or system and is able to assess the organization and the need for change. It is possible that no further change is needed. Thus, the change process would cease. However, if a change is necessary, information would be collected, possible solutions examined, and resources would be gathered. Selection and implementation of a course of action are included in the next phase of the change process. The next phase of the process is establishing the change and evolving toward acceptance of the change. In this phase, the emphasis is on combating resistance to change, thereby enabling the change to become the new norm. Following the norming of the change, the change agent evaluates the success and maintenance of the change and then separates from the organization.

Havelock stresses process of change as systematic, planned, and methodical. The change process begins with identification of the need for change and culminates with the acceptance of the change as the new norm (Figure 18.1). As relapse is always a threat, it is critical to address this challenge from the beginning of the change process (Havelock, 1973).

Rogers's Diffusion of Innovations Theory

Everett Rogers, a sociologist and scholar, expanded on Lewin's Change Theory and described types of adopters and a five-stage process to guide long-term change (Rogers, 1962, 2010). According to the Diffusion of Innovations Theory, individuals involved in change or innovation are categorized as one of the five types according to how readily they adopt a change. The distribution of these types of change recipients (i.e., innovators, early adopters, early majority, late majority, and laggards) is similar to a bell curve with

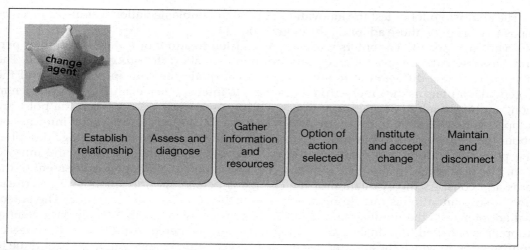

FIGURE 18.1 Havelock's theory of change.

Source: Havelock (1973).

most change recipients falling in the middle categories and the fewest at each extreme. Innovators are risk takers who are socially influential. Their financial capabilities allow them the freedom to take risks that involve the potential for failure. Early adopters have a high social standing, and their opinion is regarded with much respect as they are highly educated and financially stable. They are more discernable in their choices than innovators. The early majority are described as possessing less social leadership than innovators and early adopters, but are still relatively higher than average. For the early majority, the time frame from the introduction of the innovation to adoption is varied. Late majority adopters are behind the average adopter in the time frame for adoption. They tend to be more cynical and uncertain. Their social standing does not encourage opinion sharing, and their financial capabilities do not allow them the freedom to take risks. Laggards are the final group to adopt an innovation. They typically dislike change and distrust change agents. Laggards are often lower in social standing and financial flexibility or they may be elderly and attached to historical methods (Rogers, 2010). Diffusion of innovation is used to explain the process of change in practice such as when a change is not initially adopted but is later accepted as a standard of practice. The delay in adoption of the change may occur over the span of a few years or generations.

The Diffusion of Innovations Theory depicts a dynamic process in which change is dependent on culture, personal influence, numbers of potential adopters (change agents), and opposition resistant forces including laggards. Potential adopters or change agents foster awareness and interest in the modification. These change agents can generate the initial shift, which stimulates the change process. At that point, as more people become involved, a shift from a resistant force to a driving force is experienced (Rogers, 2010).

Rogers (2010) studied the characteristics of innovation adoption based on the perspective of potential adopters. He identified the following characteristics perceived by the adopters as important. These include seeing the following:

- The advantage of the innovation compared to current modes or methods
- The congruency or consistency of the innovation with existing modes or methods
- The adoption of the innovation as having few barriers
- The applicability of the innovation to other unintended uses

The ability to pilot or test the innovation prior to full implementation was also viewed as a positive factor by those adopting the innovation.

Over time, potential adopters will make a decision to adopt or not based on their personal assessment. However, the potential adopter may abort the process at any time. The five stages of the diffusion of innovation process explain the shift in perspective of the potential adopters as they move from awareness to interest, then evaluation, implementation, and eventually adoption (see Rogers, 2010). Awareness occurs when the potential adopter is first exposed to the innovation. The potential adopter has minimal information about the innovation and has little interest in learning more. The interest stage describes the potential adopter's curiosity and active knowledge-seeking regarding the innovation. The next stage, evaluation, is the process of the potential adopter assessment of the pros and cons. As the evaluation of the change is person specific, quantitative verification or substantiation is rare. Implementation is when the innovation is used. The potential adopter tests the innovation and acquires more knowledge about it. If the potential adopter is satisfied, the final stage of adoption stage is entered. Adoption is a process of confirmation in which the adopter decides to proceed with the innovation and continue to use it (Rogers, 2010).

The Diffusion of Innovation Theory explains several potential results of implementing an innovation. The innovation may fail to diffuse to the general population perhaps because the innovation is useful or adopted only by a particular societal subset. The adoption of the innovation may also lead to desirable or undesirable outcomes, as well as unanticipated results. As with any change, there are potential risks and consequences.

Transitional Theory

Transitional Theory is a component of the change process relating to the humanistic response, experience, and perceptions associated with change. It describes the interpersonal and intrapersonal stresses of change related to leadership challenges and the opportunities resulting from the change. In nursing, Transitional Theory has been used to explore leadership role transitions, as well as situational, developmental, health illness, and organizational transitions. In this chapter, the focus remains on organizational transitions.

Organizational transitions result from changes in the work environment. These may be broad changes or minute changes in either the internal or external environment. Organizational transition associated with change, such as leadership succession, implementation of new policy or new standards of care, structural restructuring, staff turnover, and technology applications have been widely studied (Blakeslee, Goldman, Papougenis, & Torell, 1991; Shields, 1991; Walker & DeVooght, 1989).

Bridges (2004) examined the process of transition in organizational change from the emotional and psychological perspective of the people involved in the change process. He emphasizes the emotional and psychological transitions of those involved as the greater challenge versus the organizational change process. Bridges described this process in three phases: letting go, neutral zone, and a new beginning. Understanding the leader's role in these phases, as described subsequently, facilitates effective organizational change.

The first phase, letting go, involves assisting people to manage the inevitability of loss. Regardless of whether the loss is tangible or intangible, it is important to guide and ease people through the process. The next phase, the neutral zone, is a critical phase marked by confusion. During this phase, innovation is encouraged. Again, it is vital to guide people through this psychological process by facilitating the establishment of new patterns and behaviors. The last phase, a new beginning, is marked by the development and establishment of newness. People are eager to work toward a new purpose, especially as they see the new process beginning to work. These phases can create a culture of continuous revitalization and progress within an organization (Bridges, 2004).

Tipping Point Theory

Malcolm Gladwell described change as a sudden and dramatic versus a gradual or evolutionary process. Change is the result of minor events or situations, which are "contagious" and ultimately reach climactic results. Gladwell (2002) describes this sudden and climactic change as the tipping point. He emphasizes the importance of context and perspective when dealing with change, especially changes reaching the tipping point. In terms of context and perspective, it is essential to understand and address environmental perspectives and time-sensitive issues. With this in mind, marketing or presentation is important to make a lasting impression, which entices people to change. Gladwell (2002) stresses the need to be sensitive to the culture and environment, as well as pay attention to details. He provides an example of cultural change resulting from one leader's drive to eradicate neighborhood graffiti. The seemingly insignificant act of continuously removing graffiti sent a powerful message, resulting in a major decrease in crime in that environment.

As the tipping point is reliant on a contagion and the power of groups, it is crucial to channel the power and influence of people and groups. Gladwell describes three essential functions of people that enable a tipping point to occur as the connector, maven, and salesman. Those functioning as connectors are influential and social. They know many people and have gregarious personalities. Friendliness and likability make networking and spreading information easy for connectors. The maven is very knowledgeable and eager to share knowledge with others, but does not use knowledge in a persuasive manner. Mavens act as advocates and enjoy helping others by sharing knowledge. The enthusiasm of the maven often persuades nonbelievers, often resulting in dramatic and sudden change. The salesman is charismatic and persuasive and is vital for achieving the tipping point. An example of a recent tipping point in society has been the adoption of mobile technology. Mobile technology started as a small market invention, yet has dramatically changed the face of business and cultural interactions.

Gladwell (2002) also stresses the significance and influence of people and groups, as groups amplify and boost the change process. However, large groups are challenging to direct and may experience communication barriers and difficulties, thus minimizing the leader's relationship capacity. As a result, peer influence and group unity diminish with large groups. Gladwell's research also indicates multiple small groups have greater influence and power than one large group. However, this finding may be dependent on the type of change and the environment.

Using the example of adoption of mobile technology, the effect that people and groups have on influencing change is evident. Initially, the advent of the cell phone was met with minimal purchase of the technology and minimal change to society. However, connectors discovered the varied uses for the cell phone and networked with others on these additional uses. Mavens shared the knowledge with others who might benefit, and the salesman persuaded the nonbelievers until adoption of the new technology became pervasive. More recently, the Tipping Point Theory can be used to describe and explain the rapid adoption of technologies such as Fitbit, Googlemaps, and the Weatherbug applications.

Logic Models

A logic model is a visual representation of the change process that was first introduced in the 1970s. It is an organized and visual tool used by leaders to evaluate the progress of resource and activity coordination to achieve outcomes. The components of a logic model are variable, subjective, and dynamic, with the choice of model based on the specifics of the project. Depending on the project scope and purpose, some logic models may specify assumptions, stakeholders, external influences, and environmental factors, while others may consist of minimal information. Minimally, logic models consist of three components; inputs, outputs, and outcomes (see Figure 18.2; Millar, Simeone, & Carnevale, 2001).

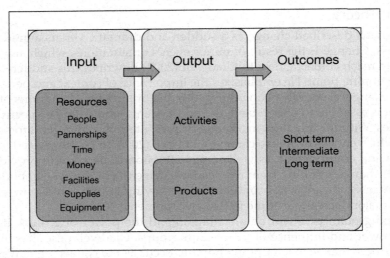

FIGURE 18.2 A basic logic model.

Sources: McCawley (n.d.); W. K. Kellogg Foundation (2004).

Inputs are the resources that are available and needed to implement the change. These inputs include people, partnerships, time, money, and physical resources such as facilities, equipment, and supplies. Output refers to the activities conducted and the processes or products developed during the change process. Outcomes are identified in varying levels of detail often depicting short-term, intermediate, and long-term outcomes. The underlying purpose of a logic model is to assess the situation and the change project and align the relationship between the plan details and the desired outcomes (Julian, 1997).

Logic models support the efficient use of resources by identifying and monitoring essential steps in a change process. This process highlights steps or resources that are unnecessary and wasteful. Once identified through the logic model, unnecessary, redundant, or wasteful steps can be eliminated. Interestingly, some logic models start with the outcome and work backward to monitor progress (Julian, 1997). Regardless of the format, logic models highlight vital steps, identify missing resources, and facilitate addressing omissions. For these reasons, logic models support efficiency.

Logic models are frequently used in project planning and research studies to map the flow of the change process to the achievement of outcomes. The structure of a basic logic model, as shown in Figure 18.2, can be adapted and expanded to meet the resources, needs, and outputs of the project. Models may include a problem statement and goal; assumptions and rationales; and external factors that influence the input, output, and outcome. The level of detail and definition of the resources is dependent on the needs of the project and the needs of those involved in the process.

⬤ COMMUNICATION FRAMEWORKS

A cornerstone of effective organizational leadership is communication. *Communication* is a complex process involving the exchange of information between stakeholders and those in the organization's internal and external environment. The complexity and chaos of organizational systems complicate communication resulting in a disconcerting and bewildering reality of organizational leadership. Leaders must be experts in basic concepts of interpersonal communication and apply these concepts on a much larger scale. The use of technology in communication further complicates the process resulting in either an opportunity or a threat.

Health care organizations and systems are described as complex adaptive systems (see Chapter 17). They are composed of multiple interdependent entities with diverse roles and functions. In complex adaptive systems, it is essential for communication to be straightforward and clear. Secrecy leads to confusion and disorganization. Being open and genuine is needed to develop healthy relationships as a leader (Zimmerman, Lindberg, & Plsek, 2008). Clear and accurate information about progress, as well as positive feedback for corrective measures, leads to confident and secure followers. Listening is also an essential component of the communication process. To be an informed leader, one must listen intently and process the information critically (Grossman & Valiga, 2013).

Communication does not end with talking and listening. Throughout the communication process, the leader must be direct, logical, and follow through with initiatives and identified concerns. This process requires courage and tenacity as a successful communication process will entail making difficult decisions and taking action. Each interaction and communication process will involve some level of risk. Grossman and Valiga (2013) emphasize the strength at which nurse leaders have historically excelled is communication.

Due to the rapid and continuous changes in technology, it is also vital to address the role of technology in communication. Whether it is considered progress or not, communication has evolved from face-to-face and paper media to electronic and digital formats. Technology has virtually eliminated communication boundaries. However, this lack of boundaries can be overwhelming and difficult to navigate and control. Text, email, and social media have replaced the verbal face-to-face communication, and as a result, there is a lack of nonverbal cues. Although quick and timely, electronic and digital communication is more impersonal than face-to-face communication and often lacks context. The absence of the verbal and nonverbal feedback loop can muddy the message and complicate the communication process. Because there are many communication options from which to choose, it is essential to choose the right format. Challenging or difficult topics are best left to face-to-face format, while email or text is more appropriate for informal, simple, or time-sensitive communication.

Interprofessional collaboration presents another challenge to communication in health care. Communicating with stakeholders and health care entities to improve patient outcomes is a challenge. Each stakeholder or entity has established informal and formal standards, regulations, and goals for patient care. Leaders must establish a system of communication to empower and manage each entity, maximize patient priorities and needs, and channel the diversity in a positive manner for optimal patient care. Developing teams for interprofessional collaboration has become an essential nursing leader function. The role of nurse leader requires expertise in managing difficult conversations and high levels of social and emotional intelligence (EI).

Difficult Conversations Model

All leaders and managers experience difficult conversations and challenges in communications. Whether the leader is dealing with an angry peer or customer, or a disgruntled superior, difficult conversations are stressful and require skillful negotiation. Rather than avoiding difficult conversations, Stone, Patton, and Heen (2010) developed the difficult conversations framework to address these challenges. This framework has been applied and studied in both personal and professional situations.

The model is based on analyzing the emotional aspects of the interaction, as well as the purpose and direction: what is being said and what is not being said. Analyzing the content and purpose of the interaction will enable the leader to respond in a constructive manner, even if he or she must admit to being wrong. The authors use three conversation types: the "what happened conversation?" the "feelings conversation," and the "identity conversation" to engage in conversation analysis (see Table 18.6).

The "what happened conversation" is based on differences and disputes regarding who is correct and who is at fault. Assuming one person is correct and another is wrong is the most

TABLE 18.6 Comparison of Basic Concepts of Communication Theories	
Theory (Theorist)	**Basic Concepts**
Difficult Conversations (Stone, Patton, and Heen)	Based on analyzing the emotional aspects of the interaction, as well as the purpose and direction: What happened conversation, feelings conversation, and identity conversation.
Emotional Intelligence (Goleman)	The ability of an individual to understand and manage his or her emotions and the emotions of others to guide thoughts and actions for goal achievement; three basic models: ability, mixed, and trait.

frequent cause for disagreement. By using knowledge inherent in Difficult Conversations Model, inaccurate assumptions can be put to rest as the leader strives to see the other's perspective. The differences in perspective are based on differences in information, experience, and interpretation. Communication is facilitated by being open to learning and understanding the other person, being inquisitive versus condemning, and by avoiding assumptions concerning the other person's intentions.

The "feelings conversation" muddies the content of the interactions because it is difficult to be objective when there are emotional ties to a particular topic. To be objective, the leader needs to think like a third party and focus on the other person's perspective.

The "identity conversation" describes the internal dialogue people have with themselves during interactions. In this type of conversation, it is important to recognize that the content of the verbal conversation may be incongruent with the nonverbal communication. A person may deny being angry, but body language and nonverbal communication may deliver an entirely different message. These conflicting messages interfere with the communication process. Active listening and interpretation of nonverbal behavior are a crucial part of relationships and interpersonal interaction (Stone et al., 2010).

Emotional Intelligence Theory

Psychologist Daniel Goleman (1998) defined EI as the ability of an individual to understand and manage his or her emotions and the emotions of others and use that understanding to guide thoughts and actions for goal achievement. The basic premise is people who have high EI demonstrate superior job performance and leadership skills over those with lower EI. The ability to understand and discriminate between different emotions enables the individual to use the information as a guide to behaviors and actions. Thus, the individual with high EI uses emotions as tools to facilitate interactions (Goleman, 1998).

EI Theory uses three basic models to describe EI: ability, mixed, and trait. *Ability* is used to describe emotions as tools to assist individuals to understand social interactions. The person should be emotionally perceptive and use emotions to facilitate goal accomplishment (Mayer, Salovey, & Caruso, 2004). The *mixed* model is the most general explanation of EI as described by Goleman (1998). It is based on analysis of leadership competencies and skills. The *trait* model explains EI in the construct of perceptions of personality traits and abilities. The trait model differs from the other models in that personality traits instead of cognitive ability are the focus (Petrides, Pita, & Kokkinaki, 2007).

The mixed model of EI outlines five concepts for leaders: self-awareness, self-regulation, social skill, empathy, and motivation. Successful leaders are aware of their emotions and can utilize them to influence their actions and behaviors. Self-regulation describes the ability to control impulses and emotions and be flexible. Social skill involves using relationships to manage and motivate others. Empathy includes assessing other's emotions and demonstrating compassion. The final concept, motivation, is simply the desire for success and accomplishment (Goleman, 1998).

EI research has found a positive correlation between successful interpersonal relationships and improved social skills and abilities (Mayer, Roberts, & Barsade, 2008). Those with high EI have adept social skills, including empathy and friendliness. They can build relationships that lead to positive perceptions by others. Although EI does not have a positive correlation with IQ, people with high EI demonstrate higher academic achievement than those with low EI. As teamwork and collaboration have become vital for professional success, an individual with high EI is more likely to be successful in today's workplace. Complex health care organizations and systems require negotiation and relationship skills. Although higher education and specialized training are attractive for a potential employer, evaluating an individual's EI gives insight into the employee's ability to succeed in a collaborative culture.

Grossman and Valiga (2013) emphasize EI skills such as self-reflection, insight, and sensitivity training for nursing leaders. To act as a patient advocate and provide high-quality care, nursing leaders must understand emotions and perceptions. The nurse leader must be able to address bias and perceptual interpretations in decision making and in supporting patient care. Health care is frequently an emotionally charged environment; nurses must be able to navigate this environment for optimal patient outcomes. EI facilitates the leader in navigating the changing health care environment.

⊙ MENTORING FRAMEWORKS

The delicate balance of mentoring someone is not creating them in your own image, but giving them the opportunity to create themselves.
—Steven Spielberg

Mentoring is an essential component of organization leadership. For organizational sustainability, resilience, and future growth, organizational leaders must be responsible for developing their workforce, as well as developing future leaders. Just as prominent leadership styles have evolved, so have styles of mentoring. Mentoring is a broad concept defined as a relationship between two people, wherein the mentor is more experienced than the mentee. Thus, the mentor shares experiences, knowledge, and provides insight to assist the mentee. Research has shown mentoring relationships to be effective and valuable (Specht, 2012). See Research Box 18.3 for a study on mentoring new faculty.

The concept of precepting is frequently confused with mentorship. Precepting occurs when as an expert shares technical skills and knowledge with a novice. In clinical situations, which are complex and potentially critical, precepting is an essential leadership role involving teaching novice nurses and other health care providers. The concept of coaching is also confused with mentorship as it mirrors several related concepts including goal setting and planning. Both mentoring and coaching are based on the premise of an experienced person developing a meaningful relationship with a less experienced person. Coaching is designed to be individualistic and specific to personal learning needs, preferences, and attributes. The coaches' role is to facilitate and nurture independence, whereas the primary role of a mentor is to lend their experience and expertise to the mentee. In modern applications, coaching is frequently associated with performance-based improvement strategies, while mentoring is more of a voluntary and emotional relationship (Garvey, Stokes, & Megginson, 2014).

> **BOX 18.3 Research Application Mentoring Relationships for Novice Nursing Faculty**
>
> This study examined the quality and effect of mentoring on novice nursing faculty. Novice faculty experience challenges with role transition from clinical practice to the academic arena. Novice faculty who were mentored experienced significantly less role conflict and ambiguity than those who were not mentored. The mentee's perception of mentoring quality was also directly correlated with their levels of role ambiguity and conflict. Thus, the novice faculty with higher quality mentoring experienced less role conflict and ambiguity than those who rated the quality of their mentoring experiences lower (Specht, 2012).

Mentoring describes a formal and often assigned role and process, or it may be an informal relationship based on mutual selection, directed by personal goals and objectives. Mentoring may be long term and span an entire career, or it may be short term based on acquiring a specific skill. The mentor may be a manager of the mentee or a peer. This chapter provides a review of several popular mentoring frameworks.

The GROW Model

The GROW Model was developed in the early 1980s by three professional coaches from the United Kingdom, Alan Fine, Sir John Whitmore, and Graham Alexander (InsideOut Development, "History," n.d.). GROW is an acronym that describes four components of mentoring decision making. Since its creation, each developer has added slight modifications to the model, particularly in the terminology used for the fourth component.

The first component, "G" represents the "Goal" the individual seeks to accomplish. "R" stands for the "Realities" that that influence the context for the decision making. The "O" represents the "Options" available and considers the obstacles that influence those options. According to Fine and Merrill (2010), the fourth component "W" refers to the "Way forward" or the action plan that will be implemented. Whitmore labeled the final component "Will," which focuses on "what" the mentee "Will" do (Performance Consultants International, 2014). Accordingly, determining what actions will be taken is based on the goals, realities, and obstacles in the situation. Alexander (2010) used the term "Wrap up" to encompass a variety of processes that can occur during the final component of the model. These wrap-up processes vary depending on the answers to the previous components. Therefore, "Wrap-up" may involve exploring implications of the obstacles identified, recognizing sources of support available and needed, making a commitment to the action plan, or determining if the goal was achieved.

For each component of the decision-making process, the mentor guides and stimulates the mentee's awareness and insight through focused questioning. Once the first component of the model (i.e., goal) has been identified, the mentor helps the mentee identify "realities" by recognizing current problems, challenges, or situations that impact the ability to achieve the goal. The third component involves considering "options" and it is influenced by the realities or obstacles identified. The fourth components (way forward, will, or wrap-up) focus on clarifying, and narrowing options, and or identifying the next steps in the action plan.

The GROW model was influenced by sports psychology and is based on the premise that performance is facilitated by more than merely obtaining knowledge. Performance also relies on removing internal barriers. Discovery of internal barriers can be achieved by reflection and asking about the Reality and Options inherent in the situation. Although the model was originally developed for coaching individuals, its applications have expanded to the corporate and systems levels to facilitate decision making in the mentoring process.

Hudson's Five-Factor Mentoring Model

Hudson's Five-Factor Mentoring Model is concerned with mentoring the mentee in specific subject areas. The model was developed based on a study by Hudson, Skamp, and Brooks (2004) that identified a statistically significant five-factor model. The first factor that encompasses all others is the personal attributes of the mentor. Six key attributes identify the desirable personal attributes. The first involves being supportive of the mentee; the second, being attentive to the needs of the mentee; and third, being comfortable with providing subject-specific mentoring. The remaining three attributes focus on actions in which the mentor needs to engage with the mentee regarding teaching specific subject matter. These include imparting positive attitudes, developing self-confidence, and fostering positive self-reflection practices related to teaching specific subjects.

The remaining four factors in the model are interrelated: system requirements, pedagogical knowledge, modeling, and feedback. The mentee needs to understand the educational system requirements, which included the curriculum, the educational system policies, and expectations. Understanding educational program accreditation and national curricular standards is a system requirement. Knowledge of pedagogy or teaching strategies is also essential for an effective mentoring experience. Eleven attributes and practices relevant to pedagogical knowledge have been identified. These can be organized using the familiar steps of the nursing process, beginning with assessing the learners and their knowledge. Next is to develop a plan for teaching including timetabling (scheduling/organizing), preparation for teaching, and integration of content knowledge into the lesson. Implementation involves using teaching strategies, employing effective classroom management methods, sharing viewpoints, developing questioning skills, and assisting in problem solving. The evaluation process involves several of the previously mentioned practices including assessment of student knowledge and using effective questioning techniques.

The next factor, modeling, is achieved by observing the mentor's teaching and interactions with students. Attributes and practices associated with positive role modeling include the mentor enthusiasm, effective teaching, well-designed lessons, effective classroom management, and model syllabi. These attributes and practices facilitate the mentee's development of effective teaching practices.

The final factor in Hudson's model is feedback, which is facilitated by specific mentor activities. The mentor makes teaching expectations clear, reviews the mentee's lesson plan, and observes the mentee's teaching, provides verbal and written feedback based on observation of the mentee's teaching, and assists the mentee in evaluating his or her teaching practices. Feedback should be formative or ongoing and summative at the end of a teaching term. Hudson (2004) combined the five factors of the model to generate a definition of mentoring in teacher education as "the process of demonstrating and articulating personal attributes, system requirements, pedagogical knowledge, modeling, and feedback for the development of a mentee's teaching practices" (pp. 6–7).

Apprenticeship Model of Mentoring

The Apprenticeship Model of Mentoring combines formal education and training with an embedded learning experience. The mentee is paired with an experienced mentor who guides the mentee through a participative experience. A hands-on approach in which the mentee is learning on the job is key. The mentee is able to experience every aspect of the job including social, cultural, and cognitive aspects (Vandermaas-Peeler, Nelson, Ferretti, & Finn, 2011).

This mentorship model was developed for the purpose of mentoring undergraduate students in the process of research and publication (Vandermaas-Peeler et al., 2011). Students are paired with an experienced faculty member who mentors the student. As students progress in the program and gain experience and knowledge, they eventually aide others and assist in the process of student development. In the Apprenticeship Model, each student participates in every aspect of research and publication with the faculty mentor.

A primary factor of this model is the development of the faculty and student relationship. The faculty member provides support and challenges based on the needs and development level of each student. The model uses a personal approach to achieve mutual connections and benefits. The faculty and students describe the relationship in terms of tangible rewards of publications or presentations and intangible rewards of positive relationships and mastery of knowledge and skills (Vandermaas-Peeler et al., 2011).

The faculty and the students describe the long-term benefits of this relationship. This model promotes connections for the development of future contacts and professional collaborations. As the student's professional development progresses, established relationships are the basis for continued support. Faculty members serve as mentors and role models, thus encouraging these behaviors in their students for future generations as well (Vandermaas-Peeler et al., 2011).

This model has been proven effective in a variety of educational programs, from psychology to archeology (Vandermaas-Peeler et al., 2011). Application of the model in these diverse settings and disciplines enhances the generalizability of the Apprenticeship Model of Mentoring to a multitude of disciplines or organizations.

Model of Caring Mentorship for Nursing

Wagner and Seymour (2007) developed a Model of Caring Mentorship for Nursing based on long-term empowering relationships versus the traditional preceptor models used in nursing clinical education. Through continual support, empowerment, and caring, experienced nurses can lead the less experienced or disenfranchised nurses. This mentoring relationship is founded on caring concepts that promote learning and increase job satisfaction.

The model defines mentoring as comprising a multitude of duties and roles including precepting, supervising, facilitating, teaching, guiding, coaching, counseling, advocating, networking, sharing, and supporting. Mentoring is defined as a holistic role that occurs in a formal and informal manner. It is inclusive of both personal and professional advising. It is a long-term relationship based on trust, mutual respect, and communication. Wagner and Seymour (2007) expanded the concept of mentoring to include caring concepts.

Caring is a humanistic relationship between people founded on self-awareness and sharing of self with others to promote human dignity. The caring relationship is one of honesty and trust, as well as concern for others. It is a demonstration of compassion and conscience. Wagner and Seymour (2007) believed the concepts of caring and mentoring mirrored each other. Thus, they developed a model of mentorship based on principles of caring.

The model is depicted as a spiral to represent a person's self-concept (the past, present, and potential future) and his or her interaction with the world. The interaction between two entities (the carer and the cared-for) in the model is recognized. The model also describes two elements: the internal reflection of caring and actions of caring stemming from internal reflection. The elements are not finite or limited, but are based on a continuum of caring (Wagner & Seymour, 2007).

The Model of Caring Mentorship for Nursing portrays mentoring as a set of learned skills, including self-reflection, professional knowledge, communication and social skills, and knowledge of the mentoring process. Although mentoring is a professional responsibility, the mentoring process requires organizational support and on-going professional development. For mentoring to be successful, it must be well-planned and supported through continuing education and reimbursement plans. It is a time-consuming process for dedicated and positive professionals, yet requires consistent planning and coordination (Wagner & Seymour, 2007).

Five-Phase Mentoring Relationship Model

Cooper and Wheeler (2010) created the Five-Phase Mentoring Relationship Model for the purpose of improving retention, job satisfaction, and role development. The core concept of this model is the relationship between the mentor and mentee. Five phases of this model, which describe the relationship and its focus, are: purpose, engagement, planning, emergence, and completion. In this model, the monitor–mentee relationship is time-consuming and requires effort and dedication. This model was designed to assist both parties in this process.

Phase 1, *purpose*, provides the informational foundation for the relationship. It is the process of exploring intentions and reasons for the relationship based on goals, plans, and interests. This phase focuses on the examination of why there is a need or desire for this relationship. With this foundation, both parties can find a suitable match for a mentoring relationship.

Phase 2, *engagement*, signals the initiation of the mentoring relationship. This phase results from a formal invitation or practice, such as a new employee mentoring program, or it may result from an informal meeting or networking opportunity. Regardless of the process, the decision to proceed with the mentoring relationship must be a mutual decision.

Phase 3, *planning*, constitutes the process of plan development with specific goals and time lines. Expectations are reviewed, and measurements of success are selected. This phase establishes meaningful exchange and communication strategies. Being proactive to clarify expectations minimizes disagreements and confusion while establishing a culture of trust and respect.

Phase 4, *emergence*, is a long-term process of relationship growth. The mentor is providing support and advice, while the mentee is actively involved. The mentor and mentee are both engaged in the relationship with ongoing evaluation. Both the mentor and the mentee reflect on their relationship and make adjustments or changes as needed.

Phase 5, *completion*, is designated as the time to commend each other on the tasks and goals achieved while redefining each other's roles and responsibilities. During this phase, the relationship becomes equal and reciprocal. The mentor and the mentee celebrate each other's successes, as the relationship moves to an "as needed" basis (Cooper & Wheeler, 2010).

Each mentoring framework provides a unique perspective that emphasizes specific concepts and processes. See Table 18.7 for a comparison of key concepts. Familiarity with these frameworks will provide the mentor and mentee with structure and guidance useful in developing and sustaining a mentoring relationship.

TABLE 18.7 Comparison of Basic Concepts of Mentoring Frameworks

Mentoring Theory	Basic Concepts
GROW Model (Fine, Whitmore, and Alexander)	G = Goal the individual seeks to accomplish R = Realities influencing the context for decision making O = Options available and obstacles that influence options W = Way forward—or the action plan, or What the mentee "Will" do, or Wrap up—the processes occurring during the final component of the model.
Five Factor Mentoring Model (Hudson)	Concerned with mentoring the mentee in specific subject areas. Five-factors: mentor's personal attributes, system requirements, pedagogical knowledge, modeling, and feedback.
Apprenticeship Model of Mentoring (Vandermaas-Peeler, Nelson, Ferretti, and Finn)	Combines formal education and training with an embedded learning experience. Hands-on approach in which the mentee is learning on the job.
Model of Caring Mentorship for Nursing (Wagner and Seymour)	Long-term empowering relationship, holistic role based on trust, mutual respect, and communication.
Five-Phase Mentoring Relationship Model (Cooper and Wheeler)	Core concept of this model is the relationship between the mentor and mentee, five phases of this model are purpose, engagement, planning, emergence, and completion.

CONCLUSION

Organizational systems leadership is as complex and chaotic as the organizational system itself. The organizational leader must skillfully facilitate internal and external influences, as well as cultural perceptions, to optimize the function of the organization or system. It is a complicated and continual process to organize multiple entities and stakeholders to accomplish common goals. System leadership requires the application of varied theoretical concepts to guide the organization's vision and strategic plan. From development and planning to change and maintenance, organizational leadership is paramount for organizational and system success. The frameworks presented are generalizable and easily adaptable to any organizational culture or plan.

The use of change and leadership frameworks to guide nurses in leading and managing change follows the evolution of nursing practice through the application of evidence-based strategies. These frameworks provide an evidence-based guide for the change process. Choosing change and leadership frameworks should be based on the applicability to the particular project or population, and an assessment of the organization's system and culture. Regardless of the population or organizational system, cultural assessment is a crucial component of choosing the most appropriate framework. Successful change is a direct result of utilizing culturally congruent change and leadership frameworks as guides.

KEY POINTS

- Leadership is not attached to a position, nor is it limited to those with positions of authority.
- A democratic leader guides a group toward common goals by engaging the group members and encouraging member participation.

- The basis of autocratic leadership style is authority and control. The leader is powerful and dominates the group members.

- The basis of the laissez-faire style of leadership is faith and trust. The leader relies on the team to work independently without strict oversight or direction.

- Servant leadership is the conscious desire to put others first, including their needs and priorities. The servant leader is humble, values and trusts others, and shares power and authority with the community or organization.

- Contingency and situational theories use a variety of leadership styles depending on the situation or event.

- The concept of transformational leadership involves positive empowerment, motivating others to meaningful action. The transformational leader is charismatic and attracts others to work toward a common cause.

- The focus of transactional leadership is to maintain the current environment through the use of rewards and punishments.

- The Theory of Quantum Leadership addresses organizational concepts of complexity and chaos and views the disorganization and lack of order as a positive organizational attribute.

- Leadership frameworks explain and guide vision and strategy for organizational goal achievement.

- Management theories are focused on the day-to-day functions and tasks required for organizational function and efficiency.

- The Scientific Management Theory is based on concepts of mass production and standardization and focuses on the systematic and efficient use of labor.

- Bureaucracy Theory explains rules and regulations for complex organizational structure. It provides a hierarchical and organized approach to addressing quality, cost control, and workforce concerns.

- Lewin developed a well-known and commonly used change theory describing three dynamic stages of change: unfreezing, moving, and refreezing.

- Havelock's Theory of Change is based on the initiation and implementation of change by an outside entity or change agent.

- Rogers's Diffusion of Innovation Theory describes a five-stage process to guide long-term change.

- Transitional Theory is concerned with the humanistic response, experience, and perceptions associated with change. It describes the interpersonal and intrapersonal stress of change and the challenges and opportunities resulting from the change.

- Tipping point describes change as the result of minor events or situations that continue to build and ultimately reach a climactic result.

- A logic model is a visual representation of the change process used to assess and align the relationship between the plan details and the desired outcomes.

- Communication is a complex process involving all stakeholders in the internal and external environment. It is influenced by the chaos of the organizational system.

- Difficult conversations model explains how to address the challenge of conversation analysis in three types of conversations: the *what happened* conversation, the *feelings* conversation, and the *identity* conversation.

- EI is the person's understanding of emotions both of self and others and uses this understanding to guide actions toward the achievement of goals.

- The Imposter Phenomenon is when leaders and high achievers believe their professional success is due to luck and chance.

- Mentoring is a broad concept defined as a relationship between the mentor and mentee in which the mentor shares experiences, knowledge, and provides insight to assist the mentee.

- The GROW model is based on the premise that performance is facilitated by more than knowledge; it also relies on removing internal barriers.

- Hudson's Five-Factor Mentoring Model is concerned with mentoring the mentee in specific subject areas. The five factors are the personal attributes of the mentor, system requirements, pedagogical knowledge, modeling, and feedback.

- The Apprenticeship Model of Mentoring combines formal education and training with an embedded learning experience. The mentee pairs with an experienced mentor who guides the mentee through a participative experience.

- Model of Caring Mentorship for Nursing is based on long-term empowering relationships relying on continual support, empowerment, and caring provided by experienced nurses.

- Five-Phase Mentoring Relationship Model focuses on improving retention, job satisfaction, and role development. The five phases of this model are: purpose, engagement, planning, emergence, and completion.

REFERENCES

Alexander, G. (2010). Behavioral coaching: The GROW model. In P. Jonathan (Ed.), *Excellence in coaching: The industry guide* (2nd ed., pp. 83–93). Philadelphia, PA: Kogan.

Bass, R., & Riggio, R. (2014). *Transformational leadership* (2nd ed.). New York, NY: Routledge.

Blakeslee, J. A., Goldman, B. D., Papougenis, D., & Torell, C. A. (1991). Making the transition to restraint-free care. *Journal of Gerontological Nursing, 17*(2), 4–8.

Bridges, W. (2004). *The way of transition: Embracing life's most difficult moments*. Cambridge, MA: Da Capo Press.

Chaudhry, A., & Javed, H. (2012). Impact of transactional and laissez faire leadership style on motivation. *International Journal of Business and Social Science, 3*(7), 258–265.

Clance, P., & Imes, S. (1978). The imposter phenomenon in high achieving women: Dynamics and therapeutic intervention. *Psychotherapy: Theory, Research, and Practice, 15*(3), 241–247.

Cooper, M., & Wheeler, M. M. (2010). Building successful mentoring relationships. *The Canadian Nurse, 106*(7), 34–35.

Dahl, R., Shapiro, I., & Cheibub, J. (2003). *The democracy sourcebook*. Cambridge: Massachusetts Institute of Technology Press.

Daniel, J., Bhardwaj, U., & Arora, S. (2015). A co-relational study to assess the relationship between the leadership styles of the nurse managers and job satisfaction of the staff nurses working in a selected hospital of New Delhi. *Journal of Nursing Science and Practice, 5*(1), 10–17.

Fine, A., & Merrill, R. R. (2010). *You already know how to be great: A simple way to remove interference and unlock your greatest potential*. New York, NY: Portfolio Penguin.

Fitzsimons, D., James, K., & Denyer, D. (2011). Alternative approaches for studying shared distributed leadership. *International Journal of Management Studies, 13*(3), 313–328. doi:10.1111/j.1468-2370.2011.00312.x

Garvey, B., Stokes, P., & Megginson, D. (2014). *Coaching and mentoring: Theory and practice* (2nd ed.). Los Angeles, CA: Sage.

Gladwell, M. (2002). *The tipping point: How little things can make a big difference*. New York, NY: Warner Book Group.

Goleman, D. (1998). *Working with emotional intelligence.* New York, NY: Bantam Books.

Greenleaf, R. (2015). *The servant as leader* (Rev. ed.). Indianapolis, IN: The Greenleaf Center for Servant Leadership.

Grossman, S., & Valiga, T. (2013). *The new leadership challenge: Creating the future of nursing* (4th ed.). Philadelphia, PA: F. A. Davis.

Havelock, R. (1973). *The change agent's guide to innovation in education.* Englewood Cliffs, NJ: Educational Technology Publications.

Hersey, P. (1985). *The situational leader.* New York, NY: Warner Books.

Hersey, P., & Blanchard, K. (1977). *Management of organizational behavior: Utilizing human resources.* Englewood Cliffs, NJ: Prentice Hall.

Hudson, P. (2004). *From generic to specific mentoring: A five-factor model for developing primary teaching practices.* Paper presented at the AARE Conference Melbourne, Australia. Retrieved from http:// eprints.qut.edu.au/971/1/hud04076.pdf

Hudson, P., Skamp, K., & Brooks, L. (2004). Development of an instrument: Mentoring for effective primary science teaching (MEPST). *Science Education, 89*(4), 657–674. doi:10.1002/sce.20025

InsideOut Development. (n.d.). History of GROW model. Retrieved from http://www.insideoutdev .com/site/history_grow_model

Julian, D. (1997). The utilization of the logic model as a system level planning and evaluation device. *Evaluation and Program Planning, 20*(3), 251–257.

Koontz, H., & Heinz, W. (1990). *Essentials of management* (5th ed.). New York, NY: McGraw-Hill.

Krogh, G., Nonaka, I., & Rechsteiner, L. (2011). Leadership in organizational knowledge creation: A review and framework. *Journal of Management Studies, 49*(1), 240–277.

Lewin, K. (1951). *Field theory in social science: Selected theoretical papers.* New York, NY: Harper & Row.

Lewin, K., Lippitt, R., & White, R. (1939). Patterns of aggressive behavior in experimentally created social climates. *Journal of Social Psychology, 10*(2), 271–301.

Mayer, J. D., Roberts, R. D., & Barsade, S. G. (2008). Human abilities: Emotional intelligence. *Annual Review of Psychology, 59,* 507–536.

Mayer, J. D., Salovey, P., & Caruso, D. (2004). Emotional intelligence: Theory, findings, and implications. *Psychological Inquiry, 15*(3), 197–215.

McCawley, P. F. (n.d.). *The logic model for program planning and evaluation.* University of Idaho Extension (Doc. # 400 10-01) (pp. 1–5). Retrieved from http://www.cals.uidaho.edu/edComm/pdf/CIS/ CIS1097.pdf

Millar, A., Simeone, R., & Carnevale, J. (2001). Logic models: A systems tool for performance management. *Evaluation and Program Planning, 24,* 73–81.

Olum, Y. (2004, July). *Modern management theories and practices.* Paper presented at the 15th East African Central Banking Course at Kenya School of Monetary Studies, Kenya. Retrieved from http:// unpan1.un.org/intradoc/groups/public/documents/AAPAM/UNPAN025765.pdf

Performance Consultants International. (2014). The GROW model. Retrieved from http://www .performanceconsultants.com/grow-model

Petrides, K. V., Pita, R., & Kokkinaki, F. (2007). The location of trait emotional intelligence in personality factor space. *British Journal of Psychology, 98*(Pt. 2), 273–289.

Porter-O'Grady, T., & Malloch, K. (2014). *Quantum leadership: Advancing innovation, transforming health care* (4th ed.). Burlington, MA: Jones & Bartlett.

Rogers, E. (1962). *Diffusion of innovations.* New York, NY: Free Press of Glencoe.

Rogers, E. (2010). *Diffusion of innovations* (4th ed.). New York, NY: Simon & Schuster.

Scheiber, L. (2012). *Next Taylorism: A calculus of knowledge work.* Frankfurt, Germany: Peter Lang.

Shields, C. (1991). *Happenstance: Two novels in one about a marriage in transition.* New York, NY: Integrated Media.

Specht, J. (2012). Mentoring relationships and the levels of role conflict and role ambiguity experienced by novice nursing faculty. *Journal of Professional Nursing, 29*(5), 25–31.

Stone, D., Patton, B., & Heen, S. (2010). *Difficult conversations: How to discuss what matters most.* New York, NY: Penguin Group.

Taylor, F. W. (1911). *The principles of scientific management.* New York, NY: Harper & Brothers.

Vandermaas-Peeler, M., Nelson, J., Ferretti, L., & Finn, L. (2011). Developing expertise: An apprenticeship model of mentoring undergraduate research across cohorts. *Perspectives on Undergraduate Research Mentoring, 1*(1), 1–10.

Vergauwe, J., Wille, B., Feys, M., De Fruyt, F., & Anseel, F. (2015). Fear of being exposed: The trait-relatedness of the imposter phenomenon and its relevance in the work context. *Journal of Business and Psychology, 3,* 565–581.

Wagner, A. L., & Seymour, M. E. (2007). A model of caring mentorship for nursing. *Journal for Nurses in Staff Development, 23*(5), 201–211; quiz 212.

Walker, K., & DeVooght, J. (1989). Invasion. A hospital in transition following the 1983 Grenadian intervention. *Journal of Psychosocial Nursing and Mental Health Services, 27*(1), 27–30.

Weber, M. (1968). Bureaucracy. In G. Roth and C. Wittich (Eds.), *Economy and society: An outline of interpretive sociology* (pp. 956–969). Berkeley: University of California Press.

W. K. Kellogg Foundation. (2004). *Using logic models to bring together planning, evaluation, and action: Logic model development guide.* Battle Creek, MI: Author. Retrieved from http://www.smartgivers.org/uploads/logicmodelguidepdf.pdf

Woods, A. (2010). Democratic leadership: Drawing distinctions with distributed leadership. *International Journal of Leadership in Education, 7*(1), 3–36.

Zimmerman, B., Lindberg, C., & Plsek, P. (2008). *Edgeware: Insights from complexity science for health care leaders* (2nd ed.). Irving, TX: Veterans Health Administration.

19

Frameworks for Evaluation

Rose Utley

True genius resides in the capacity for evaluation of uncertain, hazardous, and conflicting information.
—Winston Churchill

KEY TERMS

AGREE Model
CIPP Model
Clinical Integration Model
cluster evaluation
conceptual use
CONSORT Guidelines
COPA Model
Donabedian's Structure–
    Process–Outcomes
    Model
Duff's Quality Caring
    Model
Educational Systems
    Analysis Model
evaluand

formative evaluation
Health Care Quality
    of Life Outcomes
    Model
instrumental use
Kirkpatrick 4 Level
    Evaluation Model
meta-evaluation
outcome evaluation
participatory evaluation
Precede-Proceed
    Model
PRISMA guidelines
process evaluation
program evaluation

Promoting Excellence in
    Nursing Education (PENE)
    Pross Evaluation Model
PSDA Model
Quality Health
    Outcomes Model
Quality Implementation and
    Evaluation Model (QIE)
quality improvement
SQUIRE Model
STROBE guidelines
Systems Engineering
    Initiative for Patient Safety
    (SEIPS) Model
theory-based evaluation

LEARNING OBJECTIVES

1. Differentiate types of evaluation and evaluation processes.
2. Compare evaluation frameworks used for quality improvement (QI) in terms of emphasis, processes, and key concepts.
3. Describe and differentiate evaluation frameworks used for QI, educational program evaluation, individual performance, and project quality evaluation.
4. Identify evaluation frameworks useful for education, clinical practice, and program development.

Evaluation is concerned with assessing the effectiveness of an organization, program, or service; or identifying strengths and weaknesses inherent in an organization, program, service, or an individual's performance. Evaluation processes are used in organizational accreditation reviews when conducting a needs assessment to determine if a new product, program, or service is warranted, when conducting personnel reviews, engaging in conflict resolution, or when generating professional compliance reports. All evaluation processes share certain commonalities including the use of systematic processes to answer questions and data collection focused on organizations, processes, programs, services, resources, or individuals. Evaluation processes also share a common purpose of enhancing knowledge and informing decision making in the real world (Preskill & Russ-Eft, 2005, pp. 1–2).

As with research, theory-based evaluation (TBE) practices are preferred for building knowledge. Evaluation theory holds a unique position as a field of study in its own right; a field of study that is determined and motivated by the needs from any and all other fields of study. "Evaluation is a practice-driven field ... driven by both the needs of the evaluation practitioners and by their inventiveness" (Shadish, 1998, p. 13). A common thread shared in evaluation is that it is based on the values held by the individuals or groups engaged in evaluation activities. Values influence the processes utilized and determine the outcomes established and evaluated.

In evaluation theory, the subject or object being evaluated, also called an *evaluand*, can be the individual, a program, or a system. Two broad categories of evaluation theory described in the literature are process and outcome evaluation. *Process evaluation* is used to understand the intervention or understand the change process used in research or program implementation. Through the use of measurable objectives, *outcome evaluation* determines if the program outcomes have been achieved. According to Griffiths and King (1991), evaluation must have a purpose and must have the potential for action. It should be ongoing and provide a means for continual monitoring, diagnosis, and change. Although process evaluation often receives less emphasis than outcome evaluation, process evaluation is essential for understanding why and how an intervention or change initiative worked or did not work.

TYPES OF EVALUATION FRAMEWORKS

Evaluation frameworks may be categorized based on purpose, processes used, and levels. In this section, these categories are explored followed by models developed for QI, educational programs, individual performance, and frameworks for project quality.

Evaluation Purpose

TBE is process evaluation that depicts a "plausible and sensible model of how the program is supposed to work" (Bickman, 1987, p. 4). It relies on theory to understand the intervention or change process and seeks to explain how the program caused the outcomes (Coryn, Noakes, Westine, & Schröter, 2011). Core principles of TBE include developing a plausible theory from existing theories or research, using the theory to generate and prioritize evaluation questions, and conducting all phases of the project. In addition, the constructs or variables measured and the relationships between them should stem from the identified theory (Coryn et al., 2011). TBE typically involves the use of a theory of change and a logic model, which links the assumptions and outcomes. Identifying key services, desired outcomes, and making a hypothesis about the relationships between them enables the nurse to develop a program model or theory. In TBE, the selected theory or model can then guide all aspects of a project from planning through evaluation (B. L. Green & McAllister, 2002).

The purpose of evaluation, especially educational and program evaluation, is also related to the timing and the end results for the learners or stakeholders. *Formative evaluation* can be ongoing or conducted intermittently at any time prior to final measurement of outcomes. The findings from a formative evaluation provide feedback enabling the processes used during project implementation to be modified if needed. *Summative evaluation* is conducted to determine if the outcomes have been achieved. It occurs at the end of a program or on completion of a project. Both formative and summative evaluation processes can be used within the same program as each serves a different purpose. Using both evaluation processes strengthens the rigor of the change process and increases the likelihood that outcomes will be reached within the planned time frame.

The process of *meta-evaluation* or the systematic review of an evaluation can also be formative or summative. Formative meta-evaluation involves reviewing the evaluation plan, whereas summative meta-evaluation involves evaluation of the processes used and the outcomes achieved after actions have been taken. The process of systematic meta-evaluation is an important mechanism for ensuring the quality of the evaluation findings.

Evaluation Processes

Participatory evaluation describes a process of collaboration between the project manager or researcher and stakeholders who are directly affected by the program, change, or intervention. In participatory evaluation, stakeholders actively engage in developing all phases of the program and its implementation. Participatory methods are used in all phases of a project including conceptualization, planning, implementing, interpreting results, and measuring outcomes. When conducting participatory evaluation, the project manager and stakeholders determine relevant questions to ask to guide the evaluation process from the initial planning stage to post implementation stage. Collaboration is central to ongoing monitoring of program performance.

Principles guiding participatory evaluation include: (a) having a participant focus, (b) promoting participant ownership, (c) supporting negotiation, (d) facilitating learning, and (e) encouraging flexibility (Zukoski & Luluquisen, 2002). Structures and processes are deliberately developed to provide participant focus and create a sense of empowerment and ownership in the program. While working on the program, participants negotiate how it should be conducted, how findings will be used, and what actions may be taken based on the results. The evaluation process involves the ability and willingness to learn from each other and identify and use flexible methods that complement the resources, needs, and skills of participants.

When describing outcomes of the evaluation processes, authors distinguish between two ways the evaluation findings are used. *Instrumental use* refers to any direct action that occurs because of evaluation. This would include changes in protocol, behaviors, and ongoing QI practices. *Conceptual use* refers to cognitive or affective uses of the evaluation knowledge. Topics learned about during the program, operational practices, and knowledge of program outcomes are examples.

Levels of Evaluation

The W. K. Kellogg Foundation has delineated three levels of evaluation. First is *project-level evaluation* defined as the "consistent, ongoing collection and analysis of information for use in decision-making" (2004, p. 14). This means determining what data are needed and developing a system for collecting and analyzing the information. Project-level evaluation is focused on project development and outcomes related to the project stakeholders. Project evaluation should become an integrated part of the project and provide important information about program content, program management, and service delivery decisions. The second level is *cluster evaluation* that focuses on progress made toward achieving the broad goals of a program initiative. The information collected through cluster evaluation enhances the effectiveness of grantmaking, clarifies the strategies of major program initiatives, and informs public policy debates. The third level is *program and policy-making evaluation*. Each is discussed in more detail subsequently.

Project Evaluation

The *W. K. Kellogg Foundation Evaluation Handbook* (2004) describes project evaluation as involving three subtypes of evaluation: context, implementation, and outcome evaluation. Although evaluation is most often associated with meeting short-term and long-term outcomes, determining *context evaluation* or how well the project functions within the local community is important. Context evaluation looks at contextual factors to explain why a project has been implemented the way it has, and why certain outcomes have been achieved and others have not. *Implementation evaluation* is concerned with the planning, development, and implementation of a project. It is described as the process of adapting the plan to the real-world conditions, in which unique organizational dynamics and uncertainties occur. Of course, *outcome evaluation* is conducted to determine the achievement of the short- and long-term outcomes.

Project evaluation plans should include all three subtypes of evaluation (i.e., context, implementation, and outcomes). The purpose of the project, the purpose of the evaluation, and the stage of development of the project will influence the amount of emphasis placed on each type. The use of all three types of evaluation will strengthen the project, enhance effectiveness, and facilitate sustainability of the project.

Cluster Evaluation

Cluster evaluation was developed by the W. K. Kellogg Foundation in the 1980s to meet the evaluation needs of multisite grant recipients and their funders (Sanders, 1998). It provides a means of determining how well a cluster, or group of projects, fulfilled the objectives. Typically, each site has a distinct project environment and contextual factors, such as resources, stakeholders, and processes. To draw conclusions from the collective experiences of multiple sites, there was a need for collaboration and serial networking conferences. This enabled the groups to search for patterns in the consistency and inconsistency of the processes and outcomes. The process of cluster evaluation involves collaboration among sites to answer key questions related to the nature and direction of changes experienced. Cluster evaluation also considers the context of the changes, insights gained, and determines the processes needed to maintain desired changes.

When performing cluster evaluation, the project manager is concerned with the following questions: (a) Have changes occurred in the desired direction? What is the nature of these changes? (b) In what contexts have the changes occurred and why? (c) What insights can be drawn from failures and successes? (d) What needs to be done to sustain desired changes? Collaboration between sites is necessary to establish common goals and learn from the experiences of others from diverse sites. A key strategy used in cluster evaluation is establishing networking conferences where information is shared and analyzed by all of the grantees. When effectively carried out, cluster evaluation produces information and understandings that go beyond those found in individual project evaluations.

Program and Policy-Making Evaluation

A program is "any set of organized activities supported by a set of resources to achieve a specific and intended result" (Centers for Disease Control and Prevention [CDC], 2012, para.1). *Program evaluation* is "the systematic collection of information about the activities, characteristics, and outcomes of programs to make judgments about the program, improve program effectiveness, and/or inform decisions about future program development" (CDC, 2012, para. 2).

In 1999, the CDC published the "Framework for Program Evaluation in Public Health" that identified 30 standards grouped under four criteria for good program evaluation. These four criteria are: utility, feasibility, propriety, and accuracy. *Utility* is concerned with the concepts of the target population for the program and the timing of the program. It is concerned with the questions: Who needs the evaluation? Who will benefit from the information? And, will the evaluation results be timely? *Feasibility* is concerned with logistics and practicality

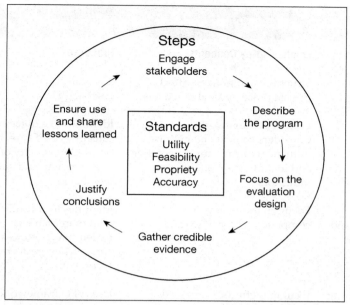

FIGURE 19.1 CDC framework for program evaluation.

CDC, Centers for Disease Control and Prevention.
Reprinted from CDC (1999).

of the program evaluation. The key question asked is: Are the planned evaluation activities realistic given the time, resources, and expertise of the evaluation committee? The criterion of *propriety* is concerned with the rights and welfare of individuals. The fourth criterion, *accuracy*, is concerned with the reliability and validity of the evaluation data.

The CDC Program Evaluation Framework also describes the step-by-step process used during evaluation (see Figure 19.1). The process begins with identifying and engaging the stakeholders who are most likely to benefit from the program. Next, the scope and purpose of the program are described. Then the evaluation design is determined, evidence is gathered, and conclusions are justified. The final criterion involves sharing the lessons learned during the program implementation and evaluation. Many skills are necessary during this six-step evaluation process. Therefore, the use of an evaluation team comprising key stakeholders and community experts is recommended. Evaluating project implementation is a vital source of information for interpreting results and increasing the power and relevance of an outcome evaluation.

Program and policy-making evaluation is a macro form of evaluation often used by the granting organization. The Kellogg Foundation conducts this level of evaluation and utilizes information synthesized from project level and cluster evaluation to make effective decisions about program funding and support. Communities also engage in program and policy-making evaluation at the local level and beyond. Taken together, the project, cluster, and program and policy-making evaluation levels provide comprehensive and multiple perspectives, and use data to strengthen and assess individual projects as well as groups of projects.

● EVALUATION FRAMEWORKS FOR QI

The remainder of the chapter covers evaluation frameworks relevant to QI. According to the Health Resources and Services Administration (HRSA), QI is the "systematic and continuous actions that lead to measurable improvement in healthcare services and the health status of targeted patient groups" (2011, p. 1). In addition to exploring QI in health care, this

TABLE 19.1 Comparison of Quality Improvement Evaluation Frameworks

Framework	Emphasis/Key Concepts	Processes
Structure–Process–Outcome (SPO)	Structural components affect clinical processes and outcomes	Assessing quality involves assessing SPO
Quality Health Outcomes	Uses SPO framework Considers context and cultural influences during implementation and identification of outcome indicators	Identifies five outcome indicator categories (self-care, health promotion, quality of life, symptom management, and perceived well-being)
Quality Implementation and Evaluation Model	Focus on the structural component of the SPO framework	Identifies four conditions that affect quality implementation (policy, patient preparedness, provider competency, performance and accountability)
Systems Engineering Initiative for Patient Safety Model	Examines effects of physical, social, and biological factors on patient safety	Uses SPO framework
Precede–Proceed Model	Five precede phase concepts: social, epidemiological, behavioral/environmental, educational/organizational, administrative/policy	Explores change from pre-intervention and post-intervention Assesses five precede phase areas then executes the proceed phase
Clinical Integration Model	Focus on facilitating coordination and quality of patient care and cost containment	Vertical integration = coordination of care between a single health care organization and the patient Horizontal integration = coordination of care across organizations

chapter covers evaluation frameworks relevant to educational programs, individual performance, and project quality. For a comparison of QI evaluation frameworks in terms of key concepts and processes, see Table 19.1.

Donabedian's Structure–Process–Outcome Model

Many approaches to quality assurance and evaluation use the structure–process–outcome (SPO) framework described by Donabedian (1966, 1980, 1988). The SPO framework identifies a direct connection between the structural aspects, clinical processes of care, and the outcomes achieved. The structural components include the organization, material resources such as technology and tools, human resources such as care providers, and clinical tasks involved in the change.

The structural components of the model interact and affect how the clinical processes such as provider's tasks and procedures are organized and performed and how clinical processes are implemented and outcomes achieved. Patient outcomes typically include satisfaction, safety, and quality of care; employee outcomes may include satisfaction, job stress, employee safety, and employee health. Finally, the organizational outcomes may include institutional profit and employee turnover rates. Assessing quality involves one or more of the aspects of SPO.

The SPO framework is often depicted in a linear fashion, showing structure as influencing processes, which influence outcomes. However, the first consideration is the influence of actions and activities of physicians and other health care workers (Donabedian, 1980). The focus is on the provider's implementation of processes and the provider's interaction with the processes.

Quality Health Outcomes Model

The Quality Health Outcomes (QHO) Model was developed in 1998 by the Expert Panel of the American Academy of Nurses (Mitchell, Ferketich, & Jennings, 1998). Using Donabedian's SPO framework, the QHO model proposes four constructs that parallel nursing's meta-paradigm concepts of person, environment, health, and nursing. The model identifies reciprocal relationships between the client, system, intervention, and outcomes; it emphasizes the need to consider context and cultural influences during implementation.

One feature of the model is the identification of categories of outcomes believed to be influenced by nursing services provided. These outcome categories are nursing activities that: help the client achieve self-care, promote health, promote quality of life, facilitate symptom management, and improve the perception of care quality.

Since its inception, the QHO Model has influenced the development of other models including one developed by Sousa (1999), which focused on Health Care Quality of Life Outcomes, and Duffy and Hoskin's Quality Caring Model (2003). In addition to being used as a framework for conducting research studies and summarizing research findings, the five outcome indicators have been used in health care reports compiled by the United States and Canada. Although the QHO Model has been most widely used in nursing, the indicators have been used in studies and reports across disciplines (Mitchell & Lang, 2004).

Quality Implementation and Evaluation Model

The Quality Implementation and Evaluation Model (QIE) is a useful guide for implementing activities to improve health care practices. It was developed to provide a theoretically-based model that could be used by institutional leadership to initiate or change organizational structures to affect performance and improve outcomes. The QIE focuses on Donabedian's structure component in the SPO model. Four conditions that facilitate quality implementation are identified in the QIE: (a) policy, (b) patient preparedness, (c) provider competency, and (d) performance and accountability. Each component is discussed subsequently.

The *policy* component necessitates examining the current institutional policy, guidelines, or protocols regarding a specific health care practice. Then current evidence-based literature is reviewed and used to modify policy to align with recommended practices. Second, patients and family require knowledge and understanding of the activities implemented to achieve the change and promote quality. Therefore, actions to promote *patient and family preparedness* are needed. The third component, *provider competency*, ensures that employees are prepared for the QI initiative. This requires three actions: communication of new policy and protocols, training in implementing the policy/protocol, and ensuring provider competency in implementing the protocol. The final component, *performance and accountability*, refers to providing mechanisms for reporting on the success of implementation and ongoing monitoring of the policy or protocol implementation.

The QIE Model provides a structure and process that can be used by nurse leaders and researchers to change aspects of the health care system and evaluate the effectiveness of changes in patient outcomes. A multisite study of the effectiveness of the QIE Model in preoperative inpatient units is presented in Box 19.1. In this study, each of the four components of the QIE Model (i.e., policy, patient preparedness, provider competency, and performance and accountability) is evaluated to determine the impact on the program.

BOX 19.1 The Effectiveness of the QIE Model

The effectiveness of the QIE Model was determined in a hospital study of evidence-based preoperative skin prep policies (Talsma, McLaughlin, Bathish, Sirihorachai, & Kuttner, 2014). Fifteen hospitals provided their preoperative skin-prep policy for review and comparison to the American Perioperative Registered Nurses (AORN) Association Guidelines. The hospitals then received feedback on any gaps in their policy and suggestions for change. Through the hospital's quarterly reports, the researchers determined the relationship between the hospital's use of the model and the adherence to the recommended skin-prep protocol. Those hospitals active in implementing the QIE Model activities showed higher use of the recommended skin prep. The QIE Model used structural components shared by the health care situation. This allowed the institution the flexibility to develop specific practice changes tailored to the institution's culture and environment.

QIE, Quality Implementation and Evaluation Model.

Systems Engineering Initiative for Patient Safety Model

The Systems Engineering Initiative for Patient Safety Model (SEIPS) builds on the concepts of physical, social, and biological factors to describe and explain how system design factors influence patient safety and how system design impacts employee and system-level outcomes. The *SEIPS Model* uses the SPO framework outlined by Donabedian, but expands the concept of structure to include mutual interactions between the organization, technology and tools, environment, tasks, and the person. The interactions between these structural factors yield outcomes reflecting patient, employee, and organizational performance in addition to safety and health, and the quality of working life (Carayon et al., 2006). These system components can contribute to safety issues and represent factors that must be managed to control for unacceptable processes and unwanted outcomes.

Besides explaining factors that impact patient safety, the model accounts for objective employee outcomes such as safety and health and subjective outcomes of stress, burnout, and work satisfaction. Organizational outcomes described in the model include financial profit, turnover, and frequency of employee injury and illness. Changes to any component of the work system (structure) will affect the overall structure and clinical processes that ultimately impact the patient, employee, and organization. Depending on the change and how it is designed and implemented, the effect can be positive or negative. In contrast to Donabedian's model, greater emphasis is placed on the systems structure or workforce design aspects.

Clinical Integration Model

Clinical integration (CI) was defined by the Federal Trade Commission in 1996 as a program designed to evaluate and modify practice patterns of physicians. It involves developing interdependence and cooperation between physicians and the health care systems to reduce cost and improve the quality of care. Since its conception, the definition has expanded to "the means to facilitate the coordination of patient care across conditions, providers, settings, and time; to achieve safe, timely, effective, efficient, equitable, and patient-focused health care" (Athena Health, 2016, para. 1).

Early applications of CI focused on cost containment by creating physician-hospital organizations (PHOs), integrated delivery networks (IDNs), mergers, acquisitions, and consolidation of physicians' practices. The goal of CI was to provide greater control over admissions and health care costs, and to improve negotiations and contracting with payers. Since that time, the CI has evolved to focus on quality care in addition to cost containment.

Current CI models do not require mergers or acquisitions, but rely heavily on health information technologies such as electronic health records for communication and tracking of health care provided. CI models occur on a continuum ranging from "vertical integration," which refers to the coordination of care between a single health care organization and the patient, to "horizontal integration" referring to the coordination of care across organizations (e.g., between hospitals, physicians, and insurers). Coordination and communication between four components (hospital, physician's office, payers, and patient) are needed for horizontal integration.

Key concepts for achieving CI include: (a) information technology, (b) payment reforms, (c) legal and regulatory factors that influence payment reforms, (d) collaborative leadership and interdependence among the hospitals, physicians, payers, and patient, and (e) clinical care coordination. A strong information technology infrastructure allows sharing of information at the point of care across specialties, services, locations, and time. Development of health information exchanges links the patient's medical records from hospitals, physician offices, and other outpatient services with diagnostic and pharmacy services. In CI, payment reforms are initiated that align the goals and incentives of different health care providers. These payment reforms promote CI by shifting from a fee-for-service system to a reimbursement system that rewards quality and cost-effective care. Legal and regulatory factors affecting reimbursement at the state and federal levels include medical liability, insurance regulations, IRS laws, and enforcement of the Civil Monetary Penalty, Starks Law, and Anti-Kickback Law (see Table 19.2).

Precede–Proceed Model

The Precede–Proceed Model was developed by Lawrence Green in 1974 for use with health promotion programs (L. W. Green & Kreuter, 2005). Development of the model was influenced by multiple disciplines including epidemiology, education, health administration, and social and behavioral sciences. Two assumptions of the model are that (a) health and health risks are caused by multiple social, behavioral, and environmental factors and (b) efforts to effect change in those factors must be multidimensional and involve the key stakeholders.

The Precede–Proceed Model provides an evaluation framework that looks at change from two perspectives: (a) the pre-intervention assessment or Precede phase, and (b) the post-intervention or Proceed phase. The Precede phase comprises five areas that are assessed: social, epidemiological, behavioral/environmental, educational/organizational, and

TABLE 19.2 Legal and Regulatory Factors Influencing Clinical Integration Models		
Legal/Regulatory Factors	**Description**	**Potential Impact on Clinical Integration Models**
Anti-Kickback Law	Payment incentives for ordering services for Medicare and Medicaid insured	May induce ordering of unnecessary services
Antitrust	Prohibits providers having market power from determining cost of services	Discourages noncompetitive reimbursement arrangements
Civil Monetary Penalty	Payments from hospitals to physicians that reward cost containment efforts	May directly or indirectly limit services provided for patients with Medicare or Medicaid

administrative/policy. Assessment within these areas results in potential diagnoses by identifying needs and issues. Social assessment involves assessing the community's perception of its own needs. From there, the epidemiological assessment involves determining which health issues are important to which segments of the population. Behavioral and environmental assessment involves further analysis of the health issues and factors that contribute to the complexity of health issues. Attitudes, values, and beliefs of the organization serve as predisposing factors that must be assessed. In addition, reinforcing factors such as rewards and factors that facilitate or support change are assessed.

After the factors in the Precede portion of the model are assessed, the Proceed portion of the model is executed. This involves planning, implementing, and evaluating the intervention or change. The evaluation includes looking at the processes used to implement change and the impact of change on the community, the health issues, and the achievement of specific outcomes.

◉ EVALUATION FRAMEWORKS FOR EDUCATION

This section describes four evaluation models each with a unique educational focus. The Pross's evaluation model was developed specifically for evaluation in academic nursing education. The CIPP Model describes a generic process for educational decision making. For evaluation of corporate training programs, Kirkpatrick's Four-Level Evaluation Model is explored. The fourth model is the Educational Systems Analysis Model (ESAM) developed to guide administrators in collection and analysis of educational data. For a comparison of key concepts and processes within these evaluation frameworks for education, see Table 19.3.

Promoting Excellence in Nursing Education, Pross Evaluation Model

According to Pross's evaluation model, having visionary, caring leadership, engaging expert faculty, and having a dynamic curriculum are major factors that affect the success of academic programs (Pross, 2010). Of these, the nature of nursing leadership is essential for nursing program success. Six components produce visionary and caring leadership. These are: (a) personal knowing, (b) strong community partnerships, (c) congruent relationships with the parent institution, (d) strategic, data-driven decisions, (e) the ability to facilitate caring environments, and (f) being grounded educationally and experientially in nursing.

Personal knowing is demonstrated by supportive and encouraging attitudes, accessible and approachable behaviors, and ability to create environments that support and encourage success. Community partnerships are essential for acquiring resources for nursing programs such as clinical sites and scholarships for student development. In addition, a strong relationship between program leaders and the institutional leadership will facilitate the acquisition of institutional resources. Pross notes that the success of a program may depend on how congruent the program and institution are in term of priorities, perspectives, and leadership styles. Data-driven decisions are made with transparency and involve continual collection and evaluation of both qualitative and quantitative data. Data that are meaningful, credible, objective, measurable, and responsive to changes in the health care system are examined and used to guide decision making. Facilitating a caring program environment benefits students by supporting the growth of others, being open, transparent, and present, as well as by pointing out strengths and providing encouragement. Finally, nursing leadership that is grounded in nursing and can communicate the perspectives and contributions of the nursing unit are needed.

Another essential component of Pross's model includes providing mechanisms for ongoing faculty development and obtaining expert faculty with curriculum and instructional expertise. Characteristics of expert faculty are: (a) internal motivation to achieve scholarship

TABLE 19.3 Comparison of Evaluation Frameworks for Education

Framework	Emphasis/Key Concepts	Processes
Promoting Excellence in Nursing Education	Leadership, faculty, and curriculum affect academic program success	Assess leadership, faculty, and curriculum to facilitate visionary, caring leadership, faculty expertise, and a dynamic curriculum
CIPP	Four types of evaluation: context, input, process, and product	Data collection within the four types of evaluation to inform decision making
Kirkpatrick's Four-Level Evaluation	Four participant-focused, progressively higher outcomes; student reaction, learning, behavior, and results	Evaluation questions are asked at each of the four outcomes levels
Educational Systems Analysis Model	Guides new academic administrators in data collection to evaluate function and performance of the institution	Collect and analyze data: external and internal institutional factors as a foundation for SWOT analysis

CIPP, Context, Input, Process, and Product Model; SWOT, strengths, weaknesses, opportunities, and threats.

and professional development goals; (b) a sense of personal knowing and collegial engagement; and (c) significant service contributions to the profession, the program, and the institution.

The final component of Pross's model is the curriculum. Four tenets of excellent curriculum are: (a) being empirically and theoretically grounded, (b) providing quality instruction and clinical placements, (c) being globally relevant, and (d) exceeding the minimum regulatory requirements. The dynamic curriculum and expert faculty are interconnected through visionary caring leadership and in combination, these factors promote excellence in nursing education programs.

Context, Input, Process, and Product Model

The Context, Input, Process, and Product Model or CIPP, was originally developed for educational decision making (Stufflebeam, 1968). However, it offers an adaptable framework for guiding the evaluation of programs, projects, personnel, products, institutions, and evaluation systems (Stufflebeam, 2003). The concepts of CIPP represent types of evaluation that correspond with the institution's goals, plans, actions, and outcomes, respectively. CIPP provides a comprehensive structure for data collection that facilitates informed decision making in a variety of projects and programs. The CIPP components are discussed subsequently.

Context evaluation helps detect needs, opportunities, and identify potential and hidden problems that could inhibit the project. Evaluation of the context involves examining the setting and the history of the institution where the intervention or change occurs. Factors such as problems, needs, assets, resources, and opportunities emerge from the context. Evaluation of goals and the sociopolitical climate provides information to facilitate planning and decision making.

Input evaluation looks at implementation plans, budget, and resources. The purpose is to assess the program's strategy, the merit of the program, and compare the work plan against current research. Then, determine the responsiveness of the program to client needs, and examine alternative strategies offered. Input evaluation uses a strategy to resolve the program problem. Data are used to determine the extent to which planned activities were carried out and to guide the staff on how to modify and improve the program plan.

Process evaluation monitors the implementation of the program or project and general operations required for ongoing institutional processes. Monitoring the project, documentation of program processes and outcomes, communication processes, and the quality of the program's implementation are the focus. In this stage, program activities are monitored, documented, and assessed by the evaluator or researcher.

The final process is referred to as *product evaluation*, which examines the achievement of outcomes and the impact of the program on the target audience and community. In product evaluation, the degree to which objectives have been achieved and the cause of the outcomes is determined. Product evaluation is also concerned with the success of the program, the quality, sustainability, and the ability of the outcomes to be achieved in other settings.

Kirkpatrick's Four-Level Evaluation Model

Kirkpatrick (2001) developed a four-level model for evaluating corporate training programs. The four levels are participant focused and outline progressively higher outcomes that the evaluator must address including student reaction, learning, behavior, and results. Beginning with the most basic level, evaluation at the *reaction* level is concerned with the learner's satisfaction with the education. Did the learner like the education? This is commonly measured using surveys, interviews, or focus groups. The next level of evaluation is concerned with student *learning*. What skills, knowledge, or attitudes changed after the education? And how much did these change? Student learning can be evaluated using exams, questionnaires, and performance testing. Evaluation of the third level, *behavior*, is concerned with whether the education has resulted in a change in behavior. Questions such as: Did the learner's knowledge transfer to the next higher level course? or, Is the learner able to apply what was learned to a work setting? are addressed at this level. The highest level of evaluation is focused on long-term results and changes within the organization. *Results* typically fall into the categories of increased productivity, increased quality, decreased turnover, and reduced costs.

Although Kirkpatrick's Four-Level Model was developed for evaluation of corporate educational programs, it is easily adaptable to general education settings. The main difference would be in the results level because the long-term outcomes in general education would differ from those of corporate education. Results for academic settings would include the pursuit of graduate education, engaging in scholarly activity, or advancing to student leadership positions within the academic setting. One application of Kirkpatrick's model in nursing education research is recounted in Box 19.2. The levels of Kirkpatrick's model were applied to the evaluation of simulation for decreasing central line infection. In general, the use of all four levels of evaluation provides a comprehensive structure for understanding the range of outcomes achieved. The model also facilitates leveling evaluation outcomes from subjective perception, knowledge, and application to long-term outcomes.

Educational Systems Analysis Model

Clark (2004) developed the Educational Systems Analysis Model (ESAM) to guide new academic administrators in data collection and in developing a comprehensive analysis of external and internal factors that affect the institution's function and performance. ESAM considers external factors or elements outside of the academic institution categorized as *environmental* and *community of interest* factors. Environmental factors include economic

---

BOX 19.2 Use of Kirkpatrick's Four-Level Evaluation Model in Education

In 2009, Orlando conducted a study using Kirkpatrick's Four-Level Evaluation Model to determine the impact of medical residents' participation in a simulation on central line insertion. Using mixed methods, data were obtained for each evaluation level. For level 1, course evaluations indicated that simulation, small group teaching, and feedback were well perceived by the students. Using pre- and posttests of knowledge, level 2 (evaluation of learning) showed significant knowledge gains and retention of learning within and between cohorts. Level 3 evaluation of data using chi-square and linear regression analyses suggested that operators' bundle compliance rate predicted their complications rate. Focus group data indicated having a nurse in the room during simulation had an unanticipated effect of reducing the number of insertion attempts by students and therefore lowered the rate complications. For level 4 (evaluation of long-term results at the institutional level), time-series analysis suggested that central line training and changes in policies and practices significantly reduced the hospital's central line-associated infection rate.

---

conditions, manpower, competition from other institutions, technology, legal, political, and regulatory influences, ethical issues, societal attitudes, and values, as well as the institutional and program reputation. These environmental factors interact with the community of interest, which comprises prospective students, employers of program graduates, alumni, donors, and the general public.

The environmental factors and community of interest interact and influence each other and also affect the internal elements of the model. The internal elements are factors within the institution or the nursing program that affect the program's function and performance. They are: (a) mission and goals, (b) organizational culture, (c) relationships, (d) structure, (e) programs and services, (f) resources, and (g) outcomes (Clark, 2004). These seven internal elements are explored further in terms of content and process. Each internal element is analyzed for content including what is done and why, and the processes used and by whom. The ESAM framework provides a foundation for evaluation of program strengths, weaknesses, opportunities, and threats, goal setting, and future program development.

EVALUATION FRAMEWORKS FOR INDIVIDUAL PERFORMANCE

Performance evaluation is often conducted for employees and students using institutionally designed tools. A common approach is to develop the evaluation tools based on job requirements, objectives, and expectations. Therefore, institutional-specific performance evaluations should reflect the roles, professional values, behaviors, competencies, and the mission and values of the institution. In this section, two evaluation models that are adaptable to a variety of institutions, (i.e., the Competency, Outcomes, and Performance Assessment Model [COPA] and Value-Added Models [VAMs]) are presented.

COPA Model

Assessment and evaluation of an individual's competence in nursing practice and education can be addressed using the COPA model. It was developed by Lenburg (1999a, 1999b) who identified eight categories of behaviors and skills nurses in educational, clinical, or leadership positions need for competence. These competencies are: (a) assessment and intervention,

(b) communication, (c) critical thinking, (d) human caring relationships, (e) management, (f) leadership, (g) teaching, and (h) knowledge integration. According to Lenburg, every significant activity or action in which nurses engage can be categorized within this framework. The model is flexible and comprehensive enough to apply to nurses from diverse educational backgrounds, diverse clinical specialties and settings, and for all nursing roles including educator, clinician, leader, and researcher.

The COPA model can promote professional development by providing a framework for self-reflection and self-assessment of one's professional practice. It can also be used in combination with formal, systems-level evaluation mechanisms to address achievement of externally established performance standards such as those determined by accrediting agencies. The model emphasizes the nurse's responsibility for engaging in self-confrontation and reflection, creating and implementing a plan for meeting competencies, seeking external evaluation of competence through peer evaluation or other employer-specified processes, and documenting evidence of competence such as in a portfolio.

Value-Added Models

The subjective nature of teacher evaluations coupled with the No Child Left Behind legislation has contributed to the use of evaluation approaches that focus on quantifiable student outcomes versus student satisfaction with a course or a teacher (Braun, 2005). One approach to objective student evaluation is referred to as Value-Added Models (VAMs). VAMs use data from student test scores, which are statistically adjusted to determine gains achieved by a teacher's students. Proponents of VAM note that analysis of the changes in student test scores from 1 year to the next enables the evaluator to objectively link the contributions of teachers and schools to student learning. Teachers are then compared to other teachers in the district based on gains achieved by their students.

Several VAMs have been developed including the Educational Value-Added Assessment System (EVAAS), Dallas Value-Added Accountability System (DVAAS), and Rate of Expected Academic Change (REACH). Each relies on purely statistical analysis of changes in student test scores from year to year, rather than on other measures of student learning or alternative data sources. The models differ in structure and underlying assumptions. Users of any of these models must confront the issues of lack of random pairings among students and teachers, the presence of confounding variables, and the tendency to make causal associations between student outcomes and teacher effectiveness.

EVAAS was developed in 1993 by William Sanders and associates for use in the Tennessee school system (Braun, 2005). Since then, it has been adopted by districts in other states. DVAAS has been employed by the Dallas school system for a number of years. It uses a value-added criterion to identify highly effective teachers as well as those in need of support. The DVAAS differs from the EVAAS in several important ways. First, it does not use student-level characteristics to adjust student test scores prior to analysis. Second, it evaluates the relationship between adjusted test scores in adjacent grades rather than combining data across more than one grade. Third, when considering the teacher's contribution to student achievement, it looks at other school-related factors that may account for student achievement. REACH is another value-added program used in California schools. It differs from EVAAS and DVAAS by looking at test-based criterion measures of student progress toward meeting a proficiency standard. As a result, a student's performance is measured against a goal rather than against the performance of other students.

Cunha and Miller (2014) note that, "While there is evidence that such test-based value-added measures can indeed capture the differential performance of institutions and teachers, several differences render the wholesale importation of the K–12 model to higher education impractical" (p. 65). First, unlike K–12, in higher education, annual standardized tests are not administered. Therefore, other outcomes such as persistence rates, graduation rates, and post-college earnings should be considered. However, these outcomes are typically measured or observed once, which limits the applicability of statistical tests that are sensitive to differences within the individual or within the individual's school experience. Other differences that must be considered are the K–12 graduates' ability to choose their educational institution and specialize their education after high school. The goals of higher education are also broader and typically involve increasing the student's economic productivity, expanding the graduate's career and lifestyle options, and enhancing informed citizenship and decision making. For a study about a value-added methodology in Texas institutions of higher education, see Cunha and Miller (2014).

◉ FRAMEWORKS FOR PROJECT QUALITY

This section covers frameworks that enhance project quality and the reporting of quality findings. Guidelines for reporting QI projects (SQUIRE Model), a framework for evaluating published clinical guidelines (AGREE), guidelines for publishing research and systematic literature reviews (PRISMA, STROBE, and CONSORT), and the Plan, Do, Study, Act cycle (PDSA) model for conducting pilot studies are described.

SQUIRE Model

The Standards for QUality Improvement Reporting Excellence or SQUIRE 1.0 was developed in 2008 to provide reliable and consistent guidelines for reporting and publishing health care improvement efforts (Davidoff et al., 2008; Ogrinc et al., 2008, 2015). Since that time, the science of evaluation and QI, and expectations for patient care quality, safety, and value have advanced. SQUIRE 2.0 was developed in 2015 to be used in a variety of situations including single settings and multisite controlled trials. In addition, SQUIRE 2.0 can be applied concurrently with other publication guidelines such as CONSORT (for randomized control trials), STROBE (for observational studies), and PRISMA (for systematic reviews).

SQUIRE 2.0 combines the IMRAD framework (introduction, methods, results, and discussion) with Bradford Hill's four questions for writing. The introduction section focuses on Hill's question, "Why was the project started?" The problem, summary of what is known about the problem, and aims are included. Explaining the rationale for the study provides a mechanism for describing the framework and concepts used in the project. The methods section answers Hill's question, "What did you do?" The context of the situation, a description of the intervention, how it was studied, the type of analysis performed on the data, and how ethical considerations were addressed are included. The next section that is essential in reporting improvement projects is the results. The results section answers the question, "What did you find?" The author reports the steps of the implementation process and identifies contextual factors that could impact the findings. Details about the process measures and outcomes achieved as well as unexpected benefits and problems are reported. The last section, "discussion," answers the question: What does it mean? This is where key findings are summarized, the results interpreted, and limitations identified.

Although SQUIRE is designed to assist with scholarly writing about evaluation studies, it requires reporting key factors in conceptualization, design, implementation, and evaluation of the study. Therefore, SQUIRE has been found useful for both planning QI studies and providing a common framework for sharing study results (Davies et al., 2015).

AGREE Model

The proliferation of health care research has resulted in the formulation of numerous clinical guidelines that are designed to consolidate findings from high-quality studies and communicate practice recommendations and standards. Thus, clinical practice guidelines have become a cornerstone of evidence-based health care. To ensure the development of quality practice guidelines, the Appraisal of Guidelines for Research and Evaluation (AGREE) tool was developed. AGREE provides a framework for assessing quality, provides rigorous methods for guideline development, and guides developers in the reporting and presentation of the guidelines.

AGREE was originally developed in 2003 by an international collaboration of developers and researchers and was revised in 2009 and updated in 2013. The updated AGREE tool consists of 23 items organized into six domains: (a) scope and purpose, (b) stakeholder involvement, (c) rigor of development, (d) clarity of presentation, (e) applicability of guidelines, and (f) editorial independence. Eleven of the 23 items were edited for clarity. One item was added under the "rigor of development" domain, which calls for the description of strengths and limitations of the body of evidence. This revised framework allows for the application of the model to "any disease area targeting any step in the healthcare continuum, including those for health promotion, public health, screening, diagnosis, treatment, or interventions" (Brouwers et al., 2010, p. 4).

Recognizing that the benefits of practice guidelines are directly linked to the quality of the guidelines, the use of AGREE II and the revised user's manual provide a mechanism for ensuring a systematic and standardized approach. AGREE II is useful for health care providers who seek to evaluate the rigor and potential applicability of practice guidelines to their own setting. It allows developers to use a systematic and organized approach to evaluate guidelines and provides policy makers with a decision-making tool to determine which practice guidelines will be used to support policy decisions. Use of the tool by nurse educators can enhance student's critical evaluation skills, as well as teach them about criteria for guideline development.

PRISMA Guidelines

Historically, the quality of reporting of research findings has been variable. To facilitate high quality and standardization in published reports of systematic reviews and meta-analysis, the Preferred Reporting Items of Systematic reviews and Meta-Analyses or PRISMA criteria were developed. In 1999, a group of international scholars compiled a set of guidelines for reporting meta-analyses of randomized controlled trials (RTC) called QUOROM or QUality Of Reporting Of Meta-analyses (Moher et al., 1999). In 2009, QUOROM was revised to include systematic reviews and was renamed PRISMA. Though designed to focus on meta-analyses and systematic reviews of RCTs, PRISMA has been used to guide reporting of non-RCT studies.

PRISMA includes a flow chart for conducting the review of literature, guidelines for reporting the findings of the review, and guidelines for research protocols. The literature review process involves four steps. First is identifying studies through database searches and other sources. Second is removing duplicates and screening and excluding studies. Third is determining the eligibility of the studies for inclusion based on full-text availability and meeting inclusion/exclusion criteria. This leads to the final step, which is including the remaining studies into the review of literature. The PRISMA guidelines include 27 items to address in reporting the findings of a systematic review or meta-analysis. The 27 items are organized under the seven sections of a research report: (a) the title, (b) abstract, (c) introduction, (d) methods, (e) results, (f) discussion, and (g) funding (Moher et al., 2009).

An international group of scholars developed the PRISMA-P (protocol) guidelines to increase the transparency, accuracy, thoroughness, and frequency of documentation of systematic review and meta-analysis protocols (Shamseer et al., 2015). They define a protocol as "a document written before the start of a systematic review describing the rationale and intended purpose of the review and the planned methodological and analytical approach" (para. 7). The PRISMA-P checklist includes 17-items that should be described in protocols of systematic reviews and meta-analyses. These are divided into: (a) administrative information, (b) introduction, and (c) methods sections.

STROBE Guidelines

STROBE stands for "STrengthening the Reporting of OBservational studies in Epidemiology," which uses established criteria for reporting observational studies. STROBE was the outcome of a collaborative initiative with epidemiologists, methodologists, statisticians, researchers, and journal editors (von Elm et al., 2007). Although observational research comprises many study designs and many topic areas, STROBE has developed a checklist for only three major types of designs: cohort, case–control, and cross-sectional studies.

A checklist of items to be included in articles reporting observational research was developed using the seven sections of a research report. These are: (a) the title, (b) abstract, (c) introduction, (d) methods, (e) results, (f) discussion, and (g) funding (von Elm et al., 2007). Many of the checklist items are the same as used in PRISMA guidelines but with variations under methods, and results that are relevant to cohort, case-control, and cross-sectional designs.

CONSORT Guidelines

CONSORT stands for CONsolidated Standards Of Reporting and is focused on increasing the quality and consistency of reporting data from RCTs and reducing the problems arising from inadequate reporting (Moher et al., 2001, 2010; Turner et al., 2012). The guidelines consist of three documents: the CONSORT statement, the checklist, and the flow diagram. The CONSORT statement is an evidence-based set of recommendations for reporting RCTs. It offers a standard way for authors to prepare publications of findings and facilitates consistent reporting of minimum criteria. It emphasizes completeness and transparency in reporting and enhances the ability to critique studies and the interpretations provided. The CONSORT statement and checklist follow the traditional research manuscript format described earlier (title, abstract, introduction, methods, result, and discussion). The methods, results, and discussion contain specific items relevant to RCTs that should be documented in the publication. The last category was renamed "other information" and includes information on funding, registration number, and where the full research protocol may be accessed.

The flow chart outlines a four-step process used in reporting individual RCTs beginning with the enrollment of subjects followed by allocation, follow-up, and analysis. The enrollment step involves identifying the number eligible to participate and describes the number meeting study criteria and the process of randomization. Next, the allocation process should describe those who received the intervention and those who did not. Follow-up should provide the number of subjects lost to follow-up. The last step, analysis, should provide the number and characteristics of those analyzed. For each step, the authors should provide the total number excluded and the reasons they were excluded. Published reports should clearly identify how each step of the process was accomplished and explain the rationale for any decisions made that affects the resulting sample.

Plan, Do, Study, Act Cycle

Plan, Do, Study, Act (PDSA) cycle describes an iterative process used to evaluate changes implemented during a pilot study, prior to full implementation. The focus of PDSA is to learn from the data and learn from observations made during the research cycle. Beginning with the "plan stage," objectives for the project in general and the PDSA cycle are determined. Who will be involved in each stage of the cycle, their responsibilities, and the time and setting for the implementation are determined. Next, the "doing stage" encompasses carrying out the plan, piloting the change, collecting data to measure how the change meets the objectives, and making observations about the implementation process. The "study stage" involves analyzing the data collected, determining whether the objectives were met, and identifying changes needed for future implementation efforts. The "act stage" includes

---

BOX 19.3 Use of the PDSA Cycle in Research

A quality improvement methodology (Plan, Do, Study, Act) was used to guide the implementation and evaluation of the Functional Disability Inventory (FDI) for the assessment of pediatric patients with chronic pain (Lynch-Jordan et al., 2010). The FDI was chosen as an outcome measure due to its established validity as an instrument for assessment of pain-related disability. The research team developed four PDSA cycles designed to evaluate specific outcomes. The first cycle was to test the practicality of FDI administration. The second cycle evaluated two methods of FDI tool administration. The third cycle determined the value of sharing FDI results with patients. The final cycle evaluated the method of documenting FDI administration.

---

making the changes identified from the study stage and repeating the cycle if further evaluation is warranted.

According to Taylor et al. (2014), the PDSA cycle offers a scientific method for rapid assessment and implementation and provides flexibility to modify the change based on feedback from the study stage. The four stages correspond to the phases of experimental research, namely, forming a hypothesis (Plan), collecting data to test the hypothesis (Do), analyzing and interpreting the data (Study), and extrapolating findings for practical use (Act). Application of the PDSA cycles in a study that involved implementing a pain assessment tool in a pediatric clinical setting is presented in Box 19.3.

 ## CONCLUSION

According to Childers (1989), evaluation is used for decision making and/or to answer research questions. Evaluation research generally follows similar phases and processes as original research, but it is also characterized by being conducted in a noncontrolled, real-world setting. TBE and the use of models as frameworks for evaluation provide consistent structure to guide the evaluation process, and provide evaluative data that can contribute to nursing science.

KEY POINTS

- Evaluation can be categorized as a process that focuses on understanding the change process or outcome.
- TBE relies on theory to understand the intervention and the change process.
- The timing of evaluation can be formative or ongoing, or summative, at the end of the program.
- Collaboration between the researcher and stakeholders during all aspects of the project is referred to as *participatory evaluation.*
- Cluster evaluation was designed to facilitate identification of patterns in data from multiple diverse sites.
- Types of evaluation frameworks can be categorized as QI, educational, individual performance, and project quality models that focus on the evaluation of clinical projects.
- QI frameworks include Donabedian's SPO, QHO, QIE, SEIPS, Precede–Proceed, and CI Models.

- Evaluation frameworks for educational projects and programs include Promoting Excellence in Nursing Education; CIPP; Kirkpatrick's Four Levels; and the ESAM.

- Individual performance can be evaluated using the COPA Model or a variety of VAMs.

- Frameworks for project quality address QI project-reporting guidelines (SQUIRE), clinician guideline development (AGREE), RCT studies (CONSORT), systematic reviews and meta-analysis (PRISMA), epidemiological research (STROBE), and the project development process (PDSA Cycle).

- Evaluation models provide guidance for project development and quality and are useful for decision making and answering project questions.

REFERENCES

Athena Health. (2016). What is clinical integration? Retrieved from http://www.athenahealth.com/knowledge-hub/clinical-integration/what-is-clinical-integration

Bickman, L. (1987). The functions of program theory. In L. Bickman (Ed.), *Using program theory in evaluation: New directions for program evaluation* (Vol. 33, pp. 5–18). San Francisco, CA: Jossey-Bass.

Braun, H. (2005). *Using student progress to evaluate teachers: A primer on value-added models*. Princeton, NJ: Educational Testing Center.

Brouwers, M., Kho, M. E., Browman, G. P., Cluzeau, F., Feder, G., Fervers, B., . . . Zitzelsberger, L. (2012, December). AGREE II: Advancing guidelines development, reporting, and evaluation in healthcare. *Canadian Medical Association, 182*, E839–E842. doi:10.1503/cmaj.090449

Carayon, P., Shoofs-Hundt, A., Karsh, A.-T., Gurses, A. P., Alvarado, C. J., Smith, M., & Flatley-Brennan, P. (2006). Work system design for patient safety: The SEIPS model. *Health Care, 15*(Suppl. 1), i50–i58. doi:10.1136/qshc.2005.015842

Centers for Disease Control and Prevention. (1999). Framework for program evaluation in public health. *Morbidity and Mortality Weekly Report, 48*(No. RR-11), 1–40.

Centers for Disease Control and Prevention. (2012). Introduction to program evaluation for public health programs: A self-study guide. Retrieved from http://www.CDC.gov/eval/guide/introduction/index.htm

Childers, T. (1989). Evaluative research in the library and information field. *Library Trends, 38*(2), 250–267.

Clark, M. (2004). Finding the way: A model for educational system analysis. *International Journal of Nursing Education and Scholarship, 1*(1), article 11. Retrieved from http://www.consort-statement.org

Coryn, C. L., Noakes, L. A., Westine, C. D., & Schröter, D. C. (2011). A systematic review of theory-driven evaluation practice from 1990 to 2009. *American Journal of Evaluation, 32*(2), 199–226.

Cunha, J. M., & Miller, T. (2014). Measuring value-added in higher education: Possibilities and limitations in the use of administrative data. *Economics of Education Review, 42*(2014), 64–77.

Davidoff, F., Batalden, P., Stevens, D., Ogrinc, G., Mooney, S., & SQUIRE Development Group. (2008). Publication guidelines for quality improvement in health care: Evolution of the SQUIRE project. *Quality, Safety and Health Care, 17*(Suppl. 1), i3–i9. doi:10.1136/qshc.2008.029066

Davies, L., Batalden, P., Davidoff, F., Stevens, D., & Ogrinc, G. (2015). The SQUIRE Guidelines: An evaluation from the field, 5 years post release. *BMJ Quality & Safety, 24*(12), 769–775.

Donabedian, A. (1966). Evaluating the quality of medical care. *The Milbank Memorial Fund Quarterly, 44*(3, Pt. 2), 166–203.

Donabedian, A. (1980). *The definition of quality and approaches to its management, Vol 1: Explorations in quality assessment and monitoring*. Ann Arbor, MI: Health Administration Press.

Donabedian, A. (1988). The quality of care. How can it be assessed? *Journal of the American Medical Association, 260*(12), 1743–1748.

Duffy, J. R., & Hoskins, L. M. (2003). The Quality-Caring Model: Blending dual paradigms. *Advances in Nursing Science, 26*(1), 77–88.

Green, B. L., & McAllister, C. (2002, April 24). Theory-based, participatory evaluation: A powerful tool for evaluating family support programs. *The Bulletin of the National Center for Zero to Three*, 1–20.

Green, L. W., & Kreuter, M. W. (2005). *Health program planning: An educational and ecological approach.* New York, NY: McGraw-Hill.

Griffiths, J. M., & King, D. W. (1991). *A manual on the evaluation of information centers and services.* New York, NY: American Institute of Aeronautics and Astronautics Technical Information Service.

Health Resources and Services Administration. (2011). *Quality improvement.* Washington, DC: U.S. Department of Health and Human Services.

Kirkpatrick, D. (2001). *Evaluating training programs: The four levels.* San Francisco, CA: Berrett-Koehler.

Lenburg, C. B. (1999a, September 30). Redesigning expectations for initial and continuing competence for contemporary nursing practice. *Online Journal of Issues in Nursing, 4*(2), manuscript 1. Retrieved from http://www.nursingworld.org/MainMenuCategories/ANAMarketplace/ANA Periodicals/OJIN/TableofContents/Volume41999/No2Sep1999/RedesigningExpectations forInitialandContinuingCompetence.html

Lenburg, C. B. (1999b, September 30). The framework, concepts, and methods of the competency outcomes and performance assessment (COPA) model. *Online Journal of Issues in Nursing, 4*(2), manuscript 2. Retrieved from http://www.nursingworld.org/MainMenuCategories/ANAMarketplace/ANAPeriodicals/OJIN/TableofContents/Volume41999/No2Sep1999/COPAModel.html

Lynch-Jordan, A. M., Kashikar-Zuck, S., Crosby, L. E., Lopez, W. L., Smolyansky, B. H., Parkins, I. S., . . . Powers, S. W. (2010). Applying quality improvement methods to implement a measurement system for chronic pain-related disability. *Journal of Pediatric Psychology, 35*(1), 32–41.

Mitchell, P. H., Ferketich, S., & Jennings, B. M. (1998). Quality health outcomes model: American Academy of Nursing Expert Panel on Quality Health Care. *Image—The Journal of Nursing Scholarship, 30*(1), 43–46.

Mitchell, P. H., & Lang, N. M. (2004). Framing the problem of measuring and improving health care quality: Has the quality health outcomes model been useful? *Medical Care, 42*(Suppl. 2), 4–11. doi:10.1097/01.mlr.0000109122.92479.fe

Moher, D., Cook, D. J., Eastwood, S., Olkin, I., Rennie, D., & Stroup, D. F. (1999). Improving the quality of reports of meta-analyses of randomised controlled trials: The QUOROM statement. Quality of Reporting of Meta-analyses. *Lancet, 354*(9193), 1896–1900.

Moher, D., Jones, A., & Lepage, L., CONSORT Group (Consolidated Standards for Reporting of Trials). (2001). Use of the CONSORT statement and quality of reports of randomized trials: A comparative before-and-after evaluation. *Journal of the American Medical Association, 285*(15), 1992–1995.

Moher, D., Liberati, A., Tetzlaff, J., & Altman, D. G., PRISMA Group. (2009). Preferred reporting items for systematic reviews and meta-analyses: The PRISMA statement. *PLOS Medicine, 6*(7), e1000097. doi:10.1371/journal.pmed.1000097

Moher, D., Plint, A. C., Altman, D. G., Schulz, K. F., Kober, T., Galloway, E. K., . . . Dias, S. (2010). Consolidated standards of reporting trials (CONSORT) and the quality of reporting of randomized controlled trials. *Cochrane Database of Systematic Reviews, 2010*(3). doi:10.1002/14651858.MR000030

Ogrinc, G., Davies, L., Goodman, D., Batalden, P., Davidoff, F., & Stevens, D. (2015). SQUIRE 2.0 (Standards for QUality Improvement Reporting Excellence): Revised publication guidelines from a detailed consensus process. Published Online First (September 14, 2015). *BMJ Quality and Safety, 25*(12), 1–7. doi:10:1136/bmjqs-2015-004411

Ogrinc, G., Mooney, S. E., Estrada, C., Foster, T., Goldmann, D., Hall, L. W., . . . Watts, B. (2008). The SQUIRE (standards for quality improvement reporting excellence) guidelines for quality improvement reporting: Explanation and elaboration. *Quality, Safety and Health Care, 17*(Suppl. 1), i13–i32. doi:10.1136/qshc.2008.029058

Orlando, J. P. (2009). *Impact study of a central lines simulation training using Kirkpatrick's four-level evaluation model* (Dissertation). Philadelphia: University of Pennsylvania.

Preskill, H., & Russ-Eft, D. (2005). *Building evaluation capacity: 72 activities for teaching and training.* Thousand Oaks, CA: Sage.

Pross, E. A. (2010). Promoting excellence in nursing education (PENE): Pross evaluation model. *Nurse Education Today, 30*(6), 557–561.

Sanders, J. (1998). Cluster evaluation. *The Evaluation Exchange, 4*(2), 7–8.

Shadish, W. R. (1998). Evaluation theory is who we are. *American Journal of Evaluation, 19*(1), 1–19.

Shamseer, L., Moher, D., Clarke, M., Ghersi, D., Liberati, A., Petticrew, M., . . . Stewart, L. A.; PRISMA-P Group. (2015). Preferred reporting items for systematic review and meta-analysis protocols (PRISMA-P) 2015: Elaboration and explanation. *British Medical Journal, 350*, g7647. doi:10.1136/bmj.g7647

Sousa, K. H. (1999). Description of a health-related quality of life conceptual model. *Outcomes Management for Nursing Practice, 3*(2), 78–82.

Stufflebeam, D. L. (1968, January). *Evaluation as enlightenment for decision-making.* Working Conference on Assessment, Sarasota, FL.

Stufflebeam, D. (2003). The CIPP model of evaluation. In T. Kellaghan & D. Stufflebeam (Eds.), *International handbook of educational evaluation* (pp. 31–62). Dordrecht, The Netherlands: Kluwer Academic Publishers.

Talsma, A., McLaughlin, M., Bathish, M., Sirihorachai, R., & Kuttner, R. (2014). The quality, implementation, and evaluation model: A clinical practice model for sustainable interventions. *Western Journal of Nursing Research, 36*(7), 929–946.

Taylor, M. J., McNicholas, C., Nicolay, C., Darzi, A., Bell, D., & Reed, J. E. (2014). Systematic review of the application of the plan-do-study-act method to improve quality in healthcare. *BMJ Quality & Safety, 23*(4), 290–298.

Turner, L., Shamseer, L., Altman, D. G., Weeks, L., Peters, J., Kober, T., . . . Moher, D. (2012). Consolidated standards of reporting trials (CONSORT) and the completeness of reporting of randomised controlled trials (RCTs) published in medical journals. *Cochrane Database of Systematic Reviews, 2012*(11). doi:10.1002/14651858.MR000030.pub2

von Elm, E., Altman, D. G., Egger, M., Pocock, S. J., Gøtzsche, P. C., & Vandenbroucke, J. P.; STROBE Initiative. (2007). The Strengthening the Reporting of Observational Studies in Epidemiology (STROBE) statement: Guidelines for reporting observational studies. *Annals of Internal Medicine, 147*(8), 573–577.

W. K. Kellogg Foundation. (2004). *W. K. Kellogg foundation evaluation handbook.* Battle Creek, MI: Author. Retrieved from http://www.wkkf.org

Zukoski, A., & Luluquisen, M. (2002, April). Participatory evaluation: What is it? Why do it? What are the challenges? *Community-Based Public Health Policy & Practice, 2002*(5), 1–6.

Sociocultural Frameworks

Kristina Henry

The world in which you were born is just one model of reality. Other cultures are not failed attempts at being like you. They are unique manifestations of the human spirit.
—Wade Davis

KEY TERMS

cultural awareness
Cultural Care Diversity
  and Universality Theory
cultural desire
cultural imprints
cultural knowledge
cultural sensitivity
cultural skill
Culturally Responsive
  Healthcare Model
Giger and Davidhizar
  Transcultural Assessment
  Model
Health Inequalities
  Imagination

Health Traditions Model
Jeffreys's Cultural
  Competence and
  Confidence Model
Justice as Fairness Theory
Kleinman's
  Explanatory Model
Papadopoulos, Tilki,
  and Taylor Model for
  Developing Cultural
  Competence
Process of Cultural
  Competency in the
  Delivery of Healthcare
  Services

Purnell Model for Cultural
  Competence
Ramsden's Cultural
  Safety Model
Social Resources
  Theory
Structural
  Functionalism Theory
Symbolic Interaction
  Theory
Transcultural Nursing
  Assessment Guide
Transcultural Nursing
  Theory-Madeleine
  Leininger

LEARNING OBJECTIVES

1. Explore the historical development and modern application of sociocultural frameworks in patient planning and care.

2. Describe sociocultural frameworks in terms of attributes, assumptions, and applicability to patient planning and care.

3. Compare and contrast sociocultural frameworks as applied to patient planning and care.

Sociological frameworks are used to describe social phenomena, including social constructs and dynamics. They provide a basis for analyzing the social world, as well as interpreting, explaining, and predicting social concepts such as culture. Some frameworks are broad and offer a general perspective, while others provide perspective to a specific social or cultural aspect.

Many nursing schools use these models to develop cultural competence in nursing students throughout the undergraduate and graduate curriculum. Excelsior College uses the Purnell Model, Georgia State uses the Giger and Davidhizar Transcultural Assessment Model (Lipson & Desantis, 2007). They have implemented these models in a variety of clinical settings and educational formats, including online, distance learning, and immersion sites.

As the basis of nursing is to provide care to all individuals, it is imperative that nurses have a comprehensive understanding of social and cultural concepts to provide patient-specific care. Social and cultural constructs influence the behaviors and actions of all individuals. To provide comprehensive and culturally competent care, nurses must be aware of the sociocultural influences on the individual. The following frameworks are used as guides to facilitate this process.

SOCIOLOGICAL FRAMEWORKS

Both nursing and sociology are concerned with understanding people and how they live and interact in the world. The impact of sociological structures and functions on health and well-being is undeniable. Therefore, in this section, several broad sociological frameworks are presented, which can enhance our understanding of the individual and family and the context in which they live and interact. These are general frameworks with a broad scope related to a wide range of social inequalities. For frameworks specific to economic conditions, inequalities, or injustices, see Chapter 15.

Symbolic Interaction Theory

The Symbolic Interaction Theory is a general sociological framework introduced by philosopher, sociologist, and psychologist George Herbert Mead. The basic premise of the theory represents individuals and their behavior as reflective of the relationships between individuals and society. Four concepts classify the interactions as communication, meanings, perceptions, and interpretations. These interactions create symbols or products that construct society, thus creating a reciprocal relationship with individuals. Society is composed of individuals, and individuals create society; neither exists without the other (Stryker & Statham, 1985).

When individuals interact, this experience yields symbols and meaning. This shared experience is reliant on individual perceptions and therefore is not the same for each participant. The interpretation of meaning and symbols will direct behavior in both future and ongoing social processes. As individuals develop, these meanings and symbols may be revised or reformatted to reflect new or different meanings (Stryker & Statham, 1985). Many researchers describe this process as fluid, emphasizing the spontaneous and creative characteristics of interactions.

Current research, using the fundamental concepts of the Symbolic Interaction Theory, has studied the connection between micro (individual) and macro (society) social processes. The concepts of habit, emotion, and self-concept have been applied to study the complexity of individuals and society as interdependent constructs. For instance, young adults are aware of the dangers of driving fast and reckless, yet statistically, they are more likely to experience car accidents due to these behaviors. Their choice to drive fast and reckless regardless of their knowledge of the danger may be based on their symbolic perception of the situation and social interpretation and desirability of being "cool."

Structural Functionalism

Herbert Spencer, a biologist, anthropologist, sociologist, and philosopher of the 1800s, studied and described society using the human body as the fundamental model (Spencer, 1896). He noted the various components of society, such as health care, education, and government, must work collectively for the entire system to function, just as the many organs and systems in the human body must work collectively to sustain life. Spencer used this analogy to describe the evolution of members of society as well; therefore, coining the term "survival of the fittest" to denote those whose collective function supports human life even through adverse conditions. As applied in the social setting, survival of the fittest means those with the most motivation, resources, or abilities will be the most successful.

Structural functionalism is a social construct composed of the interdependent components alluded to earlier by Spencer (i.e., health care, education, and government). These components form a system that functions in a state of equilibrium. When the equilibrium of the system is challenged, the components of the system must reorganize and adapt to achieve a new state of equilibrium (Wallace & Wolf, 2005). This process does not happen rapidly, but is an evolutionary process.

To apply structural functionalism to research, researchers study the interrelation, characteristics, and social needs or facts relevant to individuals and groups that constitute the structure of society. These social facts are described as laws, ethics, religion, customs, fashions, rituals, and other social and cultural rules. This also involves the study of social patterns and behaviors that may be obvious, unintentional, or undesirable (Wallace & Wolf, 2005). Women being the primary caregiver of children proves an example of an unintentional social pattern. Other examples of unintentional social patterns include the stigma or victimization of those suffering a tragedy and cycle of urban poverty.

The educational system in a society demonstrates structural functionalism in providing structure and stability. Educational systems are based on cultural norms and established socialization constructs, as well as learning and societal placement or ranking. Students often form friendships and social networks while establishing a social order based on knowledge, skills, and abilities. For example, friendships may be based on similar learning aptitudes and skills, which may persist throughout the individual's development and impact the broader social environment. These social networks provide a form of organization within a society.

Social Resources Theory

The Social Resources Theory is based on resources and capital considered necessary by society for maintaining and thriving in the environment. According to the theory, resources represent class, status, and power and are described as valuable and essential for survival. Valuable resources are further classified as personal or social. Personal resources belong to or describe individuals and include gender, age, race, religion, education, career, income, and familial resources. Social resources or social capital belong to other individuals or are ascribed to one's social network (Kwon & Adler, 2014; Lin, 1986). Examples of social resources include a friend's possessions or political connections.

This theory has been used to study the context of personal and social resources and the societal assumptions and connections in which they are based. Consideration of the role of resources in social interactions and structure is emphasized. A specific concern is, how does an individual use his or her personal and social resources to influence society and his or her own personal goals? Kwon and Adler (2014) note the theory has demonstrated applicability in a wide range of disciplines and research topics including business, social media, and management concepts. One study described in Box 20.1 examined the influence of social capital on individual performance.

Primary assumptions of Social Resources Theory are based on instrumental actions or actions with the intent to gain valuable resources. The likelihood of instrumental action success is directly correlated with current possession and application of valuable resources. Thus, if a person has political influence or knows people who have, the more likely the individual will possess a position of political influence and have access to social resources. Conversely, those with limited political influence or with limited access to others with

---

BOX 20.1 Research Application of the Social Resource Theory

Abbasi, Wigand, and Hossain (2014) examined the influence of social resources or social capital on individual performance outcomes of academic authors. They found a positive correlation between the author's social capital and research performance outcomes. In addition, they noted a direct relationship between social capital and the number of published citations by academic authors.

---

political influence will experience less success in obtaining valuable social resources. The saying, "the more you have, the more you make" is a prime example of this concept.

Justice as Fairness Theory

Political philosopher, John Rawls (1971) developed the Justice as Fairness Theory to describe the social distribution of goods. Rawls believed through cooperation and agreement, two parties competing for resources could compromise, resulting in fairness to both parties. Equality in resource distribution is a basic human right. However, inequality is acceptable only if the advantage is for those who are less fortunate (Rawls). The theory is based on two principles to address the problem of distributive justice: the liberty principle and the difference principle.

The *principle of liberty* refers to when all individuals possess equal rights to fundamental liberties. These liberties include the right to vote, run for office, freedom of speech, freedom of assembly, liberty of conscience, freedom of personal property, and freedom from arbitrary arrest. However, the right to own property or production means are not included.

The *difference principle* is founded on the concept that arbitrary factors should not determine an individual's opportunities. Thus, the family into which a person is born should not override individual characteristics or attributes for success or, in other words, a person should not be entitled to benefits through birth alone. In addition, when social and economic inequalities do exist they should benefit only those less fortunate, thus equalizing opportunities (Rawls, 1971).

⊙ FRAMEWORKS FOR CULTURAL ASSESSMENT AND COMPETENCE

Exposure to cultural diversity is not limited to the immigration of certain groups into a geographic area. Advances in transportation have afforded more opportunities for shared cultural exchanges. Likewise, developments in communication technology through telephone, Skype, and social media have blurred geographic barriers and broadened our exposure to a wide range of cultures. Nurses and other health care providers are faced with the dilemma of needing to ensure safe, effective, and respectful care in an increasingly diverse society. The need to deliver nursing care that is culturally competent hinges on the nurse's ability to assess the patient's cultural heritage and plan approaches to care that respects the patient's values and beliefs. As a profession, nursing has recognized the importance of developing skills in cultural assessment to facilitate culturally competent care. The frameworks presented in this section may be used to enhance clinical practice and promote cultural competence.

Cultural Care Diversity and Universality Theory

Anthropologist and nurse theorist Madeleine Leininger combined the concepts of nursing and anthropology to coin the term *transcultural nursing*. She studied the concepts of transcultural nursing for nearly 40 years before officially publishing the theory of Cultural Care

Diversity and Universality. She described the theory as a study of the differences and similarities of diverse patient groups and depicted the major concepts of culture that the nurse can assess in the form of the Sunrise Model.

The Sunrise Model depicts seven universal categories of factors that define cultural groups (Leininger, 2002). These factors (i.e., education, economics, political/legal, technological, religious/philosophical, kinship/social, and values/beliefs/lifeways) interact and exist in the context of the environment, language, and history of the cultural group. Cultural groups tend to identify with a set of beliefs that are passed down generationally. She asserts cultural assessment is an essential component of nursing care planning. The nurse must incorporate the client's culture to demonstrate respect and develop the nurse–client relationship. This holistic and comprehensive approach promotes the incorporation of client requests including nontraditional and spiritual therapies.

Leininger defines culture as learned routines and practices among a specific group of people based on their environment. She explains that culture influences all behaviors and decisions as it reflects values, customs, and beliefs. Language is passed from generation to generation through lived experiences and language. An individual's religion is an example of his or her cultural influence, as well as his or her perception of health and illness.

As the nurse's biases, beliefs, and attitudes directly affect the nurse–client relationship, the nurse is expected to do a self-assessment to identify potential barriers or challenges. If the nurse's culture and the client's culture have conflicting values and beliefs, this could be detrimental to the nurse–client relationship. However, the nurse could minimize the conflict by gathering information to understand the cultural differences (Leininger, 1991).

As cultural values and beliefs are long term and stable, nurses must address the cultural aspects to provide congruent care. Society comprises many diverse cultures that may conflict with health care practices. Nurses must respect as well as have knowledge and understanding of the culture to provide culturally appropriate care. The primary significance of Leininger's model is the historical basis and its use as a guide to develop specific tools for providing culturally competent care.

Giger and Davidhizar's Transcultural Assessment Model

Another model designed to assist nursing students in the assessment and implementation of culturally competent care was developed in 1988 by Giger and Davidhizar (2002). This model represents a client-specific research-based tool to guide the nurse in obtaining knowledge about the client's culture, enabling the health care provider to provide meaningful and relevant care in a timely manner. *Cultural competence* is defined as a continuous process that is more developed and in-depth than mere knowledge of the culture. It is a richer understanding of unique cultures and norms related to meaningful care and consideration, including cognitive and psychomotor skills.

Giger and Davidhizar explain culture as having acquired innate social, religious, artistic, and intellectual influences. Over time, culture develops into patterned expressions of values, beliefs, norms, and practices. Culture is unique and is passed down through generations. It guides thinking, behavior, interactions, and decision making. As culture is an intrinsic and vital characteristic, it is essential for health care providers to concentrate on culturally consistent care for optimal patient outcomes. For instance, research has shown differences exist in disease susceptibility and metabolism of drugs among different racial groups. To provide culturally competent care, the health care provider must have knowledge of these and other cultural differences and be able to address concerns in an appropriate and sensitive manner.

The foundation of the Giger and Davidhizar (2002) Transcultural Assessment Model is the six phenomena used to describe culture: communication, space, time, social organization, environmental control, and biological variations. They note *communication* refers to the verbal and nonverbal processes of human interaction and behavior. Often communication is the most significant challenge in caring for clients of diverse cultures. Communication is a tool to transmit and preserve cultural values, beliefs, and practices. Cultural practices regarding interpersonal *space* vary, with cultures defining intimate, personal, social, consultative, and public spatial distances differently. For health care providers, disruptions to a client's personal space may cause discomfort and territorial dissension, and may result in the client refusing care. Cultural groups also differ in their orientation to *time*, with some being more past, present, or future oriented. Time orientation has an impact on adherence to medical treatment and motivation to engage in future-oriented preventative care. Social organization refers to the organization within the cultural group, such as families, roles, and religion. *Environmental control* refers to the patient's belief in the ability to plan and control the environment to meet personal needs. The final phenomena to assess is *biological variation*. Identifying certain racial groups as being at higher risk for certain diseases is an example of biological variation. Overall, assessing cultural groups using these guidelines provides a comprehensive assessment of the patient and of the nurse's knowledge and competency.

Transcultural Nursing Assessment Guide

Andrews and Boyle expanded on the work of Leininger and other early leaders in transcultural nursing research. Their primary focus is on application of the theory in diverse settings to promote transcultural knowledge in the nursing care of individuals, families, groups, communities, and institutions across the life span (Andrews & Boyle, 2016). Through the use of the Transcultural Nursing Assessment Guide, they emphasize the meaningful use of cultural information and knowledge with practical utility for clinical practice in a variety of settings. With a thorough understanding of cultural perspectives, the nurse is able to incorporate the Transcultural Nursing Assessment Guide findings into the plan of care. The primary goal of Andrews and Boyle was to establish a useful framework or guide for application of transcultural care in practice.

The Transcultural Nursing Assessment Guide can be used to address transcultural care in a variety of clinical situations such as ethical decision making and pain management and in a variety of settings including community, acute care, mental health, and the health care delivery system. The assessment guide is based on the following content categories; biocultural variations and cultural aspects of disease incidence, communication, cultural affiliations, cultural sanctions and restrictions, developmental considerations, economics, educational background, health-related beliefs and practices, kinship and social networks, nutrition, religion and spirituality, and values orientation (Andrews & Boyle, 2016). See Table 20.1 for sample questions or assessment criteria related to each area of content. Although the table provides sample questions and assessment content, the questions and assessments should be adapted to the patient care situation to address culturally specific content.

Culturally competent health care is an expectation in all clinical settings. As the patient's cultural beliefs and values contribute to overall health status, addressing them is vital to providing culturally competent care. The health care provider must be flexible and consider the patient as an equal partner. For an example of the use of the Transcultural Assessment Model to study Mexican Americans' health care perspectives, see Eggenberger, Grassley, and Restrepo's (2006) study highlighted in Box 20.2.

Purnell's Model for Cultural Competence

Cultural competence, as described by Purnell (2002), is the conscious and dynamic process of modifying care to meet the cultural needs and desires of the patient. To do this, the health care provider must be educated about general and specific attributes of diverse cultures. This education is an ongoing process to eliminate cultural bias and promote respect for the cultural group served by the health care provider. As culture is a dominant factor and influence

TABLE 20.1 Andrews and Boyle's Transcultural Nursing Assessment Guide	
Transcultural Nursing Concepts	**Sample Questions**
Biocultural variations and cultural aspects disease incidence	Do you have any distinctive physical characteristics of your cultural group?
	What health conditions are common in your cultural group?
	Are there any socio-environmental diseases more prevalent in your cultural group?
	Are there any diseases to which your cultural group is more resistant?
Communication	How do you prefer to be addressed?
	What is your primary language? Do you speak other languages?
	What language do you prefer? Do you need an interpreter?
	Do you prefer spoken or written communication?
	Do you have specific nonverbal or verbal communication beliefs?
	Are there any cultural restrictions/requirements regarding your care provider?
Cultural affiliations	Where were you born? Where were your parents born?
	Where do you live? For how long? Where have you lived in the past?
	With what cultural group do you affiliate?
	What is your preferred term for your cultural group?
	Do you belong to any cultural organizations?
Cultural sanctions and restrictions	How do you express emotion or spirituality?
	How do you define modesty?
	Do you have any restrictions related to surgery, body exposure?
Developmental considerations	Are there any growth and developmental characteristics specific to your cultural group?
	What is your perception of aging?
	What are your beliefs about death? birth? illness?
	Are there any significant factors to be aware of when assessing specific age groups?

(*continued*)

TABLE 20.1 Andrews and Boyle's Transcultural Nursing Assessment Guide (*continued*)	
Transcultural Nursing Concepts	**Sample Questions**
Economics	Do you have health insurance?
	Who is the principal wage earner?
	Do you have other forms of income?
	Describe your home environment.
Educational background	What is your highest educational level completed?
	What is your preferred learning style?
Health-related beliefs and practices	What do you think caused your illness? What do you call your illness?
	How would you describe your self-image?
	What is your religious affiliation?
	What activities or behaviors do you do to promote health?
	Do you use a cultural healer? Do you practice any cultural healing methods? Who cares for you when you are sick?
Kinship and social networks	What is the composition of your family?
	Who makes up your social network?
	What are the roles of your family members?
	What influence does your culture have on lifestyle and quality of life?
	Do you participate in any cultural organizations?
Nutrition	What types of food do you normally eat?
	Describe your meals and meal times. What do you consider a "healthy" diet? Who prepares your meals and how?
	Do you have any eating or nutritional disorders?
	Do you have any religious mandates regarding your food?
	Do you observe any specific nutritional practices?
	What types of home or folk remedies do you use?

(*continued*)

TABLE 20.1 Andrews and Boyle's Transcultural Nursing Assessment Guide *(continued)*

Transcultural Nursing Concepts	Sample Questions
Religion and spirituality	How do you view your religious beliefs and practices when you are healthy and when you are sick?
	Do you practice religious rituals related to health and illness?
Values orientation	What are your views and attitudes about health and illness?
	Is there a stigma on your illness?
	How do you perceive change?
	What are your views on body image?
	What are your views on education and work?
	How do you relate to people outside your cultural group?

Source: Andrews and Boyle (2016).

BOX 20.2 Research Application of the Transcultural Assessment Model

Researchers used the Transcultural Assessment Model developed by Giger and Davidhizar to study the Mexican American health care perspective (Eggenberger, Grassley, & Restrepo, 2006). They interviewed Mexican American women to understand the cultural impact on health care. The interviews resulted in theme analysis of family, religion, control, attitudes, and lifestyle practice. As this is a growing population and the Centers for Disease Control and Prevention defines this population as medically underserved, this study provides relevant and timely information to provide culturally competent care.

in the health of a patient, addressing the unique cultural values and beliefs when providing care will ultimately improve patient outcomes.

Purnell (2002) developed a clinical assessment tool for nursing students, which has been adapted for use by other health care providers and other student groups. The model is based on diverse frameworks and evidence from communication, family development, anthropology, sociology, psychology, anatomy and physiology, biology, ecology, nutrition, pharmacology, religion, history, economics, political science, linguistics, art, music, and organizational systems literature. Purnell (2002) describes these fields as essential components of cultural characteristics, thus vital for development and application of the model.

The model is shown as concentric circles with the outer rim depicting society, followed by the community, the family, and the individual as inner circles. The individual circle comprises 12 interrelated cultural domains that impact the individual (see Box 20.3). The cultural domain of *overview and heritage* is concerned with the person's country of origin and

---

BOX 20.3 Purnell's Model for Cultural Competence: Factors Relevant to the Individual

- Overview and heritage
- Communication
- Family roles and organization
- Workforce
- Biocultural ecology
- High-risk behaviors

- Nutrition
- Pregnancy and childbearing
- Death rituals
- Spirituality
- Health care practices
- Health care practitioner

Source: Purnell (2002).

---

residence, general description of the land, economic, political, occupational, and educational status. The communication domain is concerned with the primary language, dialects, and willingness to participate and nonverbal or contextual communication. The next domain addresses the importance and centrality of the family, which varies between cultural groups. Assessment of family roles and family organization provides information about gender roles and hierarchy, priorities, development, and social status within the family group. Beliefs about the workforce, individual autonomy, acculturation, assimilation, and gender roles within the workforce are also important. Purnell also emphasized assessment of domains that have a direct impact on physical health. These include the person's biocultural ecology or their ethnic, racial, and genetic heritage, engaging in high-risk behaviors such as smoking or alcohol; nutritional intake and practices related to pregnancy and childbearing. Other domains of interest include the person's beliefs about death and dying, spirituality, and religious practices that are valued. The final two domains include the person's views and practices regarding acute and preventative healthcare, the culture's valuing of self-care, and the sick role and the perception and use of various types of health care providers.

Nurses can apply this model as a component of the patient assessment and use it to develop cultural competence specific to the patient's values and preferences in each domain. Using this tool provides essential knowledge of the client to foster culturally sensitive and competent care. Thus, the health care provider can use this cultural competence tool for self-assessment and discovery. The National Association of School Nurses provides information and resources for the use of this model. See link for available resources subsequently.

Health Traditions Model

Spector (2009) developed the Health Traditions Model to describe the holistic approach to mind, body, and spiritual health. She defines health as the balance of the mind, body, and spirit and illness as an imbalance. Spector describes the holistic approach as addressing complex cultural influences such as ethnicity and religion as *essential* components of health care, not merely complementary or alternative. Summaries of various ethnic and cultural perspectives have been published, which can be used as guides for assessment by health care providers. Although she emphasizes care is not "one size fits all," she believes the informed health care provider is more aware and able to specialize care. To provide holistic care, the provider must relate care to the context in which the individual is living, such as housing, costs, and politics (Spector).

In the Health Traditions Model, Spector identifies five steps or processes in the ongoing development toward cultural competency. These processes are: assessing one's personal heritage, the heritage of others, determining health, health beliefs, and practices, and assessing the modern and traditional health care culture and system. Personal heritage is assessing and analyzing your background and personal identification, including your family and community. Considering the heritage of others involves the assessment and analysis of the patient, the patient's family, and the patient's community. Health, health beliefs, and practices are concerned with examining the traditional beliefs associated with health care such as complementary or homeopathic remedies. The modern health care culture and system involve the topics and concerns related to costs, access, or other matters related to health care delivery. The final step identified by Spector concerns traditional health care systems and the investigation of health care delivery for the majority of people in the culture being examined. Although the Health Traditions Model is time intensive to use, it offers the flexibility of having applications to individuals, families, and the cultural community.

Health Inequalities Imagination Model

The Health Inequalities Imagination Model developed by Hart, Hall, and Henwood (2003) is organized around six basic constructs: cultural knowledge, cultural encounter, equalities awareness, equalities analysis, equalities skills, and equalities action. Cultural knowledge focuses on the willingness to adapt and understand a different worldview; gain of knowledge about epidemiological, biological, and psychological factors relevant to other individuals and groups; and advocate for them on a local and national level. Cultural encounter focuses on the continual process of interaction and communication with diverse populations. The concept of equalities awareness highlights barriers to accessing health care services, the processes of empathizing with others' values and beliefs, self-reflection on personal bias and judgments, and the ability to successfully cope with these understandings. Equalities analysis is the critical examination of the health care inequality based on system reinforcement, as well as the development of creative approaches to counter inequalities. Development of equalities skills involves application of culturally competent, patient-specific care with an emphasis on congruent communication without stereotypes or assumptions. Equalities action involves interprofessional collaboration to challenge the health care inequality.

Hart et al. (2003) developed a call to action for health care professionals to be change agents in addressing health care disadvantages or inequalities. They stressed the importance of developing and maintaining clinical competence through self-reflection and proactive knowledge seeking to address health care disparities. This proactive process of knowledge acquisition involves analyzing and questioning the facts, theories, experiences, beliefs, values, and resources of cultural norms. Engaging in critical analysis will ultimately question the status quo and result in health care that is attentive to health care inequality.

The foundation of this model is the personal and professional desire to improve health care equality. It is not enough to be politically correct. One must genuinely acknowledge and address diversity and the promotion of health care equality.

The Papadopoulos, Tilki, and Taylor Model for Developing Cultural Competence

The model designed by Papadopoulos, Tilki, and Taylor (1998) describes cultural competence as a continual developmental process for an individual. Cultural competence is evolutionary and changes through interactions, learning, and context. This ongoing and dynamic process is reflected in the framework and description of the concepts for application by health care providers. This model was designed in a cyclical fashion representing four stages: cultural awareness, cultural knowledge, cultural sensitivity, and cultural competence (Papadopoulos et al., 1998). Figure 20.1 depicts the cyclical process of cultural competence.

The first stage of the cycle begins with developing basic *cultural awareness*. Cultural awareness is initiated with a self-analysis of personal beliefs, values, and bias. It involves analysis of the meaning and influence of cultural identity as essential components of an individual's health. This stage requires the individual's personal examination of cultural identity and heritage. The second stage, *cultural knowledge,* is the process of learning about various cultures and their health beliefs and actions. This may be accomplished either through personal contact or scholastic inquiry. Through analysis of cultural similarities and differences, one is able to identify and acknowledge health inequalities. *Cultural sensitivity* is the third stage and views health care providers as equal partners in care characterized by a nondominant relationship of trust and respect, with true collaboration. The focus of this stage is on communication and cooperation to develop interpersonal relationships. The fourth stage, *cultural competence,* focuses on the application of acquired knowledge and skills, including confronting racism, inequalities, and other forms of discrimination and implementing culturally competent care. From assessment to diagnosis and evaluation, the care plan and process must reflect cultural competence (Papadopoulos et al., 1998). Figure 20.1 provides a visual representation of the model.

Jeffreys's Cultural Competence and Confidence Model

Jeffreys's Cultural Competence and Confidence (CCC) Model describes cultural competence as a minimal requirement of practice and promotes achieving optimal cultural competence for health care providers. Through continued active learning and supporting diversity while empowering others, health care providers will be able to provide the maximum level of culturally compatible care. The CCC Model is based on interrelated and multifaceted factors in the process of reaching optimal cultural competence (Jeffreys, 2016).

The model identifies a seven-step approach to achieving optimal cultural competence. Each step comprises skill development and leads to self-efficacy and confidence in caring for diverse clients. These steps include self-assessment, active promotion, systemic inquiry, decisive action, innovation, measurement, and evaluation. Through the use of these seven steps, nurses analyze historical, current, and future cultural influences. This analysis and understanding identifes barriers and challenges to optimal patient care, thus leading to transformation of patient care to address these issues (Jeffreys, 2016).

The conceptual foundation for the CCC Model is cognitive, practical or psychomotor, and affective skill development. Jeffreys defines transcultural self-efficacy (TSE) as the health care provider's self-confidence related to providing care for culturally diverse clients. Combining

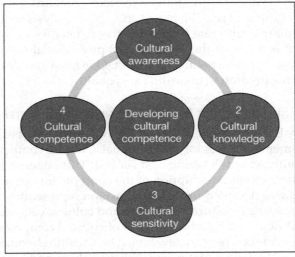

FIGURE 20.1 The Papadopoulos, Tilki, and Taylor Model for developing cultural competence.

Source: Adapted from Papadopoulos, Tilki, and Taylor (1998).

skills and TSE enables the health care provider to offer culturally congruent care. The transcultural nursing skills and TSE may be acquired through formal educational experiences (Jeffreys, 2016).

The CCC Model describes the health care provider who lacks transcultural nursing skills and TSE as someone who avoids incorporating cultural considerations when providing care and therefore provides ineffective care. However, those who are overly confident in their skills and TSE may also be unprepared. Therefore, both circumstances require early identification and intervention through formal educational processes and using the TSE tool (Jeffreys, 2016).

As diversity increases in the United States, it is imperative for nurses to acknowledge the impact of cultural imprints on health care beliefs and practices. These *cultural imprints,* defined as the "integrated systems of beliefs, values, paradigms, structures, processes, language and symbols that influence the behaviour of groups of people" (Australian Quality Council, n.d., p. 4), are unique to each cultural group. The absence of cultural imprints on health care practices minimizes the patient role as a partner in health care, as well as contributes to the lack of access and resources for diverse populations. Therefore, identifying cultural imprints, challenges, and barriers will minimize health care disparities and improve patient outcomes.

Ramsden's Cultural Safety Model

Irihapeti Ramsden, a Maori nurse from New Zealand, developed the *Cultural Safety Model* that highlights the process of caring for those who are deemed foreign in a homogenous society. The inequality in power and resources, as well as the lack of knowledge of the foreign culture, ultimately leads to unsafe health care practices when the patient is demeaned, alienated, or disempowered from accessing appropriate care (Papps & Ramsden, 1996). This model is based on the experiences of the Aboriginal people in New Zealand in which social and political influence and policies reflected imbalanced health care.

The Cultural Safety Model is linked to the Critical Social Theory (see Chapter 15) as it shares many similar attributes. Recognizing sociopolitical, economic, and power influences on the health care system and care delivery is critical in providing safe care. Cultural safety is based on providing culturally respectful and specific care. Nurses need to analyze their personal attitudes and values and establish trust and communication with the patient. The nurse–patient relationship is based on respect and validates the patient's value. This meaningful exchange empowers patients and transforms the societal culture (Papps & Ramsden, 1996).

In modern history, the Cultural Safety Model may be applied to care providers of Syrian refugees. As the Syrian people seek refuge throughout Europe, they will require health care. Applying this theory will not only assist the providers in providing care respectful of the patient's culture but will encourage the provider to analyze the sociopolitical influences that will impact the patient as well. For example, the trauma of leaving their homeland, feelings of powerlessness and dependency, and language barriers are just a few of the concerns providers must address to deliver safe health care.

Fadiman (2012) in her book *The Spirit Catches You and You Fall Down: A Hmong Child, Her American Doctors, and the Collision of Two Cultures* provides another example of the application of the Cultural Safety Model. It is a story of Hmong refugees transplanted to California and their experiences with the U.S. health care system. This story provides evidence of conflicts between traditional health care with healers and Western health care practices. See Research Application Box 20.4 for a synopsis of the book.

Culturally Responsive Healthcare Model

The Culturally Responsive Healthcare Model was developed by Culhane-Pera, Vawter, Xiong, Babbitt, and Solberg in 2003 as a result of their experiences with Hmong patients. The model is based on a health care provider recognizing profound differences in a patient's

> **BOX 20.4 Research Application of the Cultural Safety Model**
>
> Anne Fadiman provides a prime example of the application of the Cultural Safety Model in *The Spirit Catches You and You Fall Down: A Hmong Child, Her American Doctors, and the Collision of Two Cultures* (2012). It is a story of Hmong refugees transplanted to California and their experiences with the American health care system. The story explains the experiences and perspectives of a Hmong family who has a daughter with extensive health care needs, as well as the health care provider's experiences and perspectives. The experiences of the child and family, as well as the health care providers, are the result of a lack of cultural competence. Thus, the communication and trust between both parties were compromised. Ultimately, the care the child received was compromised with devastating results.

beliefs, personal concepts, and the use of communication tools to address them and provide sound, ethical health care. The model describes the foundation of culturally competent care as identifying and directing care based on cross-cultural ethical variances.

The Hmong people practice primarily traditional health care with healers. Their migration to the United States established major conflicts for health care providers practicing Western health care standards. The traditional health care methods of the Hmong were in direct opposition to the Western health care practices used by providers. The resulting conflicts and moral dilemmas led to the development of Culturally Responsive Healthcare Model. This model supports the importance of accommodating cultural beliefs to build trust and health care relationships. Blending the traditional Hmong beliefs with the provider's Western health care practices represents a comprehensive approach to culturally responsive care (Culhane-Pera et al., 2003).

Healing by Heart by Culhane-Pera et al. (2003) describes divergent perspectives, values, and beliefs resulting in the need to blend practices for culturally congruent care. They contend that by combining both traditional health care and Western health care, patient outcomes will improve. The model is founded on providing culturally specific care based on knowledge, skills, and attitudes. The model outlines interconnected content areas that can provide a guide for learning about diverse cultures including politics, economics, social and family structure, religion, geographic location, refugee flight or immigration history, relationship with other groups, cultural change, acculturation, and access to health care systems. Study of these content areas is useful in expanding the nurse's awareness of cultural influence on health beliefs and practices. They can also provide a structure for self-reflection regarding personal health beliefs and practices. Identifying similarities and differences between the nurses and the patient's personal beliefs and practices assists nurses in addressing their responsibility to learn about the cultural groups for whom they are caring. The nurse must examine cross-cultural values in health care by asking if the patient would choose traditional healing practices over modern health care. Through this assessment process, nurses develop skills to analyze and respond to cultural conflicts in health care choices and can foster culturally responsive attitudes, communication skills, and knowledge related to a variety of diverse cultural perspectives and clinical situations (Culhane-Pera et al., 2003).

Explanatory Model

Patients and providers with differing cultural backgrounds often have different perspectives and health care priorities. The patient experience is complex and a result of endless interdependent factors such as perceptions, attitudes, education, culture, family, daily stress, and society, while the provider is focused on symptom analysis, treatment, and alleviation. These conflicting perspectives led to the development of the Explanatory Model (Kleinman, 1976).

Kleinman (1976) designed an Explanatory Model to assist health care providers to understand illness and health concepts from the sociocultural perspective. The model examines cultural influences and the reality and experience of illness for research purposes in clinical settings to provide adequate health care. Kleinman encouraged the study of patient and provider perceptions through the cultural context as a method to enhance health care delivery (Kleinman, 1976).

The Explanatory Model is used in the clinical setting as a tool for providers to examine and interpret the patient's experience. An accurate interpretation assists the provider to develop patient-specific interventions. Kleinman's model is based on open-ended questions used to investigate the specific nature of the health or illness experience. The provider asks the patient what he or she thinks caused the problem and why, the effects of the illness on the patient, chief problems the illness causes, and how severe it is. The provider also asks how long the patient believes these effects will last and what the patient believes would be an adequate treatment. This line of questions culminates in determining the desired outcome of treatment (Kleinman, 1976).

Kleinman's Model is a flexible and valuable tool that allows the health care provider to incorporate patient-specific cultural and social beliefs into the care plan. The premise of the model is to clarify conflicts between provider perceptions and patient perceptions. The results will guide chosen interventions and patient education by acknowledging and incorporating conflicting values and interests of both parties in a holistic manner. An established relationship between the provider and the patient will enhance the results (Kleinman, 1976). Through this process of perspective analysis, the patient will be a partner in the health care process. The patient and provider will negotiate a plan of care that encompasses the cultural beliefs and values of the client with the perspectives and beliefs of the provider. This meaningful care supports patient participation and collaboration, thus improving patient outcomes.

● CONCLUSION

The frameworks presented in this chapter represent sociocultural phenomena applicable to nursing practice. As society and culture are embedded in health care beliefs and values, it is essential for nurses to address these constructs in the process of providing care. If social and cultural concepts were absent from nurse care planning, a void would exist in human care, resulting in incomplete and fractured health care. Nursing care must address all aspects of the individual and provide a holistic approach, to ensure optimal patient outcomes. The frameworks presented in this chapter are used as guides to facilitate this process.

The sociocultural frameworks presented are broad and may be applied to diverse settings and circumstances. From social influence to social justice, these frameworks provide a foundation for analysis and research. The basic concepts of the sociological frameworks are summarized and compared in Table 20.2. The cultural frameworks presented are useful for developing cultural competence and addressing inequities in patient care based on cultural confusion. The basic concepts of the cultural frameworks are summarized and compared in Table 20.3.

A nation's culture resides in the hearts and in the soul of its people.
—Mahatma Gandhi

TABLE 20.2 Comparison of Basic Premises of Sociological Frameworks

Theory (Theorist)	Basic Premise
Symbolic Interaction Theory (George Herbert Mead)	• This is a general sociological framework that describes the relationship between an individual and society.
	• When individuals interact, this shared experience yields symbols and meaning.
	• The fluid interpretation of meaning and symbols will direct behavior and future or ongoing social processes.
Structural Functionalism (Herbert Spencer)	• Society is a social construct composed of interdependent parts forming a system, which functions in a state of equilibrium.
	• When the equilibrium is challenged, the parts of the system must reorganize and adapt to achieve a new state of equilibrium.
Social Resources Theory (Lin)	• It is used to study the context of personal and social resources in societal assumptions and connections, including the role of resources in social interactions and structure.
Justice as Fairness Theory (Rawls)	• It is based on compromise, resulting in fairness to both parties.
	• It identifies two principles to address the problem of distributive justice: the liberty principle and the difference principle.

TABLE 20.3 Comparison of Premises of Cultural Competence Frameworks

Theory (Theorist)	Basic Premises
Model for Cultural Competence (Larry Purnell)	• Cultural competence is a conscious and dynamic process of modifying care to meet the patient's cultural needs and desires.
	• It depicts society, community, family, and individual aspects.
	• Cultural domains of the individual include overview and heritage, communication, family roles and organization, workforce, biocultural ecology, high-risk behaviors, nutrition, pregnancy and childbearing, death rituals, spirituality, health care practice, and health care practitioner.
Health Inequalities Imagination Model (Hart, Hall, and Henwood)	• Health care professionals need to be change agents and address health care inequalities.
	• It is based on six basic constructs: equalities awareness, cultural knowledge, equalities skills, cultural encounter, equalities analysis, and equalities action.

(continued)

TABLE 20.3 Comparison of Premises of Cultural Competence Frameworks (*continued*)	
Theory (Theorist)	**Basic Premises**
Model for Developing Cultural Competence (Papadopoulos, Tilki, and Taylor)	• Cultural competence is a continual developmental process; it changes through interactions, learning, and context.
	• Four stages of competence are: cultural awareness, cultural knowledge, cultural sensitivity, and cultural competence.
Cultural Competence and Confidence Model (Jeffreys)	• Cultural competence uses a seven-step approach of self-assessment, active promotion, systemic inquiry, decisive action, innovation, measurement, and evaluation.
	• Each step comprises skill development and leads to self-efficacy and confidence in caring for diverse clients.
Ramsden's Cultural Safety Model (Papps and Ramsden)	• It highlights the process of caring for those who are deemed foreign in a homogenous society.
	• Inequality in power and resources and lack of knowledge of the foreign culture lead to unsafe health care practices.
Culturally Responsive Healthcare Model *Healing by Heart* (Culhane-Pera et al.)	• Foundation of culturally competent care is identifying and directing care based on cross-cultural ethical variances.
	• Blending traditional health care with Western health care practices represents a comprehensive approach to culturally responsive care.

KEY POINTS

- The Symbolic Interaction Theory describes individuals and their behavior as reflective of society and human interactions. Theses interactions are communication, meanings, perceptions, and interpretations of the individual. When individuals interact, this experience yields symbols and meaning.

- Structural Functionalism framework is explained as a social construct composed of interdependent parts forming a system that functions in a state of equilibrium. When the equilibrium is challenged, the parts of the system must reorganize and adapt to achieve a new state of equilibrium. This does not happen rapidly but in a slower, more evolutionary process.

- The Social Resource Theory has been used to study the context of personal and social resources in societal assumptions and connections, including the role of the resources in social interactions and structure.

- Justice as Fairness Theory is based on two parties competing for resources. It is based on two principles of distributive justice: the liberty principle and the difference principle.

- Madeleine Leininger's Cultural Care Diversity and Universality Theory asserts cultural assessment is an essential component of nursing care planning. She proposed the Sunrise Model to depict imporant cultural factors to assess.

- The Giger and Davidhizar's Transcultural Assessment Model includes six phenomena to describe culture: communication, time, space, social organization, environmental control, and biological variations. They define cultural competence as a continuous process more developed and in-depth than mere knowledge of the culture.

- Andrews and Boyle's primary focus was to establish a useful framework for application in diverse settings. Their model involves promoting transcultural knowledge in the nursing care of individuals, families, groups, communities, and institutions across the life span.

- Cultural competence is described by Purnell as a conscious and dynamic process of modifying care to meet the cultural needs and desires of the patient.

- Spector's Health Traditions Model identifies five steps in the ongoing development toward cultural competency: personal heritage; the heritage of others; health; health beliefs and practices; modern health care culture and system; and traditional health care systems.

- The Health Inequalities Imagination Model describes six basic constructs: equalities awareness, cultural knowledge, cultural encounter, equalities skills, equalities analysis, and equalities action.

- The Papadopoulos, Tilki, and Taylor Model for Developing Cultural Competence describes cultural competence as a continual developmental process that is evolutionary and changes through interactions, learning, and context. The model includes four stages: cultural awareness, cultural knowledge, cultural sensitivity, and cultural competence.

- Jeffreys's CCC Model describes cultural competence as a minimal requirement of practice. Optimal cultural competence for health care providers is achieved through a seven-step approach: self-assessment, active promotion, systemic inquiry, decisive action, innovation, measurement, and evaluation.

- Ramsden's Cultural Safety Model highlights the process of caring for those who are deemed foreign in a homogenous society. The inequality in power and resources, as well as the lack of knowledge of the foreign culture, ultimately leads to unsafe health care practices.

- The Culturally Responsive Healthcare Model is based on experiences with Hmong patients.

- The Explanatory Model allows the health care provider to incorporate patient-specific cultural and social beliefs into the care plan.

REFERENCES

Abbasi, A., Wigand, R., & Hossain, L. (2014). Measuring social capital through network analysis and its influence on individual performance. *Library & Information Science Research, 36*(1), 66–73.

Andrews, M. M., & Boyle, J. S. (2016). *Transcultural concepts in nursing care.* Philadelphia, PA: Wolters Kluwer Health/Lippincott Williams & Wilkins.

Australian Quality Council. (n.d.). Cultural imprints. Retrieved from http://wiki.tafensw.edu .au/ sydney/myleadership/images/c/ce/Cultural_Imprints.pdf

Culhane-Pera, K. A., Vawter, D. E., Xiong, P., Babbit, B., & Solberg, M. M. (2003). *Healing by heart: Clinical and ethical case stories of Hmong families and Western providers.* Nashville, TN: Vanderbilt University Press.

Eggenberger, S. K., Grassley, J., & Restrepo, E. (2006). Culturally competent nursing care: Listening to the voices of Mexican-American women. *Online Journal of Issues in Nursing, 11*(3), 7. doi:10.3912/OJIN.Vol11No03PPT01

Fadiman, A. (2012). *The spirit catches you and you fall down: A Hmong child, her American doctors, and the collision of two cultures*. New York, NY: Farrar, Straus, and Giroux.

Giger, J. N., & Davidhizar, R. (2002). The Giger and Davidhizar Transcultural Assessment Model. *Journal of Transcultural Nursing, 13*(3), 185–188; discussion 200.

Hart, A., Hall, V., & Henwood, F. (2003). Helping health and social care professionals to develop an 'inequalities imagination': A model for use in education and practice. *Journal of Advanced Nursing, 41*(5), 480–489.

Jeffreys, M. R. (2016). *Teaching cultural competence in nursing and health care: Inquiry, action, and innovation* (3rd ed.). New York, NY: Springer Publishing.

Kleinman, A. (1976). Culture, illness, and care: Clinical lessons from anthropologic and cross-cultural research. *Annals of Internal Medicine, 88*(2), 251–258.

Kwon, S., & Adler, P. (2014). Social capital: Maturation of a field of research. *Academy of Management Review, 39*(4), 412–422.

Leininger, M. (1991). *Culture care diversity and universality: A theory of nursing*. New York, NY: National League for Nursing.

Leininger, M. (2002). Culture care theory: A major contribution to advance transcultural nursing knowledge and practices. *Journal of Transcultural Nursing, 13*(3), 189–192; discussion 200.

Lin, N. (1986). Conceptualizing social support. In N. Lin, A. Dean, & W. Ensel (Eds.), *Social support, life events, and depression* (pp. 17–30). New York, NY: Academic Press.

Lipson, J. G., & DeSantis, L. A. (2007). Current approaches to integrating elements of cultural competence in nursing education. *Journal of Transcultural Nursing, 18*(1 Suppl), 10S–20S; discussion 21S.

Papadopoulos, I., Tilki, M., & Taylor, G. (1998). *Transcultural care: A guide for healthcare professionals*. Wiltshire, UK: Quay Books.

Papps, E., & Ramsden, I. (1996). Cultural safety in nursing: The New Zealand experience. *International Journal for Quality in Health Care, 8*(5), 491–497.

Purnell, L. (2002). The Purnell Model for cultural competence. *Journal of Transcultural Nursing, 13*(3), 193–196; discussion 200.

Rawls, J. (1971). *A theory of justice*. Cambridge, MA: Belknap Press.

Spector, R. E. (2009). *Cultural diversity in health and illness* (7th ed.). Upper Saddle River, NJ: Pearson.

Spencer, H. (1896). *The principles of sociology*. New York, NY: Appleton.

Stryker, S., & Statham, A. (1985). Symbolic interaction and role theory. In G. Lindzey & E. Aronson (Eds.), *Handbook of social psychology* (Vol. 1, pp. 311–378). New York, NY: Random House.

Wallace, R., & Wolf, A. (2005). *Contemporary sociological theory: Expanding the classical tradition*. Upper Saddle River, NJ: Pearson.

Application of Frameworks to Nursing Roles

It is a beautiful thing when a career and a passion come together.
—Anonymous

Throughout the previous chapters, we have explored philosophies, models, theories, and taxonomies within conceptual categories that are relevant to nursing roles and research. We have noted the ways in which these frameworks are useful for nurse educators, clinicians, leaders, and researchers. In this part, we approach the application of frameworks to nursing roles from both micro- and macro-levels. On the micro-level, how nurses within each role use frameworks related to individuals and families, and to communities and organizations are discussed. On a macro-level, the use of frameworks for providing structure for each practice area and how each practice area uses these frameworks are examined.

Each of the four nursing roles (educator, clinician, leader, and researcher) are explored in separate chapters. However, we realize that there is overlap in these four roles. For example, nurse educators are often involved performing clinician functions when teaching students to provide clinical care and may engage in leadership responsibilities in managing and monitoring educational programs and curriculums. Educators may also engage in research as planners, developers, data collectors, and disseminators. Examination of the clinician, nurse leader, and researcher roles reveals similar overlap in functions depending on the nurse's responsibilities and work setting. While recognizing the overlap among nursing roles, we focus on ways that frameworks are used by nurses whose primary role is an educator, clinician, leader, or researcher and the ways each area of practice is supported by and uses frameworks.

Application of Frameworks to the Nurse Educator Role

Rose Utley

Teaching is the profession that creates all others.
—Author unknown

 KEY TERMS

Boyer's Model of Scholarship
competencies
criteria
faculty evaluation triad
standards

 LEARNING OBJECTIVES

1. Describe the history of the nurse educator roles and knowledge development in academic and professional development settings.

2. Explain how nurses in academic and professional development educator roles use frameworks focused on individuals and families.

3. Explain how nurses in academic and professional development educator roles use community and organizational-focused frameworks.

4. Explore the theoretical knowledge inherent in the competencies, standards, and criteria for academic and professional development nursing roles.

5. Recognize the theoretical knowledge inherent in the competencies, standards, and criteria for nursing program accreditation.

In this chapter, the importance of frameworks in establishing the foundational knowledge needed for academic nurse educators (ANEs) and nurse professional development educators (NPDE) is explored. In addition, the use of frameworks in the educator's scope and standards of practice and frameworks that underlie curriculum development and program accreditation in nursing education are discussed.

The importance of theoretical knowledge for the nurse educator role is explored on both the macro- and micro-levels. On a micro-level, the day-to-day use of frameworks in teaching is highlighted. The ways in which nurse educators use the frameworks related to individuals, families, communities, and organizations are examined. On the macro-level, the theoretical foundations of the competencies and standards for ANE and NPDE practices are explored, with competencies being defined as measurable or observable aspects related to knowledge, skills, attitudes, and behaviors critical to successful job performance, and *standards* being the norms or expected levels of attainment. In areas of specialty practice, the nurse's performance as an ANE or NPDE is guided by standards and competencies that identify the knowledge, skills, and qualifications needed to function in the specialization. The scope and standards of practice for the ANE (National League for Nursing Certification Commission: Certification Test Development Committee, 2012) and the NPDE (National Nursing Staff Development Organization [NNSDO] & American Nurses Association [ANA], 2010) have been delineated. These documents outline the standards or level of quality expected in ANE an NPDE practice and integrate a variety of frameworks. Also at the macro-level, the importance of frameworks that support program accreditation criteria and curricular initiatives for baccalaureate and graduate education programs is explored.

◉ HISTORY OF THE ANE ROLE

In 1872, the first school of nursing was developed in the United States (American Association for the History of Nursing, 2007). Nurse educators in these aspiring programs were often recent graduates themselves and were charged with overseeing the care provided by students. They held no advanced educational preparation. The expectation was for students to provide service to the hospitals and, in turn, students gained knowledge through providing direct care.

Medical progress in the early to mid-1900s provided an impetus for nurses to value research and advance their education. During this time, antibiotics were discovered, new surgical techniques were being performed, and immunizations and other therapies were gaining more widespread use. These events and others shifted the knowledge base required in nursing. Coupled with the increased demand for nurses created by World War I (WWI) and later World War II (WWII), there was the impetus to advance nursing education from hospital- to university-based programs. By 1950, the National League for Nursing Education had become a strong voice for nurse educators and all levels of nursing programs.

With the advancement in the education of nursing instructors and the movement to university-level education came the additional expectations of scholarship in the form of research and the performance of university service. Today, the emphasis on teaching, research, and service, known as the *faculty evaluation triad*, forms the basis for academic nursing practice as we know it today (Utley, 2011).

Boyer's Model of Scholarship

In 1990, Boyer further popularized the faculty evaluation triad of teaching, scholarship, and service by expanding the notion of scholarship. Originally conceived as solely the endeavor of researchers, Boyer initially conceptualized scholarship as having four components: (a) discovery, (b) integration, (c) application, and (d) teaching. Later, a fifth type of scholarship was added called the scholarship of *engagement*. The academic educator role incorporates one or more of Boyer's types of scholarship, depending on the type of institution, the educator's rank, and length of tenure. Each type of scholarship is described in the following section.

The *scholarship of discovery* is equated with traditional research and involves all phases of original research from planning, data collection, data analysis, and dissemination. The *scholarship of integration* involves interpreting the findings of research within a broad context beyond a single specialty or discipline and, making connections across disciplines. Those engaged in the scholarship of integration focus on understanding by asking: What does this mean? The *scholarship of application* is aligned with "doing" and "being" engaged. It encompasses applying knowledge derived from research to solve problems. In academic nursing, this has been equated with applying current evidence-based practices (EBP) into the nurse's clinical and teaching practice. Other ways to demonstrate the scholarship of application are by participating in scholarly service activities in which research knowledge is used, such as a member of editorial boards or grant review teams. The fourth type of scholarship, referred to as the *scholarship of teaching*, recognizes the importance of knowledge and conveying that knowledge readily to others. The scholarship of teaching requires the teacher to update knowledge of pedagogy (i.e., the science of teaching), as well as knowledge of specific subject matter. The teacher is engaged in learning and shares his or her understanding and enthusiasm for knowledge with students. Regarding the *scholarship of engagement*, Boyer noted, "The academy must become a more vigorous partner in the search for answers to our most pressing social, civic, economic, and moral problems" (Boyer, 1996, p. 13). Engagement has since been defined as a type of scholarship that integrates the other four types and involves the academic community in reciprocal civic initiatives with the broader community to enhance knowledge and understanding (Barker, 2004).

ANE Competencies and Certification

With nursing faculty fully entrenched in academia, the National League for Nursing (NLN) developed the first national certification examination for ANEs in 2005 along with the scope of practice for ANEs (NLN, 2005). The second edition of the scope of practice document incorporated the results of a nurse educator practice analysis, to modify the job-related responsibilities of the ANE role (NLN, 2012). The certification exam validates the educator's knowledge in eight competencies that encompass the scope of practice for ANEs. These include four competencies directly related to teaching activities: (a) facilitate learning, (b) facilitate learner development and socialization, (c) use assessment and evaluation strategies, and (d) develop and evaluate curriculum and programs. The four remaining competencies facilitate and enhance the educators teaching and role development. These are: (a) be a change agent and leader, (b) engage in continual quality improvement in teaching, (c) engage in scholarship, and (d) function in the academic setting. Each of these competencies is based on theory and research (Halstead, 2007; Utley, 2011). The underlying theory related to each competency is highlighted in the following.

The first competency, *facilitate learning*, is the core of the ANE's teaching practice (NLN, 2005, 2012). It is grounded in educational and learning theories, many of which were discussed in Chapter 7. To facilitate learning, the ANE relies on assessing the learner's needs, assessing the influence of cultural, gender, age, and experience on learning, and using and teaching learners to use reflective and critical thinking skills. The ANE uses a wide range of educational and learning models, taxonomies, and philosophies, to assess the learners and their environment and implement effective teaching strategies. These strategies will vary depending upon the attributes of the students (e.g., age, experience, gender, culture, and motivation), the type of nursing program (practical, associate, baccalaureate, graduate), the learning environment (online, hybrid, or face to face), and the focus of the content.

The second competency involves *facilitating the learner's development and socialization* into the nursing role (NLN, 2005, 2012). The ANE's focus is on facilitating the student's development in all domains of learning, including cognitive, psychomotor, and affective. To accomplish this, learning styles; teaching styles; taxonomies for cognitive, affective, and psychomotor learning (Chapter 7); communication (Chapter 18); and behavioral change (Chapter 4) are used.

I like to think that I continuously strive to clarify for myself my own philosophy of nursing. I think evolution of beliefs occurs due to experience and education.
— Victoria L. Curtis, BSN, RN

Knowledge and skill in *using assessment and evaluation strategies* are essential for meeting competency three. Assessment of learning outcomes is based on established learning objectives that use one or more of the three learning domains. For cognitive learning, Bloom's original cognitive taxonomy (Bloom, Engelhart, Furst, Hill, & Krathwohl, 1956) or the revised cognitive taxonomy by Krathwohl (2002) can be used. Learning outcomes for the affective domain can be developed using Krathwohl, Bloom, and Masia's affective taxonomy (1973), whereas Dave's (1970), Harrow's (1972), or Simpson's (1972) psychomotor taxonomies can be used for establishing psychomotor learning objectives. Another component of this competency is the design and development of tools for assessing and evaluating student learning. Evaluation tools are often grounded in learning frameworks such as cognitivism, constructivism, and humanism, among others (Chapter 7).

In the fourth competency, the ANE is involved in *curriculum design and evaluation of program outcomes* (NLN, 2005, 2012). Similar to the objectives for student learning, curriculum outcomes may be categorized, leveled, and evaluated using cognitive, affective, and psychomotor domain taxonomies described earlier. In addition, the ANE may use evaluation frameworks for collecting assessment and evaluation data on program outcomes. The curriculum design of a nursing program may be guided by learning methods such as andragogy, experiential learning, humanism, social learning theory, or by a specific nursing theory such as Orem's self-care or Watson's carative processes.

Sources of data for curriculum and program evaluation are obtained through formative and summative feedback as discussed in Chapter 19. The type and level of evaluation feedback can be guided by Kirkpatrick's Four-Level Evaluation Model, which identifies progressively higher and more objective levels of student evaluation (Chapter 19). The educator may also use program assessment models such as Pross's Promoting Excellence in Nursing Education Model or the Context, Input, Process, Product (CIPP) model to guide the overall assessment and evaluation processes of a curriculum or program change (Chapter 19). When curriculum or program revisions are needed, change can be used on a micro- or personal level to guide the change process (Chapter 4) and on a macro-level to guide organizational and systems-level change (Chapters 17 and 18). Change can be used to identify individual and organizational resources, barriers, and processes as well as guide the application of specific change strategies.

Competency five acknowledges the ANE's involvement as a *change agent and leader* in the educational process (NLN, 2005, 2012). Depending on the educator's experience, educational preparation, and academic rank, the nature and scope of change and leadership activities will vary. Development of skills as a change agent and leader in the educational setting can be enhanced by awareness and knowledge of behavioral change frameworks (Chapter 4) as well as system-level change frameworks discussed in Chapter 18. General Systems Theory, Critical Systems Thinking, Complex Adaptive Systems, and Organizational Systems are discussed in Chapter 17. Leadership frameworks relevant to organizational systems as described in Chapter 18 can guide the educator in meeting the demands of leadership within the academic community and professional organizations.

Engaging in *continuous quality improvement* is the focus of competency six (NLN, 2005, 2012). This competency involves personal improvement in the ANE role and quality improvement of the academic program. Specific actions may include designing and implementing educational policies and procedures grounded in ethical principles (Chapter 8) and assuming a mentoring role and applying mentoring concepts (Chapter 18). Assessment and evaluation activities needed for continuous quality improvement can be guided by evaluation frameworks such as Donabedian's Structure, Process, and Outcome Model and the CIPP Model presented in Chapter 19.

The ANE's *engagement in scholarship,* as noted in the seventh competency, is essential to the role of the ANE and for quality improvement. Many academic institutions use Boyer's

Model of Scholarship as a framework for evaluating the ANE's role performance. As previously noted, Boyer identified five types of scholarship as the scholarship of discovery, application, integration, teaching and learning, and engagement. As Boyer (1990) pointed out, teaching is a scholarly activity. The ANE demonstrates the scholarship of teaching by sharing and disseminating knowledge with students. Therefore, nurse educators have opportunities in either clinical or classroom instruction to demonstrate the scholarship of teaching. When the scholarship of teaching is combined with the other scholarship categories, a useful framework for developing scholarship is formed, which can be modified to fit each teacher's expertise and the needs of the institution. The type and intensity of scholarship activities engaged in will vary depending on the ANE's duties, rank, educational preparation, type of academic program, and institutional expectations regarding scholarship.

The final ANE competency is to *function within the educational environment* (NLN, 2005, 2012). This competency relies on knowledge of the social, political, economic, and institutional forces that influence nursing education and the institution's functioning. Understanding the organization's mission, philosophy, values, and leadership practices facilitates effective functioning in the educational environment. Understanding theories, philosophies, and models related to role theory (Chapter 14), organizational systems (Chapter 17), and systems leadership (Chapter 18) can be useful for framing and sensitizing the ANE's perspectives and guiding the ANE's interaction within the academic community.

HISTORY OF THE NPDE ROLE

The NPDE role was formalized with the publication of the *Nursing Professional Development: Scope and Standards of Practice* (ANA, 2010). Before the development of the NPDE role, several national initiatives motivated the development of the nurse's teaching role in providing patient care. One initiative was the Patient's Bill of Rights adopted by the American Hospital Association (AHA) in 1973 that ensured patients would receive understandable information about their medical diagnosis, treatment, and prognosis. The patients rights were later modified and renamed the patient care partnership (AHA, 2003). Later, the Pew Health Professions Commission published recommendations that affected the nurse's role in health education (1995 and 1998). The majority of the Pew recommendations concerned the provision of patient and staff education by nurses.

After the formalization of the NPDE role, other national initiatives highlighted the need for the continual professional development of nurses. In 2006, a campaign to reduce the incidence of medical errors was implemented. The initiative called the 5 Million Lives Campaign, relied heavily on patient and family education to reduce patient injury and risk (McCannon, Hackbarth, & Griffin, 2007). The Patient Care Partnership document mentioned earlier, identifies six attributes patients should expect in their hospital care (AHA, 2003). Two of these expectations (i.e., involvement in care and preparing for discharge) integrate the importance of the patient having sufficient knowledge of care and treatment options while in the hospital and upon discharge. To meet these expectations, patient education efforts by staff nurses and NPDEs received more attention.

Initially, the educational focus of the NPDE was to provide disease-oriented patient education. Eventually, this shifted to emphasizing prevention-focused education and finally to health-focused education (Grueninger, 1995). Today the charge of the NPDE is to provide professional education, development, and role socialization of nurses and other health care professionals within a health care agency (NNSDO & ANA, 2010). The training provided by the NPDE focuses on the delivery of safe, quality, and evidence-based care.

To prepare nurses and others to educate patients and family members, the NPDE utilizes a train-the-trainer approach. This approach has resulted in a change from simply giving information for disease and prevention-oriented education to emphasizing personal change and empowerment in providing health-oriented education. Over the years, the NPDE role has evolved to incorporate informatics, educational technology, EBPs, interprofessional education, and collaboration. The NPDE's involvement as a mentor, change agent, leader, and collaborator relies on integrating technology, EBP, and interprofessional education.

NPDE Scope and Standards

The 2010 *Nursing Professional Development: Scope and Standards of Practice* is based on a systems model with inputs, throughputs, outputs, and a feedback loop structure (NNSDO & ANA, 2010). The inputs include the learner and the NPDE. The throughputs comprise seven development and educational processes that contribute to the professional growth of practicing nurses and other learners. Throughputs directly related to the NPDE's teaching involve (a) providing orientation to the work setting, (b) developing, facilitating, coordinating, and conducting competency programs, (c) providing in-service education, and (d) developing, implementing, coordinating, and evaluating professional continuing education activities. The remaining three processes focus on supportive activities for the learners and the NPDE. These are: (a) career development and role transition activities, (b) research and scholarship, and (c) participation in academic partnerships between nursing schools and health care facilities.

The seven development and education processes rely on complementary concepts of EBP and practice-based evidence (PBE) that provide additional throughputs into the NPDE practice model. EBP is the application of "scientific knowledge such as research, scientific principles, and theory related to educational methods and practice" (NNSDO & ANA, 2010, p. 5). The goal of PBE is to determine the most effective practice for day-to-day use within a specific context or group. The use of EBP and PBE relies on understanding human development (Chapter 6), learning (Chapter 7), evaluation processes (Chapter 19), culture influences (Chapter 20), and roles (Chapter 14).

Knowledge of behavioral change (Chapter 4), organizational change (Chapter 17), and leadership (Chapter 18) assists the educator in carrying out the role functions of the NPDE. Also, depending upon the work setting, the NPDE may teach staff about nursing care practices using care and caring frameworks (Chapter 5), health and illness frameworks (Chapter 9), interpersonal relationships (Chapter 10), human needs (Chapter 11), and cultural competence and preferences (Chapter 20).

The system outputs section of the NPDE practice model identifies three outcomes of practice: (a) change, (b) learning, and (c) professional role competence and growth. The NPDE pursues professional role competence and growth on a personal level by seeking certification as an NPDE and by promoting clinical certification and continued growth of the health care staff. These outcomes protect the public, help ensure the quality of care, and provide feedback that impacts the input and throughput sections of the model.

With knowledge comes understanding, and with understanding comes growth.
—Sue Hudson, BSN, RN

NPDE Core Competencies

The NPDE specialty is based on four core competencies: (a) career development, (b) education, (c) leadership, and (d) program and project management. Each of these competencies relies on clusters of theoretical knowledge. The *career development competency* incorporates theoretical knowledge of interpersonal relationships (Chapter 10) and communication (Chapter 18). The *education competency* involves "applying nursing and learning theoretical and conceptual foundations as a basis for developing NPDE program" (NNSDO & ANA,

2010, p. 14). It also involves assessing learning styles and the needs of diverse learners (Chapter 7) and applying evaluation frameworks to determine program outcomes (Chapter 19). The *leadership competency* involves using philosophies and models to support ethical decision-making (Chapter 8), facilitating group processes by applying principles of group dynamics (Chapter 10), functioning as a change agent (Chapter 4), functioning as a leader (Chapter 18), and using outcome evaluation methods (Chapter 19). The final NPDE *competency of program and project management* uses knowledge of program planning and evaluation frameworks (Chapter 18) and incorporates budgetary principles (Chapter 15) to achieve successful program implementation.

APPLICATION OF FRAMEWORKS TO TEACHING PRACTICE

Both the ANE and NPDE will find the frameworks in Part II and Part III relevant to teaching practice. The ANE is responsible for teaching content related to these conceptual areas in undergraduate and graduate nursing curriculums and uses learning frameworks when teaching the content. Similarly, the NPDE may teach content related to these conceptual areas and use theoretical knowledge of learning processes, learning styles, when educating staff.

Content areas relevant to and emphasized in nursing education include (but are not limited to) the conceptual areas covered in Part II that focus on frameworks relevant to individuals and families. The ANE and NPDE may also use the teaching strategies and ideas presented in Chapter 2 to convey the importance of using theory to diverse learners. Knowledge of the community and organizational aspects covered in Part III is useful when working with educational and health care organizations or when initiating change or interventions on a broader scale, within communities, populations, and systems. In addition, both the ANE and NPDE may serve as mentors and thus find mentoring frameworks discussed in Chapter 18 helpful in guiding those relationships.

Frameworks Underlying Nursing Education Programs

The settings and organizational systems in which nurses provide care and teach have grown in complexity. In the U.S. health care system, the patient population has diversified, with patients' illnesses and health care needs increasing in number, intensity, and complexity (National Center for Health Statistics, 2017; Taylor & Morrison, 2011). The use of technology to assess, diagnose, treat, communicate, and document health care has proliferated. The number of medical specialties has expanded while the scope of these specialized providers has constricted, resulting in fragmented care. Health care systems, pharmaceutical companies, and medical insurance systems have formed complex interconnections and interdependencies. In teaching, this increased complexity is seen in the number of college degrees, the diversity of course offerings, the expanded use of educational technology, and high-stake testing. Combined, these complexities in health care and education require enhanced awareness, understanding, and sensitivity of the educator. This can be facilitated by gaining a broad awareness and understanding of diverse theoretical perspectives from multiple disciplines.

Nursing program accreditation agencies value the broad educational preparation of nurses as reflected in accreditation criteria. Knowledge of the arts and sciences is viewed as necessary to prepare nurses for care delivery. The NLN through the Accreditation Commission for Education in Nursing (ACEN) and the American Association of Colleges of Nursing (AACN, 2008) have outlined curriculum standards or essentials for nursing programs.

In the following section, the linkage between theoretical knowledge and professional standards, competencies, and curricular initiatives is explained. The expectations for nursing knowledge that underlie the standards and competencies of accrediting agencies are identified, beginning with frameworks for nursing program standards and concluding with frameworks for content-focused curriculum initiatives.

Frameworks Underlying Nursing Program Accreditation

The ACEN and the Commission on Collegiate Nursing Education (CCNE) are the primary accreditation agencies for nursing education programs. ACEN accredits all levels of programs from licensed practical nursing through the doctoral level, whereas CCNE accredits baccalaureate through doctoral-level programs only. Each agency has established standards and *criteria* (i.e., standards, guidelines, or expectations essential to judge the quality of nursing programs). In this section, the standards and criteria that rely on frameworks discussed in this text are identified.

A variety of frameworks covered in previous chapters support the standards for ACEN accreditation as outlined in Table 21.1. ACEN (2016) identifies six standards for all levels of educational programs followed by specific criteria for meeting each standard. The six standards for all educational programs focus on the (a) mission and administrative capacity, (b) faculty and staff, (c) students, (d) curriculum, (e) resources, and (f) outcomes. Many of the criteria specified in the curriculum standards rely on knowledge within the chapters of Part II and Part III .

Similarly, the CCNE has established accreditation standards and criteria for baccalaureate, master's, and doctoral programs (CCNE, 2013). CCNE groups the standards into three categories that are focused on program quality: (a) mission and governance, (b) institutional commitment and resources, and (c) curriculum and teaching-learning practices. A fourth standard titled "assessment and achievement of program outcomes" is focused on program effectiveness. The CCNE standards list "elements" of each standard, with elements being similar to criteria. The standards and corresponding framework chapters are highlighted in Table 21.2

Frameworks Important to Curricular Initiatives

Content in nursing curriculums is influenced by social, cultural, and health care expectations, accreditation bodies, and by professional nursing practice organizations. Several curricular initiatives and guidelines that are content specific have been developed and promoted by professional organizations. These content areas include genetics, geriatrics, quality and safety, and cultural competency. Many nursing education programs have incorporated content in these areas to enhance program quality and meet emerging demands.

Efforts to enhance knowledge and skills in genetics clinical nursing practice are supported by the ANA and the International Society of Nursing in Genetics (ISONG). In 1998, ISONG and the ANA published the first scope of practice for this specialty titled, *Statement on the Scope and Standards of Genetics Clinical Nursing Practice*, which encouraged the integration of basic genetic nursing knowledge into nursing programs. Then in 2016, the second edition of *Genetics/Genomics Nursing: Scope and Standards of Practice* was published by the ANA and ISONG. They identified six standards that followed the nursing process framework. Nurses need to be able to counsel and provide genetics-related health promotion and education that is sensitive to the patient's sociocultural values. Also included are standards of performance in ethics, education, evidence-based practice and research, quality of practice, communication, leadership, and collaboration, each of which is supported by a variety of frameworks covered in this text.

Another curricular initiative involves providing quality palliative care. In 1998, the AACN published competencies for care at the end of life (EOL; AACN, "Peaceful Death," 1998). Sixteen competencies were identified that reflected not only knowledge and skills needed to provide direct care but also broad personal attitudes and critical thinking (Table 21.3). Based on these competencies, the End-of-Life Nursing Education Consortium (EOLNEC) established an educational program to improve palliative care using a train-the-trainer approach. As a result, ANEs, staff development nurses, and clinical nurses from a variety of specialties received education in EOL care that they then passed on to others. Based on AACN's competencies, a set of nine core content areas was developed (see Table 21.3 for the content areas and related framework chapters).

TABLE 21.1 ACEN Accreditation Standards and Relevant Frameworks

Program Type	ACEN Standard[b]	Related Frameworks
Licensed Practical Nurse (LPN), Associate Degree (AD), Diploma, Baccalaureate, Masters, Doctoral[a]	2.4 and 2.8 Precept and mentor faculty and student in their role	Chapter 14: Role-Related Frameworks; Chapter 17: Organizational System Frameworks (Mentoring)
All[a]	2.9 Faculty evaluation	Chapter 19: Frameworks for Evaluation (Kirkpatrick's Four-Level Evaluation, Boyer's Model)
All[a]	4. 1 Curriculum competencies and learning outcomes	Chapter 7: Frameworks for Teaching and Learning (learning domain taxonomies)
LPN, Diploma, ADN, Baccalaureate	4.4 General education courses and concepts that enhance nursing knowledge and practice	Chapters in Parts II, III, and IV
MSN	4.4 Preparation for direct and indirect nursing roles	Chapters in Parts II, III, and IV
Doctoral	4.4 Nursing practice from an EBP perspective	Chapters in Parts I and IV
All[a]	4.5 Ethnic and social diversity concepts	Chapter 16: Community and Population Health Frameworks; Chapter 20: Sociocultural Frameworks
All[a]	4.6 Educational theory, interprofessional collaboration, and research	Chapter 3: Relationship Among Theory, Research, and Practice; Chapter 7: Frameworks for Teaching and Learning; Chapter 17: Organizational System Frameworks; Chapter 24: Application of Frameworks to the Nurse Researcher Role
All[a]	4.7 Diverse evaluation methods are used	Chapter 19: Frameworks for Evaluation
All[a]	4.11 Learning activities, materials, and evaluation strategies are appropriate	Chapter 7: Frameworks for Teaching and Learning; Chapter 19: Frameworks for Evaluation
All[a]	5.1 and 5.4 Fiscal resources are sufficient and sustainable	Chapter 15: Economic Frameworks
All[a]	6.1 Achievement of end of program outcomes	Chapter 7: Frameworks for Teaching and Learning; Chapter 19: Frameworks for Evaluation

ACEN, Accreditation Commission for Education in Nursing.

[a,b]*Source*: Accrediting Commission for Education in Nursing (2016).

TABLE 21.2 AACN End-of-Life Competencies and Related Framework Chapters

	Competency[a]	Related Framework Chapters
1	Recognize factors supporting the need for improved EOL care	Chapter 15: Economic Frameworks; Chapter 16: Community and Population Health Frameworks; Chapter 17: Organizational System Frameworks; and Chapter 20: Sociocultural Frameworks
2	Promote importance of comfort care	Chapter 5: Care and Caring Frameworks; and Chapter 11: Needs-Based Frameworks
3	Effective interpersonal communication	Chapter 10: Interpersonal and Family Frameworks; Chapter 13: Psychological Frameworks; and Chapter 14: Role-Related Frameworks
4	Awareness of attitudes, values, beliefs, and cultural diversity related to EOL customs	Chapter 8: Moral and Ethical Perspectives; Chapter 9: Health and Illness Frameworks; and Chapter 20: Sociocultural Frameworks
5	Respect patient views and wishes	Chapter 5: Care and Caring Frameworks; Chapter 8: Moral and Ethical Perspectives; and Chapter 11: Needs-Based Frameworks
6	Interdisciplinary collaboration	Chapter 10: Interpersonal and Family Frameworks; and Chapter 18: Leadership Frameworks for Organizational Systems
7	Use evidence-based assessment tools	Chapter 22: Application of Frameworks to the Clinician Role
8	Use assessment data to plan care and intervene	Chapter 9: Health and Illness Frameworks; and Chapter 11: Needs-Based Frameworks
9	Evaluate impact of interventions	Chapter 11: Needs-Based Frameworks; Chapter 24: Application of Frameworks to the Nurse Researcher Role
10	Provide holistic, multidimensional care	Chapter 5: Care and Caring Frameworks; Chapter 9: Health and Illness Frameworks; Chapter 10: Interpersonal and Family Frameworks; Chapter 11: Needs-Based Frameworks; Chapter 12: Physiological Frameworks; Chapter 13: Psychological Frameworks; and Chapter 20: Sociocultural Frameworks
11	Facilitate coping of self and others with EOL experiences	Chapter 5: Care and Caring Frameworks; Chapter 8: Moral and Ethical Perspectives; Chapter 10: Interpersonal and Family Frameworks; Chapter 13: Psychological Frameworks; and Chapter 14: Role-Related Frameworks
12	Apply legal and ethical principles	Chapter 8: Moral and Ethical Perspectives
13	Identify barriers and facilitators to use of resources	Chapter 4: Frameworks for Behavioral Change; Chapter 11: Needs-Based Frameworks; Chapter 15: Economic Frameworks; Chapter 16: Community and Population Health Frameworks; Chapter 17: Organizational Systems Frameworks; and Chapter 20: Sociocultural Frameworks

(continued)

TABLE 21.2 AACN End-of-Life Competencies and Related Framework Chapters (*continued*)

	Competency[a]	Related Framework Chapters
14	Skill implementing EOL care	Chapter 4: Frameworks for Behavioral Change; Chapter 5: Care and Caring Frameworks; Chapter 7: Frameworks for Teaching and Learning; and Chapter 11: Needs-Based Frameworks
15	Apply EBP to EOL care and education	Chapter 7: Frameworks for Teaching and Learning; and Chapter 22: Application of Frameworks to the Clinician Role

AACN, American Association of Colleges of Nursing; EBP, evidence-based practices; EOL, end of life.
[a]*Source*: American Association of Colleges of Nursing (1998).

TABLE 21.3 AACN Baccalaureate Essentials and Relevant Frameworks

Essential #	Essential Title[a]	Related Theoretical Content
I	Liberal Education (science and arts)	Chapters in Part II (Frameworks for Individuals and Families) and Part III (Frameworks for Community and Organizations)
II	Organizational and Systems Leadership for Quality	Chapter 15: Economic Frameworks; Chapter 17: Organizational System Frameworks; Chapter 18: Leadership Frameworks for Organizational Systems; and Chapter 19: Frameworks for Evaluation
III	Scholarship for Evidence-Based Practice	Chapters 3: Relationship Among Theory, Research, and Practice; Chapter 8: Moral and Ethical Perspectives; Chapter 19: Frameworks for Evaluation; and Chapter 24: Application of Frameworks to the Nurse Researcher Role
IV	Information Management and Technology	Chapter 8: Moral and Ethical Perspectives; Chapter 17: Organizational System Frameworks; and Chapter 18: Frameworks for Evaluation
V	Health Care Policy, Finance, and Regulation	Chapter 8: Moral and Ethical Perspectives; Chapter 15: Economic Frameworks; Chapter 16: Community and Population Health Frameworks; Chapter 17: Organizational System Frameworks; and Chapter 20: Sociocultural Frameworks
VI	Interprofessional Communication and Collaboration	Chapter 5: Care and Caring Frameworks; Chapter 8: Moral and Ethical Perspectives; Chapter 10: Interpersonal and Family Frameworks; and Chapter 14: Role-Related Frameworks

(*continued*)

TABLE 21.3 AACN Baccalaureate Essentials and Relevant Frameworks *(continued)*		
Essential #	**Essential Title**[a]	**Related Theoretical Content**
VII	Prevention and Population Health	Chapter 7: Frameworks for Teaching and Learning; Chapter 8: Moral and Ethical Perspectives; Chapter 9: Health and Illness Frameworks; Chapter 11: Needs-Related Frameworks; Chapter 16: Community and Population Health Frameworks; and Chapter 20: Sociocultural Frameworks
VIII	Professionalism and Values	Chapters 5: Care and Caring Frameworks; Chapter 6: Human Development Frameworks; Chapter 8: Moral and Ethical Perspectives; and Chapters in Part IV: Application of Frameworks to Nursing Roles
IX	Generalist Nursing Practice (care for individuals, families, communities, populations throughout the life span)	All chapters in Part II: Individuals and Families; Chapters 16: Community and Population Health Frameworks; Chapter 20: Sociocultural Frameworks; and Chapter 22: Application of Frameworks to the Clinician Role

AACN, American Association of Colleges of Nursing.

[a]*Source*: American Association of Colleges of Nursing (2008).

Quality and Safety Education for Nurses Initiative (QSEN) was developed in 2005 to integrate quality and safety competencies into nursing education at the individual and system levels (Dolansky & Moore, 2013). Six competency areas were identified: (a) patient-centered care, (b) evidence-based care, (c) teamwork and collaboration, (d) safety, (e) quality improvement, and (f) informatics. At the individual level, students and nursing staff need to be aware of the individual's risks, needs, and physiological processes that could impact safety and quality of care. Knowledge of models related to health and illness (Chapter 9), human needs (Chapter 11), and physiological function (Chapter 13) support these areas of knowledge and competencies.

On a systems level, QSEN competencies require systems thinking, which is the "ability to recognize, understand, and synthesize the interactions and interdependencies" (Dolansky & Moore, 2013, p. 10). Although both individual and system-level thinking are needed, they note that "Greater knowledge and application of systems thinking skills by nurses have the potential to mitigate errors in practice, improve nurse priority setting and delegation, enhance problem solving and decision making, improve timing and quality of interactions with other professionals and patients, and enhance workplace quality improvement initiatives" (2013, p. 10). To facilitate system-level thinking, the chapters in Part III, which deal with community and organizational systems, would be useful. Especially relevant is Chapter 19, which covers evaluation and quality improvement models that facilitate understanding of system-level change and evaluation.

The need for geriatric-focused education in the nursing curriculum has been spearheaded by the AACN and the Hartford Institute for Geriatric Nursing. The *Recommended Baccalaureate Competencies and Curricular Guidelines for the Nursing Care of Older Adults* (2010) outlines competencies related to the nine AACN essentials. Specific content and teaching strategies that can be used for each competency are also identified. Many of the frameworks presented in this text provide content relevant to geriatrics, especially Chapters 6, 9, 11, and 20. Also, the teaching strategies identified in the competencies can be bolstered by many of the learning theories covered in Chapter 7.

Another initiative has been promoted by a joint task force of the American Academy of Nurses and the Transcultural Nursing Society to enhance cultural competency in nursing care. They have jointly produced a set of standards for cultural competence in nursing practice (Expert Panel on Global Nursing & Health, 2010). Competency eight specifically mandates that students and practicing nurses receive education and training in providing culturally competent care. Teaching nursing students about the sociocultural environment (Chapter 20) helps to sensitize the learner to culturally specific issues, needs, and approaches to providing nursing care. Knowledge of values and beliefs of diverse ethnic groups provides the nurse with the foundation needed to provide culturally sensitive care. Moral and ethical frameworks discussed in Chapter 8 can help guide the nurse's actions when cultural expectations between the patient and health care providers are not aligned.

The curricular initiatives discussed in this section highlight the changing knowledge base that nurses need for effective practice. Curricular content related to each initiative can be enhanced through greater awareness and appreciation of frameworks covered in Part II and Part III.

CONCLUSION

The frameworks used by nurse educators represent a wide array of theories, models, and taxonomies from diverse disciplines. Nurse educators use learning theories, as well as cognitive, affective, and psychomotor domain taxonomies in teaching and curriculum development (see Chapter 7). They also use evaluation frameworks such as Kirkpatrick's Four Levels of Evaluation, Competency, Outcomes, and Performance Assessment Model, or Value Added Models (see Chapter 19) to determine the achievement of learner and program outcomes. Teaching students, patients, and staff of diverse ages and cultural backgrounds is facilitated by understanding developmental (Chapter 6) and cultural factors (Chapter 20) that can help the nurse tailor the educational experiences to meet the learner's needs.

In addition to using frameworks to carry out teaching and curricular activities, ANEs are charged with teaching students content related to many of the framework categories covered in this text. Content related to care and caring, ethics, health, human needs, development, community and populations, leadership, research, and theory is recognized as valuable for nursing practice. Meeting the accreditation standards and criteria developed by the ANEC and CCNE validates the quality, cohesiveness, and comprehensive scope of the nursing program.

> *For much of my previous educational experiences in high school and college I felt like I was 'faking it to make it.' I really wanted to be interested in philosophies but I just couldn't get into them. Now that I have more experiences to apply them to I find them not only relevant but also useful and necessary.*
> —Lindsey Green, APRN-CNS, MN, RNC, CCNS

KEY POINTS

- ANEs may engage in action research to study their educational practices.
- NPDEs may engage in quality improvement initiatives that focus on improving health care outcomes.

- ANE's and NPDE's role performance is guided by standards and competencies that identify the knowledge, skills, and qualifications needed to function in the specialization.

- Teaching, research, and service, known as the *faculty evaluation triad*, form the basis for academic nursing practice.

- Boyer conceptualized research broadly as the scholarship of (a) discovery, (b) application, (c) integration, (d) teaching, and (e) engagement.

- The national certification examination for ANEs validates the educator's knowledge in eight competency areas.

- The NPDE is charged with training nurses and other health care providers to deliver safe, quality, and evidence-based care.

- The core complementary processes of evidence-based practice (EBP) and practice-based evidence (PBE) provide the foundation for the NPDE's scope of practice.

- The increased complexities in health care require enhanced awareness, understanding, and sensitivity that can be achieved by familiarity with diverse theoretical perspectives and understandings.

- The Accreditation Commission for Education in Nursing (ACEN) and the Commission on Collegiate Nursing Education (CCNE) are the major accreditation agencies for nursing education programs.

- The content emphasized in nursing curriculums is influenced by social, cultural, and health care expectations and those of professional health care organizations and accreditation bodies.

REFERENCES

Accrediting Commission for Education in Nursing. (2016). *Accreditation manual section III standards and criteria* (p. 51) Atlanta, GA: Author. Retrieved from http://www.acenursing.net/manuals/SC2017.pdf

American Association of Colleges of Nursing. (1998). *Peaceful death: Recommended competencies and curricular guidelines for end-of-life nursing care*. Washington, DC: Author. Retrieved from http://files.eric.ed.gov/fulltext/ED453706.pdf

American Association of Colleges of Nursing. (2008). *The essentials of baccalaureate education for professional nursing practice* (p. 63). Washington, DC: Author. Retrieved from http://www.aacnnursing.org/Portals/42/Publications/BaccEssentials08.pdf

American Association of Colleges of Nursing & the Hartford Institute for Geriatric Nursing. (2010). Recommended baccalaureate competencies and curricular guidelines for the nursing care of older adults. Retrieved from http://www.aacnnursing.org/Portals/42/AcademicNursing/CurriculumGuidelines/AACN-Gero-Competencies-2010.pdf

American Hospital Association. (2003). *The patient care partnership: Understanding expectations, rights and responsibilities*. Chicago, IL: Author. Retrieved from http://www.aha.org/content/00-10/pcp_english_030730.pdf

American Nurses Association. (2010). *Nursing professional development: Scope and standards of practice*. Silver Spring, MD: Author.

American Nurses Association & International Society of Nurses in Genetics. (2016). *Genetics/genomics nursing: Scope and standards of practice* (2nd ed.). Silver Spring, MD: Author.

Association for the History of Nursing. (2007). Nursing history calendar. Retrieved from http://www.aahn.org/nursinghistorycalendar.html

Barker, D. (2004). The scholarship of engagement: A taxonomy of five emerging practices. *Journal of Higher Education Outreach and Engagement, 9*(2), 123–137.

Bloom, B. S., Engelhart, M. D., Furst, E. J., Hill, W. H., & Krathwohl, D. R. (1956). *Taxonomy of educational objectives: The classification of educational goals, Handbook 1: Cognitive domain*. White Plains, NY: Longman.

Boyer, E. (1990). *Scholarship reconsidered: Priorities of the professoriate*. New York, NY: Jossey-Bass.

Boyer, E. (1996). The scholarship of engagement. *Journal of Public Service and Outreach, 1*(1), 11–20.

Commission on Collegiate Nursing Education. (2013). *Standards for accreditation of baccalaureate and graduate nursing programs*. Washington, DC: Author. Retrieved from http://www.aacn.nche.edu/ccne-accreditation/Standards-Amended-2013.pdf

Dave, R. H. (1970). Psychomotor levels in developing and writing behavioral objectives. In R. J. Armstrong (Ed.), *Developing and writing behavioral objectives* (pp. 20–21). Tucson, AZ: Educational Innovators Press.

Dolansky, M. A., & Moore, S. M. (2013, September 30). Quality and safety education for nurses (QSEN): The key is systems thinking. *The Online Journal of Issues in Nursing, 18*(3), Manuscript 1. doi:10.3912/OJIN.Vol18No03Man01

Expert Panel on Global Nursing & Health. (2010). *Standards of practice for culturally competent nursing care: Executive summary*. American Academy of Nurses & The Transcultural Nursing Society. Retrieved from http://www.tcns.org/files/Standards_of_Practice_for_Culturally_Compt_Nsg_Care-Revised_.pdf

Grueninger, U. J. (1995). Arterial hypertension: Lessons from patient education. *Patient Education and Counseling, 26*, 37–55. doi:10.1016/0738-3991(95)00750-T

Halstead, L. A. (2007). *Nurse educator competencies: Creating an evidence-based practice for nurse educators*. New York, NY: National League for Nursing.

Harrow, A. (1972). *A taxonomy of psychomotor domain: A guide for developing behavioral objectives*. New York, NY: David McKay.

International Society of Nurses in Genetics & American Nurses Association. (1998). *Statement on the scope and standards of genetics clinical nursing practice*. Washington, DC: American Nurses Association.

Krathwohl, D. R. (2002). A revision of Bloom's taxonomy: An overview. *Theory Into Practice, 41*(4), 212–218.

Krathwohl, D. R., Bloom, B. S., & Masia, B. B. (1973). *Taxonomy of educational objectives, the classification of educational goals. Handbook II: Affective domain*. New York, NY: David McKay.

McCannon, C. J., Hackbarth, A. D., & Griffin, F. A. (2007). Miles to go: An introduction to the 5 million lives campaign. *Joint Commission Journal on Quality and Patient Safety, 33*(8), 477–484.

National Center for Health Statistics. (2017). FastStats. Retrieved from https://www.cdc.gov/nchs/index.htm

National League for Nursing Certification Commission Certification Test Development Committee. (2012). *The scope of practice for academic nurse educators*. New York, NY: Author.

National League for Nursing, Certification Governance Committee. (2005). *The scope of practice for academic nurse educators*. New York, NY: Author.

National Nursing Staff Development Organization & American Nurses Association. (2010). *Nursing professional development: Scope and standards of practice*. Silver Spring, MD: Nursesbooks.org.

Pew Health Professions Commission. (1995). *Critical challenges: Revitalizing the health professions for the twenty-first century*. San Francisco: University of California, San Francisco Center for the Health Professions.

Pew Health Professions Commission. (1998). *Recreating health professional practice for a new century: The fourth report of the Pew Health Professions Commission, Center for Health Professions*. San Francisco: University of California.

Simpson, E. J. (1972). *The classification of educational objectives in the psychomotor domain*. Washington, DC: Gryphon House.

Taylor, H., & Morrison, I. (2011, Mar 24). The incredible and wasteful complexity of the US healthcare system. *The Health Care Blog*. Retrieved from http://thehealthcareblog.com/blog/2011/03/24/the-incredible-and-wasteful-complexity-of-the-us-healthcare-system

Utley, R. (2011). *Theory and research for academic nurse educators: Application to practice*. Sudbury, MA: Jones & Bartlett.

22

Application of Frameworks to the Clinician Role

Maria Kenneally and Rose Utley

He who loves practice without theory is like the sailor who boards a ship without a rudder and compass and never knows where he may cast.
—Leonardo Da Vinci

⬤ KEY TERMS

Funk's Model of Research Utilization
Iowa Model of Research-Based Practice
macro-level application
micro-level application
National Organization of Nurse Practitioner Faculties

Ottawa Model of Research Use
PICO process
Rempher's Translational Research Process
Rosswurm and Larrabee's Model of Evidence-Based Practice

standards of professional performance
standards of professional practice
Stetler's Model of Research Utilization
translational research

⬤ LEARNING OBJECTIVES

1. Describe and differentiate micro- and macro-level applications of frameworks in clinical practice.
2. Recognize the importance of frameworks used in micro- and macro-levels of clinical nursing practice.
3. Identify frameworks used by clinicians in the care of individuals, families, and communities.
4. Clarify how clinicians use frameworks at the organizational systems level.
5. Explain how the PICO process is used in evidence-based practice (EBP).
6. Compare models related to EBP and research utilization in terms of purpose and processes used.

In this chapter, we review how frameworks are applicable for clinical practice on a micro- and macro-level. On the *micro-level*, meaning day-to-day nursing practice, the use of frameworks in clinical practice is explored. How the frameworks discussed in this text can be used by clinicians providing care to individuals, families, and communities is highlighted, as well as the use of frameworks relevant to health care organizations and systems. Evidence-based practice (EBP) frameworks, which are useful in assisting the nurse in "doing" EBP are also examined. These EBP frameworks provide a guide for clinicians engaging in EBP, quality improvement, systems level change projects, and research in the workplace. On the macro-level, we look at how frameworks are reflected in professional clinical practice as a whole, specifically the *Nursing Scope and Standards of Practice* (American Nurses Association [ANA], 2015) and the standards for nursing programs developed by Commission on Collegiate Nursing Education (CCNE) and the National Organization of Nurse Practitioner Faculties (NONPF). These standards and corresponding competencies emphasize the content and underlying knowledge base within many of the frameworks explored in this text.

⊙ USE OF FRAMEWORKS IN CLINICAL PRACTICE

A major premise in this text is that the nurse's clinical practice benefits from awareness and knowledge of multiple frameworks (i.e., philosophies, models, theories, and taxonomies). These frameworks describe, explain, and predict phenomena pertinent to the patient, family, community, and health care setting. Frameworks provide perspectives that filter how the world is viewed and the nature of the observations made. A quote by Oliver Wendell Holmes, "Man's mind, once stretched by a new idea, never regains its original dimensions," conveys the impact that knowledge of frameworks can have on the individual clinician. Though the nurse's use of frameworks is not always intentional, the influence of certain frameworks is pervasive in day-to-day clinical practice referred to as *micro-level application*.

Another way frameworks influence the nurse's clinical practice is at the macro-level. *Macro-level application*, which occurs on a broader scale and influences nurses through professional expectations established in the *Nursing Scope and Standards of Practice* (ANA, 2015) and CCNE and NONPF nursing program guidelines. Both micro- and macro-level applications are important to the nurse's clinical practice regardless of specialization and to the development of the profession as a whole.

Micro-Level Uses of Frameworks in Clinical Practice

When taking care of patients, whether at the bedside, in a clinic, or in a group setting, the nurse is engaged in a continual process of generating and testing theoretical relationships. This process is demonstrated through the use of the nursing process for assessment, planning, implementing, and evaluating outcomes. Essentially, theory generation and testing occur whenever the nursing process is applied. Once the nurse assesses the patient and the care situation, data are synthesized, and a hypothesis or diagnosis about the patient's problem is generated.

As with the identification of pertinent assessment data, hypothesis generation, and the development of a plan of care, the selection of intervention strategies is affected by the nurse's awareness or scope of knowledge. Exposure to diverse theories that describe, explain, or predict phenomena of concern sensitizes the nurse to an array of concepts and variables to consider in the patient care context. When caring for a patient, the nurse mentally develops a relationship statement that links the patient problem with an intervention and the desired outcome, such as "Patient X is experiencing an increase in post-operative pain due to anxiety" (or lack of emotional support or inability to effectively use coping skills). Based on the relationship statement, interventions or actions that the nurse believes will help the situation are implemented and the effectiveness of the interventions evaluated. This describes the most basic form of theory generation and testing in nursing.

In nursing, approaches to dealing with a patient's problem are identified, interventions are implemented, and the effectiveness is evaluated. The theories used in this process can be applied individually, or in combination, depending on the situation or event. For example, when obtaining the patient's social history, the nurse may discover the patient is a smoker. The next question the nurse may ask is: "Have you ever considered quitting?" Based on the patient's response the nurse can determine the individual's readiness to change by applying Prochaska and DiClemente's Stages of Change Theory (see Chapter 4).

According to the Stages of Change Theory, there are five stages of readiness for implementing a change in behavior, and each stage can be identified by the client's statements or behaviors (Prochaska & DiClemente, 1983; see Table 22.1). The first stage, *precontemplation*, is characterized by a lack of awareness of the need for change, followed by the *contemplation* stage in which there is awareness of the need to change but also a lack of readiness to engage in change in the near future. After the contemplation stage is the *preparation* stage that describes the individual as preparing to take action stage, followed by the *action* or doing stage, and the *maintenance* of change stage. The nurse uses the theory by matching the patient's comments or behaviors to a specific stage of change. Knowledge of the patient's stage of change helps the nurse to focus on strategies and interventions relevant to that stage. In using the Stages of Change Theory, a range of lifestyle issues such as weight, exercise, or habit change may be effectively addressed.

Other frameworks commonly used by basic and advanced nurse clinicians are the Modeling and Role-Modeling Theory (MRM), Maslow's Hierarchy of Needs (Chapter 11), and Pender's Health Promotion Model (Chapter 9). The MRM Theory developed by Erickson, Tomlin, and Swain (2005) blends multiple theories that focus on common concerns in nursing including the patient's developmental level, basic needs, stress, and loss. Using the MRM Theory requires the nurse to build trust with the patient and build upon the client's strengths. The nurse promotes the patient's individualism and works with the patient to develop a plan of care that is conducive to the patient's needs.

Maslow's Hierarchy of Needs is another framework commonly used in nursing practice by both basic and advanced clinicians. The hierarchy provides a structure for prioritizing needs and understanding the patient's prioritization. Using the Hierarchy of Needs, the nurse views the patient holistically and incorporates the patient's basic needs for oxygen, food, water, and shelter with higher order needs of love and belonging, esteem, and self-actualization (Fontaine, 2009, p. 16). Before initiating patient education, the nurse considers whether the patient's basic needs have been met. If the basic needs have not been met, the patient may lack the energy, motivation, or mental focus needed during instruction. An example is found in comparing the treatment approach for a homeless and a non-homeless,

TABLE 22.1 Stages of Change Model	
Stage of Change	**Characteristics**
Pre-Contemplation	Prefers the status quo; not interested in change
Contemplation	Has thought about change; no plans to start the change process
Preparation	Knows a problem exists and is seeking information on how to make a change
Action	Practices new behavior for 3–6 months
Maintenance	The new behavior is now a normal part of life
Relapse	Returns to previous undesirable behavior

Source: Prochaska and DiClemente (1983).

middle-class adult newly diagnosed with diabetes. Diabetes education regarding diet commonly involves instruction about types of foods to consume to achieve better blood glucose control. For the non-homeless patient, this recommendation can be easily achieved, as the patient has financial resources as well as food storage and preparation resources. However, the homeless patient will have limited food choices and limited resources for purchasing, storing, and preparing recommended foods. Additional unmet needs in the homeless patient such as lack of shelter, lack of family support, lack of transportation, and inadequate hygiene place further limits on treatment options. These factors threaten the person's basic needs and inhibit the individual's ability to engage in safe and effective self-care practices.

> *Maslow's theory was one of the first theories I can say I truly understood. . . . I frequently see patients whose basic needs are not being met, and that obviously is their first priority. No amount of teaching is going to matter to them until their basic needs are met.*
> —Brian Wagoner, APRN, FNP-BC

Nola Pender's Health Promotion Model is also commonly used in clinical practice to facilitate healthy changes in lifestyle behaviors such as diet, exercise, and stress management. Nurses readily recognize that many chronic conditions are the direct result of lifestyle behaviors. Using Pender's model, the nurse assesses barriers to change and the client's beliefs about the need to change and provides strategies to address the issues identified.

Nurses also use a variety of frameworks related to communities and organizations in daily practice. Community and population health frameworks (Chapter 16) are beneficial not only for those working in the fields of community and public health but also for acute care nurses who prepare the patient for discharge. The nurse's awareness and perspective are expanded and heightened by the knowledge of community and population health frameworks. This knowledge alerts the nurse to broader health issues, risks, and influencing factors and places the patient's health in a broad and comprehensive context. Once these wide-ranging community/population health factors have been recognized and anticipated, the nurse can collaborate with the patient on strategies to deal with the pertinent issues affecting the patient's health.

Nurse clinicians also assume teaching and leadership functions within their clinical role. Nurse clinicians in leadership roles such as a mentor, charge nurse, or team leader benefit from understanding leadership styles (Chapter 18) and understanding organizational systems (Chapter 17). Clinicians also engage in the educator role when teaching patients, families, and other staff. Teaching individuals and families is facilitated by knowledge of human development (Chapter 6) and frameworks for teaching and learning discussed in Chapter 7. The clinician may also rely on knowledge of the processes inherent in group dynamics (Chapter 18) and moral and ethical frameworks (Chapter 8) when working as a team member or leader on professional committees and quality improvement projects. These frameworks provide description, explanation, and/or prediction about conceptual areas that are helpful as the nurse clinician assumes these additional role functions in education and leadership.

Micro-Level Use of EBP Frameworks

Another micro level application of frameworks is found in the use of research evidence in daily nursing practice. EBP is the incorporation of research into nursing care to improve patient outcomes (Academy of Medical-Surgical Nurses, 2014). To engage in EBP, the nurse asks a clinical question and reviews the research available. Through a review of evidence-based literature, the nurse determines if there is sufficient evidence to warrant implementation in the patient care setting.

The growing emphasis placed on quality care, safety, and cost containment in health care provides the impetus for EBP. The establishment of the American Nurses Credentialing

Center (ANCC) Pathway to Excellence and Magnet Recognition® Programs acknowledges health care organizations and long-term care institutions for positive practice environments where nurses excel and use best practices (ANCC, 2016). Hospitals that have achieved Magnet Recognition have incorporated a professional practice model (ANCC, 2016) that provides a framework for providing nursing excellence throughout the health system (Hoffart & Woods, 1996). Thus, for Magnet status, theory drives practice.

The increased emphasis on EBP, coupled with the proliferation of health care research, has also spurred the incorporation of EBP into health care systems. As a result, most nurses are learning about EBP and frameworks for implementing EBP during their formal nursing education and within their work setting. Developing skills in the use of EBP enables the nurse to become active in the change processes within their institutions.

> *Gaining knowledge of philosophies and theories is one of the most important fundamentals that an advanced practice nurse can embrace. Moreover, the ability to recognize and apply these models is essential to identifying barriers, solving problems, promoting change, and integrating evidence-based practice into health care practice.*
> —Katie Walker, MSN, APRN-CNS

Many nursing programs teach students to engage in EBP by using the *PICO process*. PICO refers to four components contained within a research question: the Patient or Population, the Intervention or area of Interest, the Comparison of interventions (if any), and the Outcomes. These four components are then woven into a clinical question such as: Is the use of X (intervention) in Y (patient or population) more effective in reducing/ preventing complications (outcome) than Z (intervention)? The terms identified for each component of the PICO question, along with surrogate terms, are then used to search the literature for relevant evidence. The PICO process provides a foundational approach that is used in many of the EBP models described here. See Table 22.2 for a comparison of the model's purpose and processes.

Funk's Model of Research Utilization

Several models have been developed to support nurses in using EBP. One of the first was the Funk Model of Research Utilization developed by a team of researchers who sought to fill in the gap between awareness of evidence and use of EBP (Funk, Tornquist, & Champagne, 1989). They synthesized the literature along with data from the Conduct and Utilization of Research in Nursing (CURN) research utilization questionnaire to develop a 29-item BARRIERS Scale. The BARRIERS Scale groups the 29 items under four categories: (a) characteristics of the adopter, (b) the organization, (c) the innovation, and (d) communication. The scale was then tested, replicated, and was determined to be psychometrically valid.

The findings from the BARRIERS Scale were then used to construct a model of research utilization, which focuses on barriers to dissemination and mechanisms to achieve outcomes (Funk, Champagne, Wiese, & Tornquist, 1991). The resulting model consists of three dissemination components: (a) evaluating the quality of the research, (b) exploring the characteristics of communication in EBP, and (c) facilitating the use of research (Funk et al., 1989). For each component, mechanisms to achieve the component are identified. The quality of each research component is based on evaluation of scientific merit, significance of the findings, and readiness for practice. Mechanisms to evaluate the quality of evidence include the literature review and surveys of clinicians and researchers. Communication of published research, through the use of non-technical language that emphasizes the description of outcomes versus statistical tests, is valued. Clear communication of the implications for practice and appropriate strategies for implementation are important criteria

TABLE 22.2 Comparison of EBP Frameworks: Purpose and Processes

Framework	Funk Model	Stetler Model	Rosswurm and Larrabee Model	Iowa Model	Ottawa Model
Purpose	Research utilization Emphasizing dissemination	Research utilization Focus on critical thinking	EBP Emphasizes clinician and researcher collaboration	EBP Facilitates decision making with algorithm	Guides translation of evidence into practice Emphasizes assessing barriers and supports
Processes	Evaluate quality of evidence Explore Communication of EBP Facilitate use	Preparation Validation Comparative evaluation and decision making Translation application Outcome evaluation	Assess need for change Link interventions to outcomes Synthesize best evidence Design a practice change Implement and evaluate Integrate and maintain change	Identify triggers Generate clinical question Does question match the organization's priorities? Search literature Evaluate evidence Does evidence support change?	Assess barriers and supports Monitor intervention and its use Evaluate outcomes

EBP, evidence-based practice.

for identifying and using research findings. The quality of research, effective communication, and use of findings are supported by guidance on how to report the project, how to describe methods and statistics used, and how to disseminate the project through presentation and publication. The final dissemination component is to facilitate utilization, which emphasizes communication between researchers and clinicians, sharing experiences during implementation, ensuring assistance with implementation issues, and providing ongoing support. Final dissemination is facilitated through communication strategies such as newsletters, consultations, and referrals. The ultimate goal of Funk's model is to make use of research by the nurse attainable and to provide support and consultation during the process of research utilization.

Stetler Model of Research Utilization

The Stetler Model of Research Utilization was originally developed by Stetler and Marram in 1976 to promote research utilization and EBP. It was initially published as the Stetler/Marram Model of Research Utilization and later was revised and renamed the Stetler Model of Research Utilization (Stetler, 1994, 2001). The purpose of the model is to help nurses move beyond merely critiquing research to applying the findings in the clinical setting. The model focuses on critical thinking and the five processes involved in using research findings.

The five processes outlined in the Stetler Model are: (a) preparation, (b) validation, (c) comparative evaluation/decision making, (d) translation/application, and (e) evaluation (Stetler, 1994, 2001). In the *preparation phase*, the nurse identifies the purpose, context, and sources of evidence and recognizes contextual factors that impact implementation. The *validation phase* involves determining the credibility of the evidence and its applicability or fit within the setting. It answers the question, Did the research study the variables in practical ways that could be used? In phase three, called the *comparative evaluation/decision-making phase*, the studies are summarized, organized, and compared. The comparisons are based on the degree of evidence, the target population, the match to the current setting, and feasibility. To determine feasibility three Rs are evaluated—risk factors, resources needed to implement, and the readiness of others to implement.

Once the comparative evaluation is complete, there are four choice points: (a) use the research findings, (b) gather more information before implementing, (c) delay the use until more evidence is obtained, and (d) reject without further consideration. If the decision is to use the research findings, then phase four, the *translation and application phase* is entered. In this phase, the use of the research and the actions needed are specified, and the level of use at the individual, group, or organizational level is identified. Application of the research needs to address variations that may be needed and determine the appropriateness of those variations. This phase also involves planning for the use of change strategies and determining options for dissemination of the project within the institution.

The fifth and final phase, *evaluation*, includes implementation of formal and informal evaluation strategies, analysis of the cost/benefits, and determining outcomes. The phases of the model combine to form a process that can be used on an individual, practitioner-oriented basis, rather than an organizational systems–level basis.

Rosswurm and Larrabee Model of EBP

The Rosswurm and Larrabee Model is based on a synthesis of literature on EBP and research utilization, use of standardized language, and change theory (Rosswurm & Larrabee, 1999). The model values qualitative and quantitative research and takes the clinician through the process of collaboration with researchers from the beginning of the assessment process through integration into practice.

Six linear processes are outlined: (a) assessing the need for change, (b) linking the interventions and outcomes, (c) synthesizing the best evidence, (d) designing the practice change, (e) implementing and evaluating the practice change, and (f) integrating and maintaining the practice change (Rosswurm & Larrabee, 1999). During the *assessment* stage, it is important to collect data about the current situation and compare it to external data. This comparison leads to the identification of the problem and provides the foundation for stage two in which potential *interventions are linked to outcomes*. The *synthesis* stage involves using the major variables to search the literature and then combine high-quality evidence to determine feasibility, benefits, and risks of the intervention. Once findings have been synthesized, a plan for the *design* of the change is developed. The design should include specifying resources needed, the implementation processes, and outcomes.

The final two stages, implement and evaluate, and integrate and maintain, call for direct action. A pilot study is recommended for the *implementation and evaluation* stage as it provides a mechanism to determine the appropriateness and effectiveness of the intervention and determines if any modifications are needed before full-scale implementation. During the final stage *integrate and maintain*, strategies are introduced that inform stakeholders and staff of the results of the pilot and the change in practice. In-service education, policy revisions, and ways to monitor ongoing progress are established. Rosswurm and Larrabee (1999) note the model has been tested in acute care nursing settings and could be easily adapted to other setting and disciplines.

Iowa Model of Research-Based Practice

The Iowa Model of Research-Based Practice was originally developed to facilitate decision making during the EBP process (Titler et al., 2001). The model was first published in 1994, then revised in 2001 to incorporate feedback from users and changes in the health care system and terminology. It uses an algorithm format with feedback loops to guide the clinician through the EBP process. An interesting feature of the model is the types of research included. In the absence of experimental research, the model allows the use of nonexperimental research evidence such as case studies.

Use of the Iowa Model begins with either a question brought about by a patient need or a problem or a question about a new practice or intervention. These problem-focused or knowledge-focused triggers shape the content of the clinical question. Clinical questions are easily generated using the PICO format described earlier.

After the clinical question has been developed, the nurse determines if the question is important to the organization's priorities, values, and mission. If relevant, then a search for literature is conducted and the quality and quantity of research is evaluated. Sufficient evidence warrants a pilot study to test the intervention in the specific setting of the facility, whereas insufficient evidence warrants a full-scale research study to garner support for implementation decision making. Once the evidence has been gathered, evaluated, and synthesized, the nurse determines if there is enough evidence to support a practice change. If there is not sufficient research evidence, then other forms of evidence, such as case studies, theory, and expert opinion may be considered, or research may be conducted to provide the evidence. When the decision to implement the research has been made, the algorithm directs the nurse to monitor the process, determine the achievement of outcomes, and disseminate the results.

Ottawa Model of Research Use

The Ottawa Model of Research Use was developed by I. D. Graham and Logan (2004), K. Graham and Logan (2004), and Graham et al. (2006) to guide the translation of research into practice. The model is based on several assumptions. First, knowledge involves complex interactions between doing research and using research. Second, the processes used in EBP are affected by the social and health care environment. Third, patients are central to the knowledge translation process. The Ottawa Model views research use as a dynamic process of interconnected decisions and actions. There are three overarching processes used in the model: (a) assessing barriers and supports, (b) monitoring the intervention and its use, and (c) evaluating outcomes.

The *assessment of barriers and supports* involves three major aspects. The first aspect is the development process for EBP and the attributes of the innovation. Second is consideration of potential adopters: the identification of their concerns, level of awareness, attitudes, knowledge, skills, and current practices. Third, assessment of the practice environment is conducted to determine sociocultural and economic influences and identify uncontrollable events.

The process of *monitoring the intervention and its use* is ongoing during the implementation and adoption phases. Implementation strategies are focused on managing barriers, transfer, and follow-up. The adoption phase looks at intention and use of the intervention and leads to *outcome evaluation* regarding the patient, staff, and the system.

Micro-Level Uses of Frameworks in Research

Whereas all RNs are expected to implement EBP in the care of individual patients, graduate students are also expected to conduct research. The DNP graduates are uniquely prepared to engage in *translational research*, which is the application of EBP to a health care system or systems. Translational research, as the name implies, is concerned with translating current evidence into clinical practice. The goal of translational research is to shorten the time between generating a body of evidence to actual implementation into practice. This involves working with key stakeholders within the system to implement and evaluate evidence-based protocols, policies, and procedures that will improve outcomes. A team approach rather than an individual's effort is needed. In contrast, those with nonclinical doctorates in PhD and EdD programs are educated to conduct original research designed to generate evidence that contributes to nursing's body of knowledge. In both clinical and nonclinical doctoral-prepared nurses, the use of the PICO process which is inherent in EBP can be the start of the research process.

Rempher's Translational Research Process

One example of a framework useful in conducting translational research is seen in Rempher's (2006) six-step process. The first step is to conduct a focus group. The focus group will look at a variety of EBP models to serve as a blueprint for moving from a concept to action. Through discussion and critical analysis of available evidence-based models, the group then moves to step two, model selection. Third, the group presents their findings to the organization to gain support to integrate a change or changes into the system. Fourth, the health care team is educated on the changes based on the model chosen. Then the model is implemented into practice. Finally, the model is evaluated to determine if it is meeting the needs of the organization.

> *Translational research is how we will affect organizational change . . . I strongly believe that is not possible without the support of a strong theoretical framework.*
> —Lindsey Green, APRN-CNS, MN, RNC, CCNS

An example of applying Rempher's six methodical steps can be noted in Penkalski and Kenneally's (2016) project titled "Provider Adherence to Evidence-Based Asthma Guidelines in a Community Health Center" (Box 22.1). The impetus for the project was the observation that the care of children with asthma varied among providers and in some cases did not follow published evidence-based guidelines. In addition to using Rempher's framework to guide the process, frameworks related to systems change, education, and evaluation were used.

BOX 22.1 Application of Rempher's Six-Step Process

The project involved implementing a new asthma treatment protocol for children at a community health clinic. Rempher's Six-Step Process was applied as follows (Rempher, 2006). A group comprising the clinic medical director, researchers, and an informatics team leader was formed. The group analyzed the most recent evidence-based guidelines for treating asthma (Step 1) and selected the Expert Panel Report 3 (EPR-3) guidelines for implementation (Step 2). The group presented its findings and the recommended guidelines to the providers at the clinic (Step 3). The next step involved educating providers on the content of the guidelines and on the changes being made to the electronic health records, which would ensure adherence to the guidelines (Step 4). Once the staff received education about the new protocol and it was integrated into the electronic health records, the protocol was implemented into practice (Step 5). A 3-month follow-up was conducted to evaluate the implementation and measure the outcomes (Step 6). Based on the results, additional recommendations were made to continue to work towards improved and consistent asthma care based on current evidence.

Macro-Level Application of Frameworks

While micro-level applications are centered on ways the individual nurse uses frameworks in daily practice, *macro-level* application is focused on how the profession uses the knowledge within the frameworks. Macro-level application is concerned with the use of frameworks to support clinical nursing education and the scope and standards of nursing practice. Therefore, the concern at the macro-level is with the broader influence of frameworks on the profession as a whole. In this section, the relationships among frameworks, the scope and standards, and competencies of nursing practice are reviewed.

Scope and Standards of Nursing Practice

On the macro-level, it is important to understand how many of the conceptual categories of frameworks discussed in this text inform the ANA *Nursing Scope and Standards of Practice* (ANA, 2015). The purpose of *standards of practice* is to provide guidelines for competent patient care and outline the expectations for professional nursing practice. Academic nursing education programs not only teach students about nursing's scope and standards but also use them to justify curriculum outcomes and help ensure quality of care for all patients (Brent, 2001). Nurses are expected to provide patient care in accordance with what a reasonably prudent nurse would do in a similar circumstance. The standards of nursing practice identify performance expectations and consist of three components:

1. Professional standards of care define diagnostic, intervention, and evaluation competencies.

2. Professional performance standards identify role functions in direct care, consultation, and quality assurance.

3. Specialty practice guidelines provide protocols of care for specific populations (Brent, 2001).

The scope and standards of nursing practice have been identified and delineated by the ANA (2015) and organized around two areas, the standards of professional practice and the standards of profession performance (Box 22.2). The *standards of professional practice* identify responsibilities for nurses regardless of specialization that revolve around the steps of the nursing process. The implementation process specifies coordination of care, health teaching, and health promotion role functions for all levels of nursing and additional expectations of consultation and prescriptive authority for nurses with graduate preparation and advanced practice status, respectively.

The *standards of professional performance* describe "competent behavior in the professional role" (ANA, 2015, p. 89). Areas of competence include education, ethics, and leadership that were addressed in Chapters 7, 8, and 18, respectively. These chapters provide the nurse with multiple frameworks to incorporate into teaching, as well as ethical philosophies, decision-making models, and leadership perspectives that can influence how the nurse performs in these realms. Performance expectations related to research are discussed in Chapters 3 and 24, and frameworks for using EBP were discussed earlier in this chapter.

Standards related to the quality of practice and the evaluation of professional practice are found in the quality improvement and evaluation frameworks discussed in Chapter 19. Theoretical knowledge related to communication and leadership standards is found in Chapters 18 and 10. Similarly, content related to group dynamics, mentoring, and collaborative leadership styles are found in Chapter 18. According to the ANA's *Nursing Scope and Standards of Practice* (ANA, 2010), "Registered nurses are accountable for their professional actions to themselves, their health care consumers, their peers, and ultimately society"

BOX 22.2 American Nurses Association Standards of Professional Practice and Performance

Standards of Professional Practice

- Assess
- Diagnose
- Identify Outcomes
- Plan
- Implement
- Evaluate Outcomes

Standards of Professional Performance

- Ethics
- Education
- Evidence-Based Practice and Research
- Quality of Practice
- Culturally Congruent Practice
- Communication
- Leadership
- Collaboration
- Resource Utilization
- Environmental Health
- Evaluation of Professional Practice

Source: American Nurses Association (2015).

(p. 10). The knowledge and perspectives contained within philosophies, models, theories, and taxonomies provide a foundation for informed nursing practice.

On an organizational level, the CCNE ensures all nursing programs from an institution of higher learning meet the same quality and integrity standards. CCNE evaluates baccalaureate and graduate-degree nursing education programs on a scheduled basis to assess the achievement of the institution in meeting its mission, goals, and expected outcomes. Accreditation of a nursing program validates that the curriculum has met predetermined standards, is based on the program objectives, and confirms achievement of curriculum objectives that support competent clinical practice.

On graduation from an accredited graduate nursing program that prepares the nurse for advanced practice, the nurse is eligible for national certification. Two certification bodies for nurse practitioner graduates include the ANCC and the American Academy of Nurse Practitioners (AANP). Each of these certification organizations outlines standards for nursing knowledge and clinical practice that are founded on theoretical and research knowledge such as the many frameworks discussed in this text.

Advanced Practice Education

The Advanced Practice Registered Nurses (APRN) Consensus Model is the result of more than 40 nursing organizations that collaborated to make APRN practice more uniform across the country (APRN Consensus Work Group & the National Council of State Boards of Nursing APRN Advisory Committee, 2008). Its purpose was to have standardized education, certification, accreditation, and licensure regulations by 2015 for APRNs. This included certified registered nurse anesthetist (CRNA), certified nurse-midwife (CNM), clinical nurse specialist (CNS), and certified nurse practitioner (CNP). However, as of 2016, the only consensus model recommendation that has taken effect is the standardized education of the APRN. Educational programs are accredited by each state Board of Nursing and adhere to the NONPF and CCNE curriculum guidelines.

To become an APRN, there are additional standards of practice that must be met over and above those put forth by the ANA. Practice standards for nurse practitioners are defined by NONPF. The competencies identified by NONPF were developed by comparing patient data sets with evidence-based standards to improve patient care (Thomas et al., 2017). The NONPF core competencies and the frameworks that support them are provided in this section and summarized in Table 22.3. The first competency is broad and relates to providing scientific foundations for practice that integrates research, theory, and practice knowledge. It acknowledges the importance of the interrelationships among theory, research, and practice for the development of knowledge. This competency is supported by knowledge of theory, research, and practice as discussed in Chapter 3. Demonstrating leadership, competency 2, by collaborating with stakeholders to foster change within a health care setting is supported by knowledge grounded in leadership frameworks (Chapters 17 and 18).

Competency 3, providing safe, high-quality care is supported by many client-focused frameworks discussed in Parts II and III of this text. These client-focused frameworks can enhance the nurse's awareness of influencing factors, risks, and attributes in patients, families, and communities receiving care. This enhanced awareness, in turn, can influence and guide the nurse to perform a more comprehensive assessment of the patient, family, and community, leading to safer and higher quality of care. Another related competency involves the analysis and translation of clinical guidelines and application of clinical investigative skills to improve patient care. The evaluation frameworks discussed in Chapter 19, coupled with the EBP frameworks discussed earlier in this chapter, can guide the nurse in applying EBP guidelines and participating in translational science.

Other NONPF competencies are concerned with ethical, legal, and social factors to promote equity in health care costs, quality, and access. The frameworks discussed in Chapters

TABLE 22.3 NONPF Core Competency Areas and Related Educational Content

Core Competency Area	Educational Content (*Related Framework Chapters*)
1. Scientific Foundations	Analysis of evidence (*Chapter 3: Relationship Among Theory, Research, and Practice*)
	Integrates sciences and humanities (*Chapter 6: Human Development Frameworks; Chapter 9: Health and Illness Frameworks; Chapter 11: Needs-Based Frameworks; Chapter 12: Physiological Frameworks; Chapter 13: Psychological Frameworks; Chapter 20: Sociocultural Frameworks*)
	Translates research and integrates theory, research, and practice (*Chapter 3: Relationship Among Theory, Research, and Practice; Chapter 24: Application of Frameworks to the Nurse Researcher Role*)
2. Leadership	Advanced leadership and change agent (*Chapter 4: Frameworks for Behavioral Change; Chapter 18: Leadership Frameworks for Organizational Systems; Chapter 23: Application of Frameworks to Leadership Roles in Nursing*)
3. Quality	Evaluates care processes, financing, and organizational structure (*Chapter 5: Care and Caring Frameworks; Chapter 15: Economic Frameworks; Chapter 17: Organizational System Frameworks; Chapter 19: Frameworks for Evaluation*)
4. Practice Inquiry	Leads in translation of knowledge, analyzes clinical guidelines (*Chapters 3: Relationship Among Theory, Research, and Practice; Chapter 19: Frameworks for Evaluation*)
5. Technology and Information Literacy	Assess client's educational needs and coach in behavioral changes (*Chapter 4: Frameworks for Behavioral Change; Chapter 7: Frameworks for Teaching and Learning*)
6. Health Policy	Analyzes social, cultural, and economic factors that influence ethical policy development (*Chapter 8: Moral and Ethical Perspectives; Chapter 15: Economic Frameworks; Chapter 16: Community and Population Health Frameworks; Chapter 20: Sociocultural Frameworks*)
7. Health Delivery System	Analysis of the organization, apply knowledge of complex systems, facilitate system change to meet cultural needs (*Chapter 17: Organizational System Frameworks; Chapter 18: Leadership Frameworks for Organizational Systems; Chapter 20: Sociocultural Frameworks*)
8. Ethics	Uses ethical principles in decision making and evaluates ethical consequences (*Chapter 8: Moral and Ethical Perspectives*)
9. Independent Practice	Provides the full spectrum of health/illness care to individuals and families (*Chapter 4: Frameworks for Behavioral Change; Chapter 9: Health and Illness Frameworks; Chapter 10: Interpersonal and Family Frameworks; Chapter 11: Needs-Based Frameworks; Chapter 12: Physiological Frameworks, Chapter 13: Psychological Frameworks; Chapter 22: Application of Frameworks to the Clinician Role*)

NONPF, National Organization of Nurse Practitioner Faculties.

Sources: NONPF (2012); Thomas et al. (2017).

these broad and far-reaching concerns. Ethical competencies include ethical decision making for individuals, populations, and systems of care. Several ethical decision-making models adaptable to a variety of ethical dilemmas were discussed in Chapter 8. Frameworks to inform the clinician about social factors related to health care costs, quality, and access issues were presented in Chapters 15 and 20.

NONPF also includes competencies focused on health care delivery systems and evaluation of the organizational structure to determine how health care delivery can be improved. Frameworks covered in Chapter 17 can provide guidance on evaluation of organizational structure and systems. The last competency is to function as a licensed independent practitioner providing a full spectrum of health services to patients and families. This competency implies knowledge of patient and family interpersonal relationship dynamics and health care needs that were addressed in Chapters 10 and 11. Overall, these competencies guide the curricular structure of advanced practice nursing programs to help ensure the programs prepare clinicians to provide safe, effective, evidence-based care.

● CONCLUSION

The ANA provides the foundation for which the nursing profession as a whole formulates its competencies. CCNE and NONPF further define the educational standards upon which basic and advanced practice nursing programs are built. One key standard is the use of theory including frameworks from nursing as well as those borrowed from other disciplines. These frameworks provide a basis for implementing nursing care and for using evidence-based guidelines to care for patients, families, and communities. These frameworks broaden the clinician's perspective, enhance knowledge, and sensitize the nurse's understanding of the patient and patient care environment.

● KEY POINTS

- The clinician's practice benefits from awareness and knowledge of multiple frameworks.
- Use of frameworks on a day-to-day basis is referred to as *micro-level application*.
- *Macro-level application* focuses on how frameworks support and inform the nurse's educational program and scope of practice.
- Theory generation and testing occur on a basic level whenever the nurse uses the nursing process.
- Selection of interventions is influenced by the clinician's scope of knowledge. Exposure to diverse frameworks broadens the nurse's scope of knowledge.
- Knowledge of community and population health frameworks alerts the nurse to broader issues beyond acute care such as health risks and sociocultural, economic, and environmental factors that influence health.
- Micro-level uses of frameworks in clinical practice include applying frameworks individually or in combination to the patient care situation and engaging in EBP.
- PICO is a systematic process that can be used to engage in EBP.
- Use of the PICO process establishes clinical research questions and identifies search terms for the review of literature.
- Funk's Model of Research Utilization categorizes barriers to EBP as characteristics of the adopter, the organization, the innovation, and the communication processes.

- Stetler Model of Research Utilization focuses on five processes: preparation, validation, comparative evaluation/decision-making, translation/application, and evaluation.

- Rosswurm & Larrabee's Model of EBP involves six processes: (a) assess the need, (b) link the intervention to the outcome, (c) synthesize the best evidence, (d) design a practice change, (e) implement and evaluate, and (f) integrate and maintain the practice change.

- Iowa Model of Research-Based Practice uses an algorithm format with feedback loops to guide the EBP process and integrates the use of PICO.

- Ottawa Model of Research Use describes three main processes: assess barriers and supports, monitor intervention use, and evaluate outcomes.

- Translational research involves the application of EBP to health care systems.

- Rempher's Translational Research Process uses six steps: (a) conducting a focus group, (b) model selection, (c) obtaining organizational support, (d) education of the health care team, (e) implementation into practice, and (f) evaluation.

- The American Nurses Association specifies the scope and standards of nursing practice as including standards for professional practice and standards for professional performance. Frameworks provided in Part II and Part III provide a foundation for implementing the standards in practice.

- The National Organization of Nurse Practitioner Faculties has established competencies and curricular guidelines, which is informed by the frameworks presented in this text related to individuals, families, populations, and systems.

REFERENCES

Academy of Medical-Surgical Nurses. (2014). Evidence-based practice. Retrieved from https://www.amsn.org/practice-resources/evidence-based-practice

Advanced Practice Registered Nurses Consensus Work Group & the National Council of State Boards of Nursing APRN Advisory Committee. (2008, July 7). Consensus model for APRN regulation: Licensure, accreditation, certification & education. Retrieved from http://nursecredentialing.org/APRN-ConsensusModelReport.aspx

American Nurse Credentialing Center. (2016). ANCC certification center. Retrieved from http://www.nursecredentialing.org/certification.aspx

American Nurses Association. (2010). *Nursing scope and standards of practice* (2nd ed.). Silver Spring, MD: Author.

American Nurses Association. (2015). *Nursing scope and standards of practice* (3rd ed.). Silver Spring, MD: Author.

Brent, N. (2001). *Nurses and the law: A guide to principles and applications.* St. Louis, MO: Saunders.

Erickson, H., Tomlin, E., & Swain, M. (2005). *Modeling and role-modeling: A theory and paradigm for nursing.* Cedar Park, TX: EST.

Fontaine, K. (2009). *Foundations of mental health nursing* (6th ed.). Upper Saddle River, NJ: Pearson.

Funk, S. G., Champagne, M. T., Wiese, R. A., & Tornquist, E. M. (1991). BARRIERS: The barriers to research utilization scale. *Applied Nursing Research, 4,* 39-45. doi:10.1016/S0897-1897(05)80052-7

Funk, S. G., Tornquist, E. M., & Champagne, M. T. (1989). A model for the dissemination of nursing research. *Western Journal of Nursing Research, 11*(3), 361–372.

Graham, I. D. & Logan, J. (2004). Innovations in knowledge transfer and continuity of care. *Canadian Journal of Nursing Research, 36*(2), 89–103.

Graham, I. D., Logan, J., Harrison, M. B., Straus, S. E., Tetroe, J., Caswell, W., & Robinson, N. (2006). Lost in knowledge translation: Time for a map? *Journal of Continuing Education in the Health Professions, 26,* 13–24. doi:10.1002/chp.47

Graham, K. & Logan, J. (2004). Using the Ottawa model of research use to implement a skin care program. *Journal of Nursing Care Quality, 19*(1), 18–24. doi:10.1097/00001786-200401000-00006

Hoffart, N., & Woods, C. (1996). Elements of a nursing professional practice model. *Journal of Professional Nursing, 12*(6), 354–364.

National Organization of Nurse Practitioner Faculties. (2012). *Nurse practitioner core competencies.* Washington, DC: Author.

Penkalski, M., & Kenneally, M. (2016). Provider adherence to evidence-based asthma guidelines in a community health center. *Journal of Doctoral Nursing Practice, 9*(3), 128–138.

Prochaska, J., & DiClemente, C. (1983). Stages and processes of self-change of smoking: Toward an integrative model of change. *Journal of Consulting and Clinical Psychology, 51*(3), 390–395.

Rempher, K. J. (2006). Putting theory into practice: Six steps to success. *American Nurse Today, 1*(2), 41–42.

Rosswurm, M. A., & Larrabee, J. H. (1999). A model for change to evidence-based practice. *Image Journal of Nursing Scholarship, 31*(4), 317–322.

Stetler, C. (1994). Refinement of the Stetler/Marram model for application of research findings to practice. *Nursing Outlook, 42*, 15–25.

Stetler, C. (2001). Updating the Stetler model of research utilization to facilitate evidence-based practice. *Nursing Outlook, 49*, 272–279. doi:10.1067/mno.2001.120517

Thomas, A., Crabtree, M., Delaney, K., Dumas, M., Kleinpell, R., Marfell, J., . . . Wolfe, A. (2017). *Nurse practitioner core competencies content.* National Organization of Nurse Practitioner Faculty. Retrieved from http://c.ymcdn.com/sites/www.nonpf.org/resource/resmgr/competencies/2017_NPCoreComps_with_Curric.pdf

Titler, M. G., Kleiber, C., Steelman, V. J., Rakel, B. A., Budreau, G., Everett, C. L., . . . Goode, C. J. (2001). The Iowa model of evidence-based practice to promote quality care. *Critical Care Nursing Clinics of North America, 13*(4), 497–509.

Application of Frameworks to Leadership Roles in Nursing

Kristina Henry

Most people think of leadership as a position and therefore don't see themselves as leaders.
—Stephen R. Covey

Leadership is a potent combination of strategy and character. But if you must be without one, be without the strategy.
—Norman Schwarzkopf

KEY TERMS

academic nurse leader
clinical nurse leader

nurse executive
policy and advocacy leader

LEARNING OBJECTIVES

1. Define and differentiate nurse leadership roles in terms of knowledge, skills, abilities, and functions.
2. Review competencies and certifications for nurse leadership roles and how they integrate knowledge of diverse frameworks.
3. Explore the application of frameworks in nurse leadership roles.
4. Compare competencies and knowledge needed to function as a nurse executive, academic nurse leader, clinical nurse leader, and policy and advocacy leader.

Leadership is a general characteristic of all nurses; however, this chapter focuses on formal nursing leadership roles such as the nurse executive, the clinical nurse leader (CNL), the academic nurse leader, and the public policy and advocacy nurse leader; and how frameworks discussed in previous chapters inform these roles. Each role is associated with a variety of career options and potential work settings. Educational preparation for these leadership roles including certification is explored, and frameworks that support the nurse leader's role performance are identified. Also, how nurse leaders use knowledge and apply frameworks within diverse leadership roles is explained in this chapter.

A commonality shared by nurse leaders, regardless of title, is to empower, inspire, and motivate others through interpersonal and communication skills. The nurse leader acts as an example to others, demonstrates integrity, and establishes the vision and culture of the team. In addition, the nurse leader recognizes and supports the value of the team in collaborating to achieve outcomes, and seeks to maximize the strengths of each member to optimize results. For a nurse leader, the team often consists of an inter-disciplinary mix of stakeholders, health care providers, business support, community, and political resources. The nurse leader's role in the team is to maintain the vision of the team, transform the team from a group of independent people to a functional entity with a purpose, and manage group conflict (Grossman & Valiga, 2013).

Nurse executives and administrators are formal leadership roles for nurses. However, as discussed in greater detail in Chapter 18, these roles and positions of authority are often confused with management roles and principles. Although there is generally some overlap in that managers may be leaders and leaders may perform management tasks, this chapter differentiates the two roles with emphasis on leadership attributes and characteristics versus management tasks and functions.

○ LEADERSHIP ROLES

In nursing, there are virtually endless avenues to demonstrate leadership roles. Regardless of the specific health care setting, one is likely to find a nurse working in a leadership capacity. In the following section, four leadership roles are discussed: the nurse executive, CNL, academic nurse leader, and policy and advocacy leader. These roles along with educational and certification criteria are discussed and framework chapters that support the competencies and expectations of each role are identified.

The Nurse Executive

The nurse executive is a visionary and administrative role focused on influencing patient care and quality. This role has some managerial functions; however, the primary role is leading, empowering, and motivating others for successful achievement of organizational goals. Work settings for the nurse executive may include acute care, community, health care businesses, or entrepreneurial activities. The business settings may include insurance companies, governmental agencies, medical supply, pharmaceutical businesses, or health care information technology corporations. In addition to operating within a range of settings, the nurse executive role may focus on a specific structure or function, such as personnel or quality improvement.

A growing role of interest to the nurse executive is the nurse entrepreneur or sole proprietor. The unique skills, attributes, and expertise of nurses are reflected in successful entrepreneurial businesses. Nurse entrepreneurs often provide training for businesses: legal, educational, or health care consultation. As an entrepreneur, the nurse demonstrates expertise in a specific area of nursing, as well as in business knowledge and acumen, and establishes the organization or nursing unit's vision, mission, and goals (Meek, 2015).

Nurse Executive Certification

The American Organization of Nurse Executives (AONE) describes the nurse executive through a set of competencies, which are not specific to the nurse's education, title, or practice settings (AONE, n.d.). These competencies are grounded in knowledge areas relevant to a variety of frameworks discussed in this text and serve several purposes. The nurse executive may use the competencies for self-assessment, or the aspiring nurse executive may use them for career preparation. Organizations and health care settings use the competencies to develop job descriptions and evaluation criteria, whereas academic institutions use these competencies to guide curriculum development in nursing leadership programs of study.

The AONE core competencies include five areas: communication and relationship management, knowledge of the health care environment, leadership, professionalism, and business skills and principles. For each of these competencies there are related frameworks that inform the nurse's practice. See Table 23.1 for an outline of the AONE core competencies.

Communication and relationship building include abilities and skills for oral and written presentations, establishing and maintaining collaborative and diverse relationships in an interprofessional environment, and skills in influencing and empowering others. (These skills rely on information in Chapters 10 and 18.) The second competency, nurse's *knowledge of the health care environment*, is enhanced by understanding organizational systems (Chapter 17), health care economics (Chapter 15), and sociocultural influences (Chapter 20). The third competency, *leadership*, is facilitated by understanding communication, mentoring, and leadership styles discussed in Chapter 18. This competency also includes the translation of evidence into practice for quality improvement processes such as patient safety and risk management. These topics are covered in greater detail in Chapters 19 and 22. The leadership competency is concerned with providing vision and innovative thinking, leading change and critically analyzing organizational concerns (Chapter 17). *Professionalism* involves accountability and professional contributions such as certification, covered in this chapter, and mentoring covered in Chapter 18. The final competency focuses on organizational and *business skills* including financial and human resource management, in addition to strategic management, information management, and information technology management (Chapters 17 and 18). These competencies represent the necessary knowledge and skills identified by AONE for the nurse executive role (AONE, n.d.).

As previously noted, promoting, achieving, and maintaining professional certification is a primary component of the professionalism competency for AONE nurse executives. AONE offers two pathways for nurse executive certification: Certified in Executive Nursing Practice (CENP) and Certified Nurse Manager and Leader (CNML). The CENP is designed specifically for nurse executives, while the CNML certification incorporates the nurse manager role. The content of the certification exams is based on the nurse executive competencies as explained above. As demonstrated, each of the nurse executive competencies is facilitated and supported by a variety of frameworks presented throughout the text.

Another option for professional certification for the nurse executive is through the American Nurses Credentialing Center (ANCC), a subsidiary of the American Nurses Association (ANA). Through the credentialing process, the ANCC fosters nursing excellence and quality health care by validating nurse knowledge and expertise (ANCC, 2017). Certification includes the Nurse Executive-Board Certified (NE-BC) or the advanced option, Nurse Executive Advanced-Board Certified (NEA-BC). Both pathways (AONE and ANCC) require an examination to validate knowledge for certification. See the AONE and ANCC organization websites for more information.

Depending on the focus of the nurse executive role, there are also many role-specific certifications. The National Association for Healthcare Quality (NAHQ) validates expertise with the Certified Professional in Healthcare Quality certification (NAHQ, n.d.). This certification is built on the knowledge of quality improvement (Chapter 19) and change processes as explained in Chapter 18. The Human Resource Certification Institute (HRCI) provides certification in Professional in Human Resources (HRCI, n.d.). Human resources certification requires the application of psychological (Chapter 13), interpersonal (Chapter 10), and business and organizational frameworks (Chapters 17 and 18).

Nurse executives apply a variety of frameworks in their everyday practice. Consistent theoretical application becomes inherent and creates the culture of the organization, as well as defines the leadership style of the nurse executive. The specific frameworks used are based on the nurse executive competencies. From communication and mentoring, to change and quality improvement, the application of specific frameworks becomes embedded into each leadership decision. Relevant models, theories, and taxonomies used by the nurse executive are found in Chapters 17, 18, and 19.

TABLE 23.1 AONE Description of Core Competencies	
Core Competency	**Description**
Communication and relationship building	Effectively communicate to diverse audiences on variety of topics through oral and written presentations
	Build collaborative and interprofessional relationships, including academic planning and partnerships
	Share vision and inspire others
	Community and stakeholder involvement
	Situational leadership skills: conflict resolution, representation, serve as resource
Knowledge of the health care environment	Knowledge of standards of practice and regulatory compliance, including ethical considerations
	Knowledge of care delivery models
	Knowledge of health care economics and policies, including legislative processes and regulations
	Nursing representation at governing body of organization
	Translation of evidence into practice
	Performance improvement processes such as patient safety and risk management
Leadership	Empowering, supporting, and exploring innovation
	Critical analysis of organizational concerns
	Visionary and reflective thinking
	Leading change
	Learning from success and failure
Professionalism	Accountability: professional certifications, participate in professional organizations, role model and mentor others
	Reflect on personal strengths and weaknesses
	Advocate for nurses and others including ethical considerations
Business skills	Budget development and management
	Resource management and negotiations
	Workforce development including recruitment, education, compensation, and evaluation processes
	Strategic outcome management: SWOT and Gap analysis, balanced scorecard and marketing
	Information management, technology analysis, and implementation

AONE, American Organization of Nurse Executives; SWOT, strengths, weaknesses, opportunities, and threats.
Source: American Organization of Nurse Executives (n.d.).

Change theories are especially helpful for leaders and managers to understand the resistance that sometimes accompanies change.
—Mary Booth, BSN, RN, DNP student

Clinical Nurse Leader

According to the American Association of Colleges of Nursing (AACN), the role of the nurse at the bedside is becoming increasingly complex. The Institute of Medicine's (IOM's) Future of Nursing Report (IOM, 2010) has recognized this fact and emphasizes the need for nurses to achieve higher levels of education to address this increasingly complex and diverse health care climate. This recommendation appears to be well supported by research. Blegen, Goode, Park, Vaughn, and Spetz (2013) note that patient outcomes improved when nurses at the bedside were prepared with a baccalaureate-level or higher degrees. Further research has shown the use of master's-prepared CNLs improves the quality and safety of patient care through the application of evidence-based practice (EBP) at the bedside (CNL Association, n.d.). The nation's largest employer of nurses, the Veterans Health Administration (VHA), has recognized the value of the CNL in patient outcomes and is planning to implement the role in all VHA institutions (AACN, 2012). Thus, health care settings across the country are beginning to redesign their care processes using the CNL as a solution to improve patient outcomes.

The CNL is a master's-prepared nurse who leads the coordination of care, risk management, and quality improvement for patients. The complex role functions of the CNL, including clinical care, risk management, team leadership, and translation of evidence to practice, require the application of diverse frameworks. As an expert at implementing evidence-based care at the bedside, the CNL facilitates communication among the interprofessional team and promotes EBP. Therefore, familiarity with frameworks for EBP described in Chapter 22 and use of quality improvement processes described in Chapter 19 supports the CNL role. The CNL also practices at the bedside and thus uses a variety of frameworks related to care of individuals and families as covered in Part II. As the CNL also leads the care team, knowledge of interpersonal communication and organizational systems (Chapter 17) and Leadership Frameworks for Organizational Systems (Chapter 18) are relevant. The CNL needs familiarity with a wide variety of perspectives in a wide range of subject areas that vary depending on the area of clinical practice. But regardless of the setting, the CNL's primary responsibilities are to organize care through evidence-based means while coordinating interprofessional collaboration processes. The complexity of this role requires a multifaceted competency development program as described in the next section (AACN, 2013).

CNL Competencies

Minimal competencies for the CNL have been described by the AACN (2013). The first educational requirement is to be a master's-prepared nurse (AACN, 2013). Programs may be designed as complete master's degree in clinical nurse leadership or a post master's certification in the CNL role. The graduate curriculum covers health care organizations and system analysis, direct care knowledge and skills, and role-specific expectations. The CNL graduate is eligible for certification through the Commission on Nurse Certification (CNC), a subsidiary of the AACN. The CNL competencies, outlined as nine essentials and corresponding frameworks chapters related to the essentials are shown in Box 23.1.

Academic Nurse Leader

The academic nurse leader may be a program director, a department head, dean, provost, or college president. As an academic leader in a nursing program, the nurse must marry the concepts of higher education such as curriculum development, teaching, scholarship, and

---

BOX 23.1 American Association of Colleges of Nursing Master's Essentials and Chapter Coverage

Essential 1: Background for Practice From Sciences and Humanities (Chapters in Part II and Part III)

Essential 2: Organizational and Systems Leadership (Chapters 17 and 18)

Essential 3: Quality Improvement and Safety (Chapter 19)

Essential 4: Translating and Integrating Scholarship into Practice (Chapters 3 and 22)

Essential 5: Informatics and Health Care Technologies

Essential 6: Health Policy and Advocacy (Chapter 23)

Essential 7: Interprofessional Collaboration for Improving Patient and Population Health Outcomes (Chapters 16 and 18)

Essential 8: Clinical Prevention and Population Health for Improving Health (Chapter 16)

Essential 9: Master's-Level Nursing Practice (Chapters in Part II and Part III)

Source: American Association of Colleges of Nursing (2013).

---

service, with nursing competencies. This is a complex process involving the application of general leadership (Chapter 18), educational frameworks (Chapter 7), and many content areas in Parts II and III of this text. The vision of the academic nurse leader is focused on maintaining quality nursing education programs that address evolving standards of nursing practice. The academic nurse leader demonstrates expertise in didactic and clinical areas and participates in nursing, academic, and professional committees and organizations.

Competencies of the Academic Leader

The National League for Nursing (NLN) describes the competencies of the academic nurse leader as a combination of all other nurse leader competencies. The academic nurse leader needs to understand policy and educational trends in nursing while integrating those into the practices and goals of the academic institution. An understanding of interpersonal relationships (Chapter 10), sociocultural influences (Chapter 20), political, economic influences (Chapter 15), and mentoring (Chapter 18) is useful in leading and implementing change in the educational arena. Academic nurse leaders need to recognize these factors and identify trends that impact the learning environment, curriculum, and the expectations and competencies of new graduates. The academic nurse leader establishes clinical partnerships within the community and between the health care organization and the community. They are accountable for mentoring new faculty as well as engaging in and promoting continued professional development (Utley, 2011).

The competencies for the academic nurse leader are the same as those of the AONE, simply applied in a different setting (AONE, n.d.). Each of the five competencies: communication and relationship management, knowledge of the health care environment, leadership, professionalism, and business skills and principles are reflected in the academic setting. However, the academic nurse leader focuses on relationship development and merging clinical expertise with academic responsibilities.

For the academic nurse leader, the methods of demonstrating the competencies will differ from the AONE due to the academic setting. Thus, for the academic nurse leader, the first competency, *communication and relationship management*, is reflected in collaboration with students, clinical agencies, and academic colleagues. The focus of the academic nurse leader is on student–nurse achievement and success. Coordination of interprofessional resources is a primary responsibility, as well as developing and maintaining clinical partnerships. Frameworks to support and facilitate this competency are found in Chapters 10, 13, and 18. The second competency, *knowledge of the health care environment*, uses organizational systems and change frameworks that are essential for curriculum development, clinical planning, and program design. Academic *leadership* also involves change management and mentoring (Chapter 18), and systems thinking (Chapter 17). *Professionalism* is reflected in participation in professional organizations, advocacy, and ethical considerations (Chapter 8). The use of *business skills* is exhibited by the academic nurse leader in budget and resource management (Chapter 15), program marketing, and grant administration (Utley, 2011).

> *In health care today, we must all be systems thinkers.*
> —Lindsey Green, APRN-CNS, MN, RNC, CCNS

As the role of the academic nurse leader is dependent on the setting and specific job description, there is not a singular identified definition or criteria for this role. A recent study indicated that leaders in higher education are currently being recruited outside of the traditional methods. As these academic nurse leader positions are increasing in complexity, the job expectations require a new and innovative skill set. The traditional leadership approach to higher education is not adaptable to the current environment. The committees tasked with hiring the academic executive are looking for candidates with a focus on communication and relationships (Chapters 10, 13, and 14). They also seek experience in translating evidence into practice (Chapter 22) and conducting evaluation activities, as covered in Chapter 19. Barden (2013) also noted the importance of communicating and implementing a strategic vision, which is identified and supported by frameworks in Chapter 18.

Educational preparation and certification for the academic nurse leader role is varied and diverse, and as a result there is no certification specifically for the role. Likewise, the educational preparation for academic nurse leader positions is variable depending on nursing state board, accreditation, and institutional requirements. The certifications available for the academic nurse leader as discussed subsequently represent the range of competencies, core knowledge, and skills used in this role. The frameworks represented in this text substantiate and support the diverse knowledge required as an academic nurse leader.

The academic nurse leader who completes the CENP and NE-BC certifications for the nurse executive must demonstrate competence in business and leadership knowledge and skills (Chapters 17 and 18). However, to validate nursing-specific academic knowledge and skills, the academic nurse leader may pursue a nurse educator certification as discussed in Chapter 21. The NLN offers the Certified Nurse Educator (CNE) credential to validate the expertise of nurse educators. Certification requires competence in teaching and would benefit from knowledge within Chapters 7, 18, and 19.

There are also certifications available to validate expertise in higher education leadership. The National Association of State Administrators and Supervisors of Private Schools (NASASPS) has implemented the Certified Higher Education Professional (CHEP) certification. This is designed for academic leaders at vocational schools, colleges, or universities and demonstrates expertise and specialization in higher education leadership, management, supervision, teaching, or admissions (see Chapters 7, 17, and 18). Information is provided by NASASPS (2016) regarding additional training and certification options.

As the role of the academic nurse administrator is complex and diverse, so are the frameworks used to guide and support the organizational structure and processes of the academic unit. However, in building and maintaining relationships with faculty, students, and constituents, the academic nurse leader may find knowledge of behavioral change (Chapter 4), roles (Chapter 14), and culture (Chapter 20) helpful. Evaluation of programs and curriculum would benefit from the knowledge of evaluation discussed in Chapter 19. The opportunities and options for application of frameworks as a nurse academic leader are potentially endless.

Policy and Advocacy Leader

Although politics may seem daunting and unpleasant, it is a critical component for health care policy development. The negotiation process among competitive entities is necessary for distribution of limited resources. When advocating for patient care at the policy and public health level, nurses may use knowledge of economics (Chapter 15), ethics (Chapter 8), and social justice frameworks (Chapter 20) to prioritize needs and improve care. With limited resources and seemingly endless needs, nurses must advocate for the most critical needs of the most vulnerable first. These decisions are morally and ethically challenging. Policy and advocacy leaders rely on ethical and social justice frameworks to guide and support decision making.

> *Finding the rationale for a decision and utilizing a theory-driven evidence-based model is necessary to provide safe and effective care.*
> —Katie Walker, MSN, APRN-CNS

Nurses who focus on health care policy advocacy do so primarily for patients or the nursing profession. These nurses play a significant role in influencing legislation and policy development for improved patient outcomes, as well as improving outcomes for the nursing profession. As most political figures lack health care expertise, it becomes critical for nurses to share their knowledge and experiences to influence decisions affecting health care. This requires the application of interpersonal (Chapter 10) and leadership frameworks (Chapter 18). Nurse leaders in policy and advocacy develop careers in a variety of settings including research organizations, legislative offices, professional nursing organizations, or health care provider organizations. They also may represent the public as an elected official on the state or national level.

Another avenue for policy and advocacy leaders is to represent the nursing profession through active involvement with professional nursing organizations such as the ANA or NLN. These nurse leaders may work at or with organizations whose purpose is to influence and develop health care policies to improve patient safety and outcomes. Professional nursing organizations, governmental agencies, and private entities all function in this capacity (Table 23.2). These organizations are able to merge the force of millions of nurses to create a source of highly effective influential power. The nurse leader's engagement with these organizations requires the application of democratic and transformational leadership and change frameworks addressed in Chapter 18. The policy and advocacy leader must also appreciate how ethics (Chapter 8), economics (Chapter 15), organizational systems (Chapter 17), and sociocultural phenomena (Chapter 20) influence health policy. Understanding these interrelated issues and the political processes involved is complex and chaotic. Thus, the application of organizational and systems frameworks (Chapter 17) such as complexity and chaos frameworks is helpful.

In addition to the nurse executive competencies, the health policy and advocacy leaders require intimate knowledge of the lawmaking process at the state and national level, as well as have the ability to develop interpersonal relationships (Chapter 10). The advocacy and policy nurse leader must be aware of trending health care legislation, as well as the roles of each government branch. This nurse leader must know the names and contact information of elected representatives, as well as develop professional relationships with influential figures. The ANA website has details of the current legislative and regulatory priorities.

TABLE 23.2 Agencies and Organizations Relevant to the Policy and Advocacy Leader Role

Governmental Agencies	Role and Priorities
Department of Health and Human Services (DHHS)	Improve and protect health of citizens through programs and services, grants and contracts, and law and regulation influence
National Advisory Council on Nurse Education and Practice (NACNEP)	Policy advisement to legislators and the Secretary of Health and Human Services
Health Resources and Services Administration (HRSA)	Focuses on improving health and access to quality programs and services for vulnerable populations
Veterans Administration (VA)	The largest employer of RNs in the United States Provides health care services and support to veterans
National Institutes of Health (NIH)	The national medical and scientific research agency focused on health care studies and innovations
Professional Nursing Organizations	**Role and Priorities**
National Council of State Boards of Nursing (NCSBN)	Coordination of boards of nursing (state based), priorities include nursing licensure and patient safety
Institute of Medicine (IOM)	Nonprofit organization that provides evidence-based research recommendations for public health and policy; membership is honorary
National League for Nursing (NLN)	Represents nurses in any academic setting to influence nursing workforce developmental policies
American Association of Colleges of Nursing (AACN)	Represents baccalaureate and graduate nursing programs, supports education for improved knowledge, skills, and abilities for nurses
American Organization of Nursing Executives (AONE)	A faction of the American Hospital Association, provides support, leadership, and advocacy for professional and patient issues and concerns
Minority nurse organizations: National Black Nurses Association, National Association of Hispanic Nurses	Represent and advocate for the interests of minority nurses
Private Entities/Foundations	**Role and Priorities**
Robert Wood Johnson Foundation	A nonprofit organization that provides grants and support for research and programs to enhance health
Kaiser Family Foundation	Non-profit public charity focusing on national and global health issues and policies; non-partisan source of information and facts

TABLE 23.3 Role Descriptions, Competencies, and Certifications for Nurse Leadership Roles

Leadership Role	Description	Competencies	Certifications
Nurse Executive	A visionary and administrative role focused on influencing patient care and quality. Primary role is leading, empowering, and motivating others for successful achievement of organizational goals.	AONE competencies: communication and relationship management, knowledge of the health care environment, leadership, professionalism, and business skills and principles	AONE and ANCC offer pathways for nurse executive certification; also role specific certifications in quality improvement or human resources.
Clinical Nurse Leader	Leads the coordination of care, risk management, and quality improvement for patients. Expert at implementing evidence-based care at the bedside and facilitating communication among the interprofessional team.	AACN's nine essentials for the CNL master's degree: 1. Sciences and Humanities Background 2. Organizational and Systems Leadership 3. Quality Improvement and Safety 4. Translating and Integrating Scholarship 5. Informatics and Health Care Technologies 6. Health Policy and Advocacy 7. Interprofessional Collaboration 8. Prevention and Population Health 9. Master's-Level Nursing Practice	CNL certification is offered through the Commission on Nurse Certification (CNC), a subsidiary of the AACN.
Academic Nurse Leader	Titles may include program director, department head, dean, provost, or college president. Combines the concepts of teaching, scholarship, and service with nursing competencies and curriculum. Focused on maintaining nursing education with evolving standards of health care.	The role combines all other nurse leader competencies. Understand policy and educational trends in nursing, cultural and relationship influences, including social, political, economic, mentoring, and technological factors and trends.	No specific certification for role.

(*continued*)

TABLE 23.3 Role Descriptions, Competencies, and Certifications for Nurse Leadership Roles (*continued*)

Leadership Role	Description	Competencies	Certifications
		AONE competencies include communication and relationship management, knowledge of the health care environment, leadership, professionalism, and business skills and principles reflected in the academic setting.	Nurse executive certifications (i.e., CENP or NE-BC) could apply. Certified Higher Education Professional (CHEP) certification from NASASPS available.
Policy and Advocacy	Focus on health care policy, advocate primarily for patients and the nursing profession. Involves negotiation and competition for limited resources.	No formal role-specific competencies.	No role-specific certification available.
		Nurse executive competencies apply. Knowledge of the lawmaking process at the state and national levels. Includes trending health care legislation and various roles of each government branch.	Nurse executive certifications would apply.

AACN, American Association of Colleges of Nursing; ANCC, American Nurses Credentialing Center; AONE, American Organization of Nurse Executives; CENP, certified nurse manager and leader; CHEP, certified higher education professional; CNC, Commission on Nurse Certification; CNL, clinical nurse leader; NASASPS, National Association of State Administrators and Supervisors of Private Schools; NE-BC, Nurse Executive-Board certified.

⬤ CONCLUSION

This chapter focused on formal nursing leadership roles such as the nurse executive, the CNL, the academic nurse leader, and the policy and advocacy nurse leader and how the nurse's functioning in those roles uses the frameworks covered in this text. The educational preparation, professional competencies, and certifications define and validate expertise in each role. Descriptions of roles, competencies, and certifications are summarized in Table 23.3. From the health system executive to the small business entrepreneur, nursing leadership roles are diverse. The frameworks used in each role are dependent on the activities, responsibilities, and goals of each role. The potential for theory application in nursing leadership roles reflects the diversity of the roles themselves.

According to the IOM report *The Future of Nursing: Leading Change, Advancing Health* (2010), nursing is an essential provider of patient care and the largest component of the health care workforce. Nurses' expertise and education, partnered with other health care providers, constitute an influential and knowledgeable group to lead and influence the health care system. The variety of frameworks presented throughout this text highlight the scope of knowledge and the ultimate strength of the nursing profession. Regardless of the specific career track, the functions of the nurse leader are to empower, motivate, and communicate. The nurse leader demonstrates integrity and vision, acts as a role model for individuals, while maximizing the strengths of the interprofessional team for overall success.

○ KEY POINTS

- The nurse executive is a visionary and administrative role focused on influencing patient care and quality. Primary role is leading, empowering, and motivating others for successful achievement of organizational goals.

- AONE describes the nurse executive through a set of competencies that include communication and relationship management, knowledge of the health care environment, leadership, professionalism, and business skills and principles.

- Nurse executives may pursue advanced degrees in business or health care administration, as well as nursing.

- AONE and the American Nurses Credentialing Center (ANCC), a subsidiary of the American Nurses Association (ANA), offer pathways for nurse executive certification.

- Nurse executives apply a variety of frameworks in their everyday practice. Application of these diverse frameworks becomes inherent and creates the culture of the organization, as well as defines the leadership style of the nurse executive.

- Frameworks can be used by the nurse executive to address competence in communication, mentoring, organizational change, and quality improvement.

- The CNL is a master's-prepared nurse who leads the coordination of care, risk management, and quality improvement for patients. The CNL is an expert at implementing evidence-based care at the bedside and facilitating communication among the interprofessional team.

- The CNL role may be implemented in any health care setting. The CNL requires expertise in clinical care, risk management, and team leadership, as well as the ability to synthesize and implement evidence-based care.

- The academic nurse leader role may be a program director, a department head, a dean, or eventually a provost or college president. As an academic leader in a nursing program, the leader must marry the concepts of higher education, such as teaching, scholarship, and service, with nursing competencies and curriculum.

- The National League for Nursing (NLN) describes the competencies of the academic nurse leader as a combination of all other nurse leader competencies. The academic nurse leader must understand policy and educational trends in nursing while integrating those into the practices and goals of the academic institution.

- AONE describes five competencies for the academic nurse leader: communication and relationship management, knowledge of the health care environment, leadership, professionalism, and business skills and principles.

- Nurse leaders in policy and advocacy focus primarily on issues relevant to patients and the nursing profession.

- As most political figures lack health care expertise, it is critical for nurses to share their knowledge and experiences to influence major decisions affecting health care.

- Nurse leaders in policy and advocacy develop careers in research organizations, legislative offices, elective offices, or health care provider organizations.

REFERENCES

American Association of Colleges of Nursing. (2012). CNL frequently asked questions. Retrieved from http://www.aacnnursing.org/CNL/About/FAQs

American Association of Colleges of Nursing. (2013). Competencies and curricular expectations for clinical nurse leader education and practice. Retrieved from http://www.aacnnursing.org/Portals/42/AcademicNursing/CurriculumGuidelines/CNL-Competencies-October-2013.pdf?ver=2017-05-18-144336-663

American Nurses Credentialing Center. (2017). Nurse executive. Retrieved from http://nursecredentialing.org/NurseExecutive

American Organization of Nurse Executives. (n.d.). AONE nurse leader competencies. Retrieved from http://www.aone.org/resources/nurse-leader-competencies.shtml

Barden, D. (2013, January 14). Seeking a different sort of leader. *The Chronicle of Higher Education.* Retrieved from http://chronicle.com

Blegen, M., Goode, C., Park, S., Vaughn, T., & Spetz, J. (2013). Baccalaureate education in nursing and patient outcomes. *Journal of Nursing Administration, 43*(2), 89–94.

Clinical Nurse Leader Association. (n.d.). What is a CNL? Retrieved from http://cnlassociation.org

Grossman, S., & Valiga, T. (2013). *The new leadership challenge: Creating the future of nursing* (4th ed.). Philadelphia, PA: F. A. Davis.

Human Resource Certification Institute. (n.d.). HRCI certification. Retrieved from https://www.hrci.org/our-programs/our-certifications

Institute of Medicine. (2010). *The future of nursing: Leading change, advancing health.* Washington, DC: National Academies Press. doi:10.17226/12956

Meek, J. (2015). Nurse entrepreneur's guide to starting a business. *Clinical Nurse Specialist, 29*(2), 78–79.

National Association for Healthcare Quality. (n.d.). CPHQ certification. Retrieved from http://www.nahq.org/certify/content/index.html

National Association of State Administrators and Supervisors of Private Schools. (2016). Certified higher education professional (CHEP). Retrieved from http://www.nasasps.org/certification

Utley, R. (2011). Function as a change agent and leader-competency 5. In R. Utley (Ed.), *Theory and research for academic nurse educators* (pp. 275–315). Sudbury, MA: Jones & Bartlett.

Application of Frameworks to the Nurse Researcher Role

Lucretia Smith

It is a good morning exercise for a research scientist to discard a pet hypothesis every day before breakfast. It keeps him young.
—Konrad Lorenz

KEY TERMS

Burke's Model for Teaching Research
Declaration of Helsinki
Eide and Kahn Ethical Framework for Qualitative Research
ethical theory
evidence-based practice
Hardicre's Ethical Research Framework
International Council of Nurses *Code of Ethics*
National Center for the Dissemination of Disability Research Framework
Nuremberg Code of Ethics
Poortman and Schildkamp's Framework
triangulation of methods
van Dijk's Framework
Zeelie's standards for research

LEARNING OBJECTIVES

1. Compare and contrast the use of research frameworks among the differing research methodologies.
2. Analyze the differences between a research theory and theory being tested by research.
3. Discuss the applications of frameworks in the areas of methodology, ethics, rigor/quality, and research dissemination analyses.

As noted in Chapter 3, theory forms both the foundation and the outcome of research. According to Bengtson, Acock, Allen, Dilworth-Anderson, and Klein (2005), the purpose of any theory is to explain or predict. The purpose of research is to support, refute, or modify those theoretical explanations or predictions. Therefore, when research is not based on theory, there is a potential for loss of continuity, loss of evidence that could support or refute theoretical concepts, loss of the importance of the research, and, as a result, loss of evidence for improving patient care.

Since research is grounded in theory, the idea of discussing theories about how to do research may seem redundant. However, if the science is to be consistent, there must be a framework (or series of frameworks) upon which the methods and concepts of research itself rests. If, as proposed earlier in this book, a theory is a statement of the relationships between concepts, and the theory is continually improved through research, then theories become the repository used by research to produce the most predictable, and most elegant, explanations for the phenomenon being studied.

Argyris (1996), in a review of theories and research in the business world, suggests it is not only possible but also probable that researchers, using the lens of specific theory, may conduct their research with unrecognized gaps. Since nursing research covers a broad scope, it behooves the nurse to use research theories to add to the evidence of best practices and in effect counterbalance the tendency to "prove" (or "disprove") specific theoretical constructs.

> *In clinical practice, we are researchers of some form. We may not be conducting a large randomized study, but we are studying aspects of our patients' health, well-being, illness, and healthcare in a rapidly changing environment.*
> —Deann Thompson, MSN, RN, FNP-C

THE MULTIPLE NATURES OF RESEARCH: EVALUATIVE FRAMEWORKS

This section of the chapter summarizes the frameworks used to evaluate research. The quality of research, its validity, trustworthiness, and generalizability should be measured. However, due to the variety of research emphasized earlier, there should not be a single framework that equates to a "one size fits all" evaluation of research. A variety of frameworks for evaluating research as well as some of the disputes regarding the evaluation of research are presented in the following.

National Center for the Dissemination of Disability Research Framework

Nursing research is as varied as the roles of nurses (American Association of Colleges of Nursing [AACN], 2006). The most common, quantitative, positivistic research, traditionally using experimental methods, is judged for quality by determining the validity and reliability in each of its steps. The National Center for the Dissemination of Disability Research [NCDDR] (2005) compiled the beginnings of a standards framework by which researchers can both judge their own research and share their testing of those standards. This framework, supported by literature review, identifies 12 characteristics that both a researcher and a consumer of research should expect to find in a well-constructed quantitative study. These principles are summarized in Box 24.1. While the NCDDR does not claim to have consensus on a specific algorithm, it does have wide support from its stakeholders that using these principles to evaluate quantitative research will increase the quality of the work. There is no claim that any set of constructs or algorithms can ensure quality.

The van Dijk Framework

In 1986, the *van Dijk Framework* was developed, which contained standards by which social research, including a large component of nursing research, should be judged. In social sciences, the types of research vary according to the segment of practice being studied. The background to van Dijk's theory was an increasingly dichotomous view of applied social research. One view insisted that all research was fundamentally alike and the differences between experimental research and applied social research could be bridged by simply adding rules that define quality to the indicators of experimental rigor. The other side of the argument held that the differences were so great that a completely different scientific canon should be applied.

BOX 24.1 Principles for Quality Research

- Pose important empirical question
- Questions relate to theory
- Appropriate methods
- Solid reasoning
- Sufficient information to replicate study
- Transparent and objective design and methods
- Thorough sample description
- Reliable measurement
- Explain findings
- Acknowledge bias and its impact
- Subject research to a peer-review
- Use quality standards for reporting

Source: National Center for the Dissemination of Disability Research (2005).

Van Dijk's Framework endeavored to uphold the unity of scientific method in all quantitative and qualitative paradigms while fully acknowledging the different purposes. According to this framework, research in field settings has five characteristics: variety, contextual, eclectic/opportunistic, longitudinal/cumulative/feed-back-loop, and quick data analyses. These characteristics should adhere to seven quality standards: transparency, consistency, communication/cooperation, stimulus for change, multi-method, feedback/confrontation, and dynamic. All of the concepts are similar to, but differ from, traditional experimental characteristics and quality measures. For example, transparency and communication are similar to qualitative methodological standards that value the ability of the participant and the researcher to clearly understand and articulate the context and questions involved in research. Another similarity between qualitative and quantitative methodology is consistency, specifically between the means of data collection and the question that is being asked by the researcher. This differs from traditional research methods in that field research is, as a rule, short of both the time and resources that lengthy analyses require. Van Dijk argues that this forces a more focused research question that requires a consistent, and sometimes confrontational, form of feedback resulting in a decrease of the analyses time.

Poortman and Schildkamp's Framework

In more recent research, Poortman and Schildkamp (2012) observe the progressively divergent quality standards for qualitative and quantitative methodologies. The framework they propose argues that when the standards are different, there can be no comparability of the quality between different types of studies, nor can there be solid decision making about their comparative usefulness. The Poortman and Schildkamp Framework is a "coherent and inclusive framework of quality criteria for both qualitative and quantitative studies" (p. 1727). The framework uses quantitative language for seven criteria (controllability, objectivity, reliability, validity, construct validity, internal validity, and external validity). Then the framework suggests procedures specific to the type of research that will address the quality criterion. For example, under objectivity, the interpretation of quantitative data should include standardization while the interpretation of qualitative data should include thick description.

According to Poortman and Schildkamp's framework, mixed methods or *triangulation of methods* may be used to increase the validity or credibility and the reliability of a study, make the data more complete, and overcome the limitations of a single method. Triangulation of

---

BOX 24.2 Multi-Method Triangulation Research Issues

Casey and Murphey (2009) point out the difficulties in using more than one method of research in a single study. While much of the theory about research focuses on the quality of qualitative or quantitative methodology, there is a rising propensity to use more than one method in an effort to validate the findings of one method through the use of another, reducing bias, deepening/completing the results, and increasing the generalizability of findings. Casey and Murphey critique the thinking behind this propensity and offer a framework by which to judge the quality of multi-method or triangulated research. The critique begins with the seldom-recognized fact that both across method triangulation and within method triangulation techniques may be used. That is, qualitative and quantitative may be used, or two kinds of either qualitative or quantitative methods may be used. Both kinds are subject to the potential incompatibility of research paradigms, the possibility that the question asked cannot be answered by both techniques, and the possibility that neither decrease of bias nor increase of comprehensive or generalizable findings were achieved. The critique framework suggests that evidence of a clear and rational account of how and why triangulation was used should be present. In addition, each data collection method should be demonstrably valid, and an explanation of how triangulation was a purposeful addition to the study should be made. Finally, the type of triangulation and how it was achieved should be clear. Also, how triangulation promoted the completeness, bias containment, and validity increase should be obvious to the reader.

---

methods enhances scientific rigor by using more than one method to determine if the same results are obtained. Each method serves to validate the other. For a critique of triangulated research see Box 24.2.

◉ FRAMEWORKS FOR RESEARCH ETHICS

Research, in all disciplines, paradigms, and methodologies is obligated to attend to ethical issues. Therefore, one of the major theories that should guide nursing research is an ethical theory. Here again, the difference between testing ethical theory (Jameton & Fowler, 1989) and using ethical theory as a guide for research processes (Ignacio & Taylor, 2013) should be realised. The multiplicity of study designs has generated a need for ethical frameworks that addresses all issues of a specific design. The creation of multiple ethical frameworks has given rise to both the opportunity and the need to decide about ethical theory in terms of design, population, and purpose of individual studies (Salloch, Wäscher, Vollmann, & Schildmann, 2015).

> *Being able to handle change and maintain your values is imperative in how you practice your nursing care. When we are able to hold onto our value system within the workplace to care for our patients in the best way that we know how, it somehow makes that change a little easier.*
> —Tara Fuchs, BSN, RN

Nuremberg Code of Ethics

Prior to the Nuremberg Code there was no generally accepted code of conduct governing the use of human subjects in research. Sadly, the articulation of research ethics in the Nuremberg code was necessitated by the historical use of poor ethical judgment. Due to the lack of consent, purposeful dishonesty, intimidation, and even purposeful deaths during research studies conducted under the Nazi regime, the need for a code for ethical treatment of research participants became evident. As an outcome of the World War II war crimes tribunal, held in Nuremberg in 1947, 10 principles were identified that must be adhered to in all research on human subjects (Jewish Virtual Library, 2017). These principles are summarized in Box 24.3.

Declaration of Helsinki

The most recent widely used model of ethical research is the Declaration of Helsinki. The Declaration was originally adopted in 1964 and named after its city of origin Helsinki, Finland. It has undergone several revisions with the last in 2013 (World Medical Association, 2013). The Declaration consists of 13 general principles that are focused predominantly on the physician's responsibility and duty to the patient or research subject. Emphasis is placed on the physician's expectations to respect human subjects, protect their health and rights. Although written with an emphasis on the physician who is involved in research, all others involved in human subject research are encouraged to apply the principles.

Another section of the Declaration addresses subjects' rights and protections and aspects of the research protocol. Risks and potential benefits to the subjects must be anticipated. Subjects' privacy must be maintained and informed consent provided. The study sampling and protocol should also adhere to certain guidelines. Attempts to recruit underrepresented subjects should be made, post-trial access to an intervention found to be effective should be made available to all participants, and compensation to subjects who are harmed during the research process should be provided. The Declaration document adds to the Nuremberg Code the caveat that not only must the participants of research be protected, but ethical research means the process and results of the study are credible and accurate.

Hardicre's Ethical Research Framework

Salloch et al. (2015) suggest a framework in which the use of ethical theory in empirical work is clear and coherent, adequate for the issue at stake, and suitable for the purposes and design of the project. One such framework was developed by Hardicre (2014) to guide the researchers' ethical planning and conduct of research on an international level. The

---

BOX 24.3 Principles From the Nuremberg Code of Ethics

1. Voluntary consent of subjects to participate
2. Purpose of study will benefit society
3. Sufficient evidence exists to warrant the study in humans
4. Study is conducted to avoid inflicting unnecessary harm
5. No perceived risk of disability or death
6. Risks to subjects should not outweigh the importance of the issue
7. Preparations and facilities in place to protect subjects from harm
8. Research is conducted by qualified persons
9. Subjects have the right to withdraw from the study
10. Researcher's duty to terminate study if continuation could result in harm

Source: Jewish Virtual Library (2017).

BOX 24.4 Research Ethics and the Internet

Ellett, Lane, and Keffer (2004) identified the Internet as both an advantageous tool and a challenge to the ethical and legal parameters of nursing research. The most frequently questioned ethical principles in Internet research seemed to be privacy, confidence that participants know the risks and benefits of participation (including withdrawal without repercussion), and the nature of the relationship between the researcher and the participant. A tie between the ethical nature of the participant and the quality of the study was made. Whether the research question can be answered best using Internet technology, how exclusion criteria will be enforced, and how the reliability and validity of both the instruments and the data can be maintained were all questions that, while they are generally quality questions, bear directly on the ethical component of using the Internet to conduct research.

---

framework depicts the participant in the center of a circle of locking "pieces" that represent aspects the researcher is expected to assess. These pieces include ethics specific to national/international research conventions, nursing, health care, and research institution.

Among the national and international considerations in Hardicre's framework are the Declaration of Helsinki, Nuremberg Code, National Research Council, national/international law, government-specific research policies, product regulation agencies, and review by international health research authorities outside the researcher's country of origin. Ethical considerations for nursing and the research site include the American Nurses Association *Code of Ethics*, national nursing policies, policies of the researcher's institution, and the researcher's adherence to the role of patient advocate. If a researcher attends to each part of this model, there is a greater chance the participant will be better served and the research will be an ethical work with publishable results.

Eide and Kahn's Ethical Framework for Qualitative Research

Eide and Kahn (2008) describe ethical issues inherent to the relationships created and often sustained in the process of conducting qualitative research. Using qualitative methodology, they propose a framework for the ethical assessment of qualitative research that is based on two models. The first supporting model is the International Council of Nurses *Code of Ethics for Nurses* (see Chapter 8), which notes that a researcher is responsible for patient health, not only to avoid harm but also to act if a patient is in need of the expertise of the researcher. The second model, Swanson's Theory of Caring in Nursing (see Chapter 5), stresses five components that Eide and Kahn maintain are necessary for ethical patient-researcher relationships. These components are: maintaining belief, knowing, being with, doing for, and enabling.

The speed of technological advancements has outpaced the development of specific ethical decision-making approaches that should be applied to these emerging technological situations. For an example of the use of Eide and Kahn's framework for ethical thinking, regarding the use of the Internet as a data-collection tool, see Box 24.4.

⬤ FRAMEWORKS RELATED TO RESEARCH RIGOR AND COMPETENCY

While ethical theory suggests that research should be performed in a rigorous and competent manner, theory specific to those attributes helps to clarify and guide studies generated in all research paradigms. Nurses are becoming increasingly aware of the necessity of creating research-based knowledge upon which to build evidence-based practice (EBP).

Nursing education has created frameworks for the kinds of research to meet the "evidence" requirement for EBP (AACN, 2006). In addition, competencies for conducting and consuming research have been developed (Burke et al., 2005; Zeelie, Bornman, & Botes, 2003). This section reviews those frameworks and the recently developed Clinical Research Nursing Scope and Standards for Practice

Burke's Model for Teaching Research

Both understanding and use of EBP begins in undergraduate education and continues through all levels of nursing education (Burke et al., 2005). Burke et al., seeing the lack of preparation for the critique and use of research in the curriculum of most nursing programs, proposed a model for education that is composed of leveled research competencies.

Burke's model proposes research competencies for each year of BSN education. It begins with demonstrating access to research information and ends with evaluation of research for its applicability to practice. According to this model, nursing curricula at the master's level should enable the student to synthesize findings and critically evaluate the treatment plans that are based on those findings. At the clinical doctorate level, the Doctor of Nursing Practice graduate is expected to design and implement EBP in the form of protocol. PhD graduates should be able to evaluate the need for research, conduct original research, and disseminate research.

Nursing Scope and Standards for Clinical Nurse Researcher

Clinical research nursing is defined by the International Association of Clinical Research Nurses (IACRN) as a specialty practice that incorporates five domains: human subjects' protection, study management, care coordination and continuity, contribution to clinical nursing science, and clinical practice (IACRN & ANA, 2015). A clinical research nurse (CRN) differs from a nurse researcher in academic preparation and scope of practice. A nurse researcher is a doctorally prepared nurse who is focused on expanding and clarifying nursing knowledge. The nurse researcher plans and conducts the research study, leads the research team (which includes the CRN), and evaluates and disseminates findings. The CRN, at the direction of the nurse researcher, addresses the five domains of practice within the research practice setting (Hastings et al., 2012). Therefore, part of the CRN's practice is in facilitating the research study and part is in clinical practice and coordination of care of subjects who are participating in a study.

In 2015, the IACRN, in conjunction with the American Nurses Association (ANA), developed the Clinical Research Nursing Scope and Standards of Practice. Fashioned after other scope and standards documents, it outlines standards of practice and standards of performance for the role. The standards of practice follow the nursing process and include assessing, diagnosing, identifying outcomes, planning, implementing, and evaluating care. The standards of professional performance for clinical research nursing include 11 standards of which ethics, EBP, and research are especially relevant to the frameworks discussed in this text.

In addition to the research ethics frameworks just discussed, the CRN may find one or more of the ethical decision-making frameworks discussed in Chapter 8 helpful. For example, metacognitive process of reflection, reasoning, and review described in the Nurses Ethical Reasoning Skills Model (NERS) can be used to guide the processes used in ethical decision making. In the Symphonological Bioethical Theory, also discussed in Chapter 8, the emphasis is on understanding the agreements between the nurse and patient as well as the context of the situation. This perspective would be especially relevant to the relationship between the CRN and the research patient. Determining the congruence between the nurse's and the patient's ethical perspectives and the ethics and values inherent in the research protocol will help reduce conflicts that may arise during implementation of the research protocol.

Even nurses not specifically designated as CRNs are expected to understand the principles of finding and using evidence upon which to base their practice. For example, in 2005, Parkin and Bullock reviewed the addition of a research standard to the standards of care already present in a U.K. hospital. According to the standards of care framework familiar to most nurses, "nurses undertaking research ... will be facilitated through the research process in order to achieve high-quality research" and "will be supported ... to increase [the nurse's] awareness and disseminate research into practice, advancing evidence-based patient care" (p. 421). Facility-specific models are suggested. However, much work remains for the creation and testing of a useable framework for quality clinical nursing research.

Zeelie's Standards for Research

The work of Zeelie et al. (2003) used the clinical research criteria proposed by Bowden (1995) to create standards for research. Bowden specified eight attributes by which clinical research should be judged. Clinical research should, (a) be foundational to quality assurance, (b) define quality, (c) provide directional outcomes, (d) be sensitive to the context, (e) be acceptable to colleagues and users, (f) be measurable, (g) be written, and (h) include criteria for evaluating achievement.

Zeelie et al. used Bowden's criteria and applied Muller's phases of standard development (i.e., formulation, quantifying, and testing) to develop standards for quality research that could be used in nursing education programs. Using qualitative methods, they sampled nurse educators, managers, clinicians, researchers, and nursing students regarding their perceptions of nursing research education. From the data, they identified 26 standards and multiple criteria for research education, which encompassed characteristics of structure, process, and outcomes. These standards are listed in Table 24.1.

Florczak's Framework

In general, judgment about the rigor of quantitative research is accomplished by evaluating the adherence of its parts to the generally accepted standards of research. These standards are concerned with the choice of sample, fulfillment of methodological assumptions, choice of analytical tools, analysis, and dissemination of findings. These methodological assumptions impact the reliability and validity of the study.

While multiple guidelines have been suggested for establishing rigor in quantitative research, Florczak (2011) began a dialog for the creation of a framework that would guide the rigor of nurses pursuing knowledge within the quantitative paradigm. She suggests that the trend in the literature is to lend scientific merit to certain buzzwords (e.g., randomized controlled trial) without having either the information or the framework to analyze the quality or rigor of the specific study. Beginning with two concepts, population and sampling, and questioning the effectiveness of rapid critical appraisal, she begins a dialog encouraging the creation of a framework by which nurses should judge their (and others') research for rigor.

McBrien's Framework for Rigor in Qualitative Research

McBrien (2008) outlined a framework specific to the use of qualitative work in clinical settings. He suggests its use would increase the rigor of qualitative work. Specific methods included in McBrien's framework are member checking/peer debriefing, development of an audit trail, reflexivity, and triangulation.

Member checking and peer debriefing deal with the recurring problem of divergent interpretations of data in qualitative work. Member checking seeks to include the participant's view of the researchers' interpretation of the data. Peer debriefing is the review of the

	TABLE 24.1 Zeelie's Standards for Research		
	Standard		**Standard**
1	Ensure quality education and research	14	Educators and students are competent in research related roles
2	Demonstrate needed knowledge, skills, attitude, and values	15	Evaluation of education in nursing research is operationalized
3	Research education based on strategic plan	16	Building research capacity is essential
4	Research education program is systematic, planned, integrated, and value added	17	Student support for research program is implemented proactively
5	Uses contextually appropriate didactic concept	18	Educators and students perceive self as competent
6	Research curriculum is responsive to society needs	19	Systematic audit used to monitor and evaluate processes
7	Assessment is focused on mission and goals	20	Networking is promoted and valued
8	Environment supports quality research outcomes	21	Quality assurance measures incorporate satisfaction
9	Educators meet research requirements	22	Ongoing relevance of the research program
10	Research skills and competencies are acquired by graduates	23	Nurses are active in all aspects of scholarship
11	Institutional policy guides education of nursing research	24	Accountability is promoted
12	Support systems for students available	25	Excellence is overall goal
13	Financial support for conducting research and education		

Source: Zeelie, Bornman, and Botes (2003).

interpretation and categorization of data by field experts. The *development of an audit trail* can be described as documenting the rationale for decisions made in methodology and interpretations. The use of an audit trail addresses the criticism that qualitative research fails to provide a clear accounting of the research procedures undertaken. The concept of *reflexivity* is a part of building an audit trail. Using reflexivity, the researcher acknowledges the impact his/her opinions and actions have on the resulting data.

McBrien suggests that qualitative research is an exercise in reaching completion. Given this suggestion, *triangulation*, or using more than one source of data, can be helpful in enhancing rigor. According to McBrien (2008), triangulation should be recognized as a method in its own right, not merely an effort to confirm the results of a single method of data collection. Using the concepts outlined by McBrien, the validity and trustworthiness of qualitative research should be more apparent.

FRAMEWORKS FOR EVALUATING PUBLISHED RESEARCH

Knowledge and skill in evaluating the quality of published research are essential to nurses engaged in EBP. One category of research that requires attention, especially in the face of the increased emphasis on EBP, is the review and analysis of multiple published research studies (i.e., meta-analysis and meta-synthesis). These studies represent the highest level of research evidence for quantitative and qualitative studies, respectively. However, they are subject to several unique problems such as a lack of or inconsistent information published in the original study and the use of different populations and methods to address a single research question. The Preferred Reporting Items for Systematic Reviews and Meta-Analyses (PRISMA) Guidelines incorporate 17 criteria to guide the evaluation of the meta-analysis studies (see Chapter 18). Another tool, the Quality Assessment Tool Studies with Diverse Designs (QATSDD), was designed to evaluate the quality of a body of research composed of diverse study designs. Sirriyeh, Lawton, Gardner, and Armitage (2012) developed and tested the 16-item QATSDD tool using literature from nursing, psychology, and sociology. They found the tool to have good validity and test–retest reliability when used for evaluating the quality of quantitative and qualitative research. While this is not technically a theory, it provides a framework for evaluating the rigor of review studies as suggested by Crossetti (2012).

In addition to the PRISMA guidelines for evaluating meta-analysis, other frameworks have been developed to guide the evaluation and reporting of findings of single research studies (e.g., CONSORT, AGREE, SQUIRE, and STROBE). Further discussion of these may be found in Chapter 18. Not only can these guidelines be used to evaluate the completeness and quality of published research, but also to guide the development and implementation of studies as well.

I have come to appreciate the nuances of the individual theories and appreciate the time and effort put forth to formulate them.
—Brian Wagoner, APRN, FNP-BC

CONCLUSION

The growing demand for EBP is both encouraging and alarming (see Box 24.5 for a critique of the current standards for evidence used in EBP). Encouraging possibilities include the increase of resources available for research to generate evidence, the increase of professional interest in doing research and in giving attention to disseminated research, and the growing expectations for quality nursing practice. The alarming possibilities could include shortcuts to the results of evidence resulting in questionable quality, and the possible decrease rather than an increase in excellence in patient care. For the profession of nursing, a lack of quality could include the denigration of theory-supported research. Using a cohesive theory of research, such as those explored here will increase the likelihood of the reliability of the research that tests the evidence and guides practice.

Rigor in qualitative work has been much debated. Several authors suggest that qualitative studies should be judged by the same frameworks that drive analysis in quantitative studies (Poortman & Schildkamp, 2012; Sirriyeh et al., 2012). Others argue qualitative work should have its own theory set by which it is judged (McBrien, 2008). Still others argue that each method within each paradigm carries the requirement for a different set of rules, and therefore requires a different theory set (Nixon & Power, 2007; Rolfe, 2006; van Djik, 1986).

BOX 24.5 Rigor and Evidence-Based Practice

Florczak (2011) suggested the current emphasis and pressure upon researchers (and potential researchers) for evidence on which to base practice undermines the rigor of the research process. She had a specific concern about using "randomized controlled trial" (RCT) as the standard by which all evidence is generated. Often a deeper look at a RCT will show the assignment of the subjects to the control or the experimental group were randomized, yet the sample itself was not selected in a randomized manner. Random assignment without random sampling does nothing to increase the validity or decrease the sampling bias, which is the purpose of randomization. Florczak also expressed concern regarding the tools or checklists being created to, supposedly, assure rigor of evidence. These checklists may decrease the depth with which the critique is executed.

● KEY POINTS

- The NCDDR Framework is supported by literature and identifies 12 characteristics for researching and consuming research.

- The van Dijk Framework is based in social research and attempts to bring together critique and valid use of multiple methods.

- Poortman and Schildkamp established standards to judge both qualitative and quantitative research.

- The history of research ethics beginning with the Nuremberg Code and the Declaration of Helsinki dictates ethical standards by which research must be conducted and reported.

- Hardicre's Framework suggests researchers should not only be aware of but also actively check the multiple codes and laws that are both within and beyond the researcher's immediate research context.

- Eide and Kahn proposed ethical concepts specific to qualitative research based on the International Council of Nurses Code of Ethics for Nurses and Swanson's Theory of Caring in Nursing.

- Rigor and competency are necessary parts of well-constructed research.

- Burke's Model for teaching research outlines the research competencies that should be present in each level of nursing education from baccalaureate through PhD.

- The clinical research nurse is responsible for facilitating the research study and engages in clinical practice and coordination of care of subjects who are participating in a study.

- Zeelie et al. proposed standards for nursing research education using Bowden's attributes of standards and Muller's phases of standard formulation.

- Florczak began a dialog based on the concern that the quality of quantitative research has been slowly denigrating due to the increased demand for more studies more quickly to support EBP.

- McBrien proposed a framework identifying attributes of validity and trustworthiness in qualitative clinical research.

- PRISMA is a series of guidelines for evaluating (and reporting) published research.

REFERENCES

American Association of Colleges of Nursing. (2006). AACN position statement on nursing research. Retrieved from http://www.aacnnursing.org/Portals/42/News/Position-Statements/Nursing-Research.pdf

Argyris, C. (1996). Unrecognized defenses of scholars: Impact on theory and research. *Organization Science, 7*(1), 79–87.

Bengtson, V. L., Acock, A. C., Allen, K. R., Dilworth-Anderson, P., & Klein, D. M. (2005). *Sourcebook of family theory & research*. Thousand Oaks, CA: Sage.

Bowden, S. (1995). How to develop a staff development indicator. *Journal of Nursing Staff Development, 11*(3), 166–169.

Burke, L. E., Schleck, E. A., Sereika, S. M., Cohen, S. M., Happ, M. B., & Dorman, J. S. (2005). Developing research competence to support evidence-based practice. *Journal of Professional Nursing, 21*(6), 358–363. doi:10.1016/j.profnurs.2005.10.011

Casey, D., & Murphy, K. (2009). Issues in using methodological triangulation in research. *Nurse Researcher, 16*(4), 40–55.

Crossetti, M. O. (2012). Integrative review of nursing research: Scientific rigor required. *Revista Gaúcha De Enfermagem/EENFUFRGS, 33*(2), 12–13.

Eide, P. & Kahn, D. (2008). Ethical issues in the qualitative researcher participant relationship. *Nursing Ethics, 15*(2), 199–207. doi:10.1177/0969733007086018

Ellett, C. M. L., Lane, L., & Keffer, J. (2004). Ethical and legal issues of conducting nursing research via the internet. *Journal of Professional Nursing, 20*(1) 68–74. doi:10.1016/j.profnurs.2003.12.005

Florczak, K. L. (2011). Rigor: Lost in the quest for evidence-based practice. *Nursing Science Quarterly, 24*(3), 202–205. doi:10.1177/0894318411409429

Hardicre, J. (2014). An overview of research ethics and learning from the past. *British Journal of Nursing, 23*(9), 483–486.

Hastings, C. E., Fisher, C. A., McCabe, M. A., & The National Clinical Research Nursing Consortium. (2012). Clinical research nursing: A critical resource in the national research enterprise. *Nursing Outlook, 60*(3), 149–156.e3. doi:10.1016/j.outlook.2011.10.003

International Association of Clinical Research Nurses. (2015). Scope and standards of practice: Clinical research nursing [Draft]. Retrieved from http://iacrn.org/resources/Documents/Scopes%20 and%20Standards%20for%20Public%20Comment.pdf

Ignacio, J. J., & Taylor, B. J. (2013). Ethical issues in health-care inquiry: A discussion paper. *International Journal of Nursing Practice, 19*(51),1856–1861. doi:10.1111/ijn.12017

Jameton, A. & Fowler, M. D. (1989). Ethical inquiry and the concept of research. *Advances in Nursing Science, 11*(3), 11–24.

Jewish Virtual Library. (2017). *Nuremberg code August 19, 1947*. Retrieved from http://www.jewish virtuallibrary.org/the-nuremberg-code

McBrien, B. (2008). Evidence-based care: Enhancing the rigour of a qualitative study. *British Journal of Nursing, 17*(20), 1286–1289. doi:10.12968/bjon.2008.17.20.31645

National Center for the Dissemination of Disability Research. (2005). What are the standards for quality research? *Technical Brief #9*. Retrieved from http://ktdrr.org/ktlibrary/articles_pubs/ncddrwork/ focus/focus9/Focus9.pdf

Nixon, A., & Power, C. (2007). Towards a framework for establishing rigour in a discourse analysis of midwifery professionalisation. *Nursing Inquiry, 14*(1), 71–79. doi:10.1111/j.1440-1800.2007.00352.x

Parkin, C., & Bullock, I. (2005). Evidence-based health care: Development and audit of a clinical standard for research and its impact on an NHS trust. *Journal of Clinical Nursing, 14*(4), 418–425. doi: 10.1111/j.1365-2702.2004.01080.x

Poortman, C., & Schildkamp, K. (2012). Alternative quality standards in qualitative research? *Quality & Quantity, 46*(6), 1727–1751. doi:10.1007/s11135-011-9555-5

Rolfe, G. (2006). Validity, trustworthiness and rigour: Quality and the idea of qualitative research. *Journal of Advanced Nursing, 53*(3), 304–310. doi:10.1111/j.1365-2648.2006.03727.x

Salloch, S., Wäscher, S., Vollmann, J., & Schildmann, J. (2015). The normative background of empirical-ethical research: First steps towards a transparent and reasoned approach in the selection of an ethical theory. *BMC Medical Ethics, 16,* 20. doi:10.1186/s12910-015-0016-x

Sirriyeh, R., Lawton, R., Gardner, P., & Armitage, G. (2012). Reviewing studies with diverse designs: The development and evaluation of a new tool. *Journal of Evaluation in Clinical Practice, 18*(4), 746–752. doi:10.1111/j.1365-2753.2011.01662.x

van Dijk, J. V. (1986). Methods in applied social research: Special characteristics and quality standards. *Quality & Quantity, 20*(4), 357–370.

World Medical Association. (2013). WMS Declaration of Helsinki: Ethical principles for medical research involving human subjects. Retrieved from https://www.wma.net/policies-post/wma-declaration-of-helsinki-ethical-principles-for-medical-research-involving-human-subjects

Zeelie, S. C., Bornman, J. E., & Botes, A. C. (2003). Standards to assure quality in nursing research. *Curationis, 26*(3), 4–11.

INDEX